LIFE SPAN MOTOR DEVELOPMENT

LIFE SPAN MOTOR DEVELOPMENT

Kathleen M. Haywood, PhD
University of Missouri—St. Louis

Human Kinetics Publishers, Inc.
Champaign, Illinois

Library of Congress Cataloging-in-Publication Data

Haywood, Kathleen.
    Life span motor development.

    Includes bibliographies and index.
    1. Growth.   2. Motor ability.   I. Title.   [DNLM:
1. Growth.   2. Motor Skills.   WE 103 H397L]
QP84.H34   1986   612'.76   86-312
ISBN 0-87322-054-4

Developmental Editor: Gwen Steigelman, PhD
Production Director: Ernest Noa
Copy Editors: Ann Morris Bruehler and Terry Jopke
Typesetter: Sandra Meier
Text Layout: Denise Mueller
Text Design: Julie Szamocki
Cover Design: Jack Davis
Printed By: Braun Brumfield, Inc.

Line drawings in chapters 3 and 4 by Dick Flood

ISBN: 0-87322-054-4

Printed in the United States of America

10 9 8 7 6 5 4 3 2 1

Human Kinetics Publishers, Inc.
Box 5076, Champaign, IL 61820

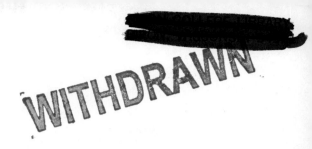

To my parents in return
for their unwaivering support

Acknowledgments

As with any work this size, many people provided valuable assistance. John Strupel, MD and Elizabeth Sweeney, BSN were kind enough to read chapter 2 for medical accuracy. Bruce Clark, PhD reviewed chapter 7 and Susan Greendorfer, PhD offered valuable suggestions on chapter 9. Mary Ann Roberton, PhD furnished materials from which many of the chapter 4 illustrations were drawn.

The photographs in chapter 2 were taken by Brian Speicher. Michael, Douglas, and Jennifer Imergoot, and Matthew and Christina Haywood posed for the pictures. Laura Haywood posed for the pictures in chapter 3. Ann Wagner typed many of the manuscript tables and figure captions and Cynthia Haywood assisted in checking the reference list. In addition, the support of Elizabeth Sweeney, Lynn Imergoot, Stephanie Ross, Cathy Lewis, and members of the Motor Development Research Consortium is gratefully acknowledged.

Contents

Preface

Change in motor behavior from infancy to older adulthood is a fascinating process to study. Just a few years ago, study in motor development was limited to children and adolescents. Today, however, motor development is an expanding area of study. Increasingly, motor development is recognized as a continuous developmental process that must include the study of motor behaviors over the entire life span. Certainly age-related changes in motor behavior and skill performance are not limited to persons under 20 years of age. It is important, then, that changes in motor development that occur throughout adulthood and older adulthood also are studied in a systematic way. *Life Span Motor Development* is intended to fill the need for a comprehensive motor development text that takes a life span view.

In 1982, several members of the Motor Development Academy of the American Alliance for Health, Physical Education, Recreation, and Dance developed a list of minimum exit competencies appropriate for student coursework in motor development. These competencies include: (a) the ability to formulate a developmental perspective, especially from a life span viewpoint; (b) knowledge of changing motor behavior across the life span; (c) knowledge of the factors affecting motor development, including physical growth and physiological change, perceptual change, cognitive change, sociocultural practices, and interventions; and (d) the ability to apply motor development knowledge. This text covers the suggested areas of knowledge; course instructors may wish to further enhance the application of motor development knowledge with supplemental activities in laboratory and clinical settings.

The text is written as an undergraduate introductory text, so little background knowledge in the movement sciences is required. Persons who are interested in motor behavior as it relates to physical education, developmental psychology, elementary education, early childhood education, special education, and gerontology should find this book instructive as well. It is assumed that most readers anticipate working with children, adolescents, and perhaps young adults. With the increasing proportion of adults in the population who are concerned with developing and maintaining an active life-style, the demand for individuals with knowledge of life span motor development will afford increased employment opportunities.

The breadth of information pertaining to motor development throughout the life span often seems overwhelming to beginning students. One way to handle the large volume of detailed information is to conceptualize how this information supports broader generalizations about motor development. A conceptual understanding of motor development is particularly useful for students whose application of this knowledge may occur in a wide array of professional settings. For this reason, *Life Span Motor Development* focuses on concepts in motor development throughout.

The book consists of nine chapters divided into two parts. Part I (chapters 1 to 5) concerns the developmental perspective on human behavior and includes changes in physical growth and aging and changes in motor performance. Part II (chapters 6 to 9) includes a consideration of the correlates of motor behaviors, that is, the factors that influence individual performance levels such as physiological, perceptual, and cognitive changes, and sociocultural influences. Featured within each chapter are several motor development concepts. After the concept is introduced and discussed, a brief summary is provided before moving on to the next concept.

The book's chapters and concepts are organized to provide a logical sequence of study beginning with parameters of physical growth and development, continuing with motor skill acquisition, and progressing to correlates of motor development. Other than in chapters 3, 4, and 5, which concern specific developmental periods, the discussion covers the entire life span. Concepts within the chapters are supported by discussions of relevant research and study and by specific examples of their application in natural settings. Instructors may wish to introduce additional materials for various chapters and concepts as appropriate; because each chapter is a complete unit, the chapters may be read in a different order than presented to meet the needs of individual instructors or students without jeopardizing the integrity of the book.

The concepts emphasized in *Life Span Motor Development* should help you make knowledgeable decisions concerning motor development. I hope that as you gain an understanding and appreciation of the process of developmental change in motor behavior, you will continue to seek new information in the study of motor development.

Kathleen M. Haywood

P A R T

1

Change Throughout the Life Span

Part I begins with a discussion of the importance of the developmental perspective in the study of motor development. Five chapters in this part comprise the discussion focusing on patterns of changes throughout the life span first with changes in the body itself, then with changes in motor behavior.

In chapter 1 the life span view of development is introduced. Several critical issues in the study of development are presented and discussed. The formal study of motor development as a subdiscipline of motor behavior is also examined.

Physical growth and aging as the foundation for motor development is explored in the second chapter. Growth and age-related changes in skill performance are so closely tied that it makes little sense to study motor development without a thorough knowledge of growth and the aging process. Included in chapter 2 is a discussion of overall body growth as well as growth and aging in each of the relevant body systems. Factors that specifically affect physical growth and aging are also discussed.

In chapters 3 and 4 motor behavior from infancy through childhood is examined. Reflexes and motor milestones of early life are explored initially, followed by the processes of basic skill acquisition. The emphasis here is on understanding the mechanical principles underlying skill performance and how age-related changes in movement patterns increasingly obey these mechanical principles. Motor skill developmental sequences are noted whenever such information is available for specific skills.

The progression of motor behavior during preadolescence, adolescence, and adulthood is discussed in chapter 5 with particular attention to the effect of aging on motor development. Assessment of motor performance and the strengths and weaknesses of the available assessment tools are also addressed.

The Developmental Perspective

The learning and performance of motor skills is a lifelong challenge. Basic skills must be acquired early in life; this process begins with the achievement of postural control and the ability to grasp objects with the hands. It continues with the acquisition of locomotor skills and then manipulative skills such as throwing. During childhood, the basic skills learned earlier are refined and combined into movement sequences in order to produce complex skills. The individual continues to acquire movement sequences into adolescence as improvements are made in the ability to match motor skills to the demands of the movement tasks at hand. Throughout infancy, childhood, and adolescence our bodies are continually growing and maturing. Gradually, our perception of the surrounding world becomes keener, and mental capacity increases while mental skills improve. Social skills, too, are acquired as new social relationships are formed; with all these changes, the performance of motor skills must be accommodated and modified.

The perfection of motor skills is usually accomplished during late adolescence and young adulthood. Professional, world class, and Olympic athletes are good examples of persons who have fully developed their motor skills. Such skilled performers have maximized their motor performance based on their physical size and condition and their cognitive and social experiences. Developmental changes are most dramatic in the early years of our life span, but they do not cease with the onset of adulthood. Physiologic changes continue to occur within our bodies just as environmental experiences refine our perceptions, mental skills, and social relationships. New ways to perform skills might be attempted, but both new and well-learned skills must persistently accommodate these ever-present, though subtle, changes. This is particularly true much later in life, when physical, mental, and social change may be experienced more rapidly than in earlier adulthood.

It is clear that motor performance changes throughout our life span. This developmental process raises important questions for educators. For example, how is the potential for skilled performance influenced? Is it determined at conception by an individual's genetic make-up, or can parents and educators provide experiences during growth and developmental periods to promote skill development? Does skilled performance necessarily decline after young adulthood? The study of the developmental process with its many facets and intricacies helps us begin to unravel the answers to questions such as these.

Concept 1.1   Many changes in motor skill performance are age-related and occur throughout the entire life span.

It is traditional to think of motor development solely as the process of skill acquisition in children; that is, a progression from unskilled or low skilled performance evident in very young children, to intermediate levels of skill mastery exhibited during childhood, to relatively skilled performance demonstrated during late adolescence. Working from this perspective, a motor developmentalist studies the development of motor behavior by testing children of different ages and monitoring the course of their skill acquisition process. The presumption that motor development concerns only children and adolescents has developed because the majority of study in motor development has concentrated on the early years of the life span. However, many researchers now recognize that the study of development in general and motor development in particular should encompass the entire life span. Motor development in this text is viewed from the unique perspective that involves the process underlying behavioral change. (See chapter 1 of Endler, Boulter, & Osser, 1976, for a parallel discussion of developmental psychology.) Motor developmentalists, thus, not only describe changes but also seek to explain such changes over the course of development. This is best achieved from a life span perspective of motor development.

Challenges of the Life Span Perspective

An ever-greater portion of our population consists of older adults. Increasingly, older adults seek to improve the quality of their lives through healthful and enjoyable physical activities. Thus, from a realistic viewpoint, it no longer suffices to consider older adulthood as a period of sedentary living and illness. From a theoretical level, it is recognized that development does not stop at puberty with the cessation of physical growth, nor at the age of 21, nor at any other landmark of young adulthood. Changes in motor behavior, both substantive and qualitative, occur during older adulthood, too. Because the earliest developmental research focused on the motor behavior of children, many aspects of motor behavior in older adulthood are largely unexplored, and specific scientific knowledge of motor skill changes is sparse. Better knowledge and understanding of the motor behavior of older adulthood is an important challenge for motor developmentalists.

A fuller appreciation of motor development can be gained from a life span perspective, even for individuals who anticipate working only with children or only with adolescents. Consider, for example, that children and older adults are often similar in their motor behavior. Both groups are relatively slower in their reaction time to a visual stimulus than young adults. Are the causes of this difference in behavior the same for children and older adults? No, they are not. Children and older adults cognitively process information about the visual stimulus in different ways. This question of differential causes of behavior will be discussed in more detail throughout the text.

Behavior is the product of many influences. Our understanding of behavior is based on the integration of these influences—psychological, sociological, biological, physiological, cognitive, mechanical, and so on. Similarly, our greatest understanding of motor development is based on the integration of many behavior changes within a phase of development. It is impossible to study all behavioral influences at one time. Even though the discussions in this text may focus for a time on one particular aspect of behavioral change, the goal of developmentalists is to explain behavioral change over the life span from a global viewpoint. A broader range of cause-and-effect is encountered from this viewpoint, which in turn provides the basis for a more complete understanding of the factors involved in behavioral changes. More importantly perhaps, a life span perspective enables students of motor development to better understand motor behavior and the influence educators might have upon optimal motor development throughout life.

Summary 1.1—The Life Span Perspective

The view of motor development discussed in this text emphasizes a perspective on motor behavior that relates to the processes underlying change throughout the life span. The study of motor development involves both the description and the explanation of change in motor behavior. Ultimately, motor developmentalists integrate knowledge of various biological, psychological, sociological, cognitive, and mechanical factors that influence behavior at particular levels of development. This method is quite different from studying change as a function of time, as in the case of a researcher who studies a particular motor behavior in several age-groups to identify the characteristics and components of elite, proficient performance. Because changes in motor behavior occur from infancy through adulthood and in old age as well, a broad range of cause-and-effect influences in behavioral change are considered when examining motor development from a life span perspective. Consequently, motor skill development is viewed with a knowledge of preceding processes as well as potential effects.

Concept 1.2   Development is continuous, but aspects of the developmental process are identified by special terms.

The study of the development process is facilitated by understanding the terms used within this field of study. Every area of study develops its own terminology. Sometimes the terms and their usage within a field of study make it difficult for new students to read the literature with comprehension. It is especially confusing, for example, to find that a word used in everyday conversation has a very specific or perhaps different meaning when used in scientific study. Yet, specific meanings for terms are necessary for precise communication among those interested in the topic. Terms used frequently in the study of motor development are discussed in this concept.

Terminology in Motor Development

Two of the basic concepts discussed in this text focus on the terms *growth* and *development*. Although they are sometimes used interchangeably, growth means a *quantitative increase in size*. If physical growth is involved, the increase in size or body mass results from an increase in complete biological units (Timiras, 1972). This means that growth in height, for example, is not promoted by adding a new section to each leg but by the legs (as a biological unit) growing longer. The body is a complete biological unit that increases in size. Sometimes growth also is used to refer to an increase in the magnitude of intellectual ability or in social aptitudes (Rogers, 1982). This text, however, uses the term growth in the context of *physical* growth, not social or cognitive growth. The physical growth period (change in absolute size) for humans generally spans the time between conception and approximately 19 to 22 years of age.

As a complement to growth, development implies *a continuous process of change* leading to a state of organized and specialized *functional capacity*, that is, a state wherein an intended role can be fully carried out (Timiras, 1972). Development may occur in the form of quantitative change, qualitative change, or both simultaneously. *Motor development*, then, is the sequential, continuous age-related process whereby an individual progresses from simple, unorganized, and unskilled movement to the achievement of highly organized, complex motor skills, and finally to the adjustment of skills that accompanies aging. This process is *not* limited to the physical growth period; rather, development continues through the entire life span. The term *motor*, when used with other terms such as development and learning, refers to *movement*. Hence, *motor learning* deals with aspects of learning involving body movement and is not necessarily age-related. If both the learning and performance of movement are to be addressed, the term *motor behavior* is often used.

Another term often used in conjunction with growth is *maturation* or physiological maturation. Maturation is a *qualitative* advancement in biological makeup and may refer to cellular, organ, or system advancement in biochemical composition rather than to size alone (Teeple, 1978). Typically, maturation connotes progress toward *maturity*, which is the state of optimal functional integration of the body systems and the ability to reproduce.

Physiological changes occur over the entire continuum of life, although these changes are much slower after the physical growth period. The term *aging*, used broadly, applies to the process of growing old regardless of chronological age. More specifically, aging refers to continuing molecular, cellular, and organismic differentiation. Aging changes reflect a prior state of development and foreshadow future changes such that aging is inseparable from developmental processes (Timiras, 1972).

Developmentalists have adopted terms to describe specific age periods by delineating characteristics of growth and development that set these age periods apart. Researchers have defined the age periods somewhat differently because there are rarely sharp, distinguishable divisions between the periods. Aside from events such as birth and menarche (the first menstrual cycle in girls), the age periods blend into one another, reflecting the continuous na-

Table 1.1 Chronological Ages for Various Developmental Periods

Developmental Period	Approximate Chronological Age
Prenatal	
Embryo	2 weeks to 8 weeks
Fetus	8 weeks to birth
Neonate	Birth to 4 weeks
Infancy	Birth to 1 year
Childhood	
Early childhood (preschool)	1 to 6 years
Late childhood (preadolescence)	6 to 10 years
Adolescence	
Girls	8 or 10 to 18 years
Boys	10 or 12 to 20 years
Adulthood	
Young adulthood	18 to 40 years
Middle adulthood	40 to 60 years
Older adulthood	60 years and over

ture of growth, development, and maturation. In a few cases, commonly used terms apply to more than one chronological age period as you will see by examining the time frames of the age periods listed in Table 1.1. Note also that some age periods, such as childhood, are subdivided.

Summary 1.2—Developmental Terminology

Development, then, is a complex, continuous process that involves the entire life span. In order to distinguish the many aspects of development and the subtle differences and changes in growth and development, precise terminology is used. This precise interpretation of common vocabulary is necessary to comprehend specific facts and research studies about growth as well as various theoretical viewpoints that guide the study of development.

Concept 1.3   Some issues in development remain unresolved.

It would be ideal if the scientific information educators apply in the teaching process were complete, accurate, and proven. Unfortunately, in relatively few areas of knowledge is this the case, and development is certainly not one of the "complete" areas. Although some of the cornerstone research in motor development was conducted in the 1930s, many questions central to development generally and to motor development specifically are still undergoing investigation. These major developmental questions remain unresolved for several reasons. First, scientific research on the question simply has not been conducted. Such is the case with study of the mechanical aspects of older adults' motor skill performance. Another reason is that the technology for conducting a given type of research may not exist, or the existing technology may limit the amount of research and the degree to which research is conducted. Historically, initial attempts to analyze motor skill performance via high speed filming were limited in this manner. Before digital and computer film analysis systems were available, film was meticulously analyzed by hand measurement, a time-consuming and less accurate process. Developmentalists also often examine an issue using basic assumptions from conflicting theoretical viewpoints, which is yet another reason why developmental questions cannot be resolved easily. Some developmentalists, for example, believe heredity is the major influence in development and conduct their research from this perspective; other researchers believe the environment is the major influence.

As with any area of study, it is important for students to recognize the limitations of the information currently available. Toward that end, the following discussion examines the prevailing theoretical viewpoints in development and some of the major unresolved issues that have implications for the study of motor development.

Theoretical Viewpoints

Consider the many factors contributing to development—biological, perceptual, and social factors, to name a few—that must be synthesized to form a total conceptualization of development. Is it any wonder that most developmentalists choose to study development from only one perspective at a time? In doing so, developmentalists adopt a frame of reference or *theoretical viewpoint*. While no single frame of reference can encompass all of the details of development, the adoption of a single viewpoint permits the identification and structuring of a finite set of hypotheses or questions that developmentalists can begin to test. Our knowledge in some areas is developed almost solely from one perspective. In other areas, research conducted from two different viewpoints yields conflicting results! It is helpful to know the major perspectives or frames of reference in development so that explanations of behavior can be better understood. This knowledge is especially useful when two or more explanations are in conflict.

Biological Versus Psychological Perspectives

Development is generally viewed from either a biological or a psychological perspective. In the former, the body's parts and systems are studied, sometimes at a cellular level, and sometimes at an organismic level. In the psychological perspective an individual is studied as a thinking, emotional being (Rogers, 1982) whose behavior is observed as a reflection of the developmental process. Both perspectives are important in the study of motor development. Biological (physiological) aspects of motor skill cannot be overlooked, because a full understanding of motor development requires knowledge of physical growth and of the age-related changes to the physiological demands of vigorous activity. Hence, it is necessary to adopt a biological viewpoint to study many aspects of motor development.

At the same time, it is important to understand behavior resulting from an individual's decisions and feelings. Such behavior plays an important role in the choice to be active, in the success of skill performance, and the extent of an individual's participation. So, the psychological (and social psychological) perspective must be adopted to study still other aspects of motor development. Ultimately, educators must be concerned with both perspectives, biological and psychological. For example, the reluctance of a 12-year-old boy to participate in physical activities might be traced to his small size in relation to most other boys his age. His physical size affects his social relationships and, in turn, his motivation to participate in physical activities. Teachers and parents must understand his situation from both viewpoints if they are to help him find a way to participate in healthful and enjoyable physical activities. The biological and psychological perspectives of development are complementary and consideration of both views contributes to a greater understanding of the total person.

Major Theories in Developmental Psychology

The psychological frame of reference on development, known as *developmental psychology*, includes several important theoretical approaches for studying development that have implications for motor development. Each theoretical approach could be studied in great detail; however, our discussion focuses on the implications for motor development.

Maturational Approach. Arnold Gesell's *maturational approach* (Gesell, 1954; Salkind, 1981) is an important developmental viewpoint that was influenced by *recapitulation theory*—the notion that *ontogeny*, the individual's development, recapitulates or reflects *phylogeny*, the species' development. Gesell believed that the biological and evolutionary history of a species (e.g., humans) determined its orderly and invariable sequence of development, and that the *rate* of the developmental sequence was individually determined. He explained maturation as a process controlled by internal (genetic) rather than external (environmental) factors. Environmental factors were thought to affect developmental rate but only temporarily, because hereditary factors were in ultimate control of development.

Gesell and his coworkers introduced the *co-twin control strategy* to experiments in developmental research. In this strategy, identical twins are the research subjects. One twin receives specific training (the experimental treatment), while the other twin (called the "control") receives no special training (the control treatment) and is allowed to develop as natural circumstances and opportunities dictate. After a specific period of time, the twins are measured and compared on certain previously determined developmental criteria. In an alternate version of this research technique the experimental treatment (training) is applied to the control twin at an older age, after which the twins are again compared. The co-twin control research strategy provided significant contributions to the study of development. It had particular impact on the study of basic motor skills that emerge during infancy and childhood, because developmentalists began identifying the sequence of skill development, noting variations in the rate of skill onset.

Gesell's maturational theory predicted that skill development could not be accelerated by a special training program before a child's biological development reached a point of readiness to learn the skill. Studies using the co-twin control strategy appeared to confirm this prediction, but questions remain because Gesell could not exclude the nontrained twin from all activities similar to the criterion skill. The ages of skill onset therefore were close in the twins.

To summarize, Gesell's theory emphasized hereditary factors as the major influence on development and de-emphasized the influence of the environment. The testing of Gesell's theory and others is discussed in greater detail in chapter 3.

Behavioral Theory. Another major developmental perspective is represented by *behavioral*, sometimes called *environmental*, theories. Several articulations of the behavioral perspective exist, most of which tend to view the individual as reactive, that is, subject to influence by external stimulation. Hence, stimulus-response associations are the basic behavioral units. Ivan Pavlov, John

Watson, Edward Thorndike, B.F. Skinner, and Sidney Bijou with Don Baer are among the psychologists who outlined early behavioral theories. More recently, however, the work of Albert Bandura reflects a movement by behaviorists away from the notion of a strictly passive, reactive individual. The example presented here is Bandura's social learning theory (Bandura, 1977), on which most of the research on imitation and motor performance has been based (Weiss, 1983).

In his theory, Bandura views reinforcement of a response to a stimulus as a powerful means to shape behavior, but he also attributes much of learned behavior to the *imitation* of successful (rewarded) models. In other words, *vicarious* reinforcement is as valuable as direct reinforcement. Behaviorists, in contrast to maturationalists (Gesell), emphasize environmental influences in development. Bandura moderates this behavioral tenet by stressing the concept of *reciprocity* between the individual and the environment. For example, a learner does not simply observe a model and then imitate behavior, but rather the learner first internalizes the model's behavior and then attempts to match this internal representation through progressive approximations of the model's behavior. Reinforcement (reward) is used to refine the approximations until they match the internalized behavior (Salkind, 1981). The process whereby children begin to participate and imitate others in sport is often explained from the social learning viewpoint, which will be discussed in more depth in chapter 9.

Cognitive Theory. A third developmental psychology perspective is the *cognitive*, or *organismic*, position whose chief proponent was Jean Piaget (Piaget, 1952). Piaget theorized that an individual can act upon the environment and the environment can act upon the individual, so that an *interaction* occurs between the two. This position contrasts sharply with most behavioral theories (although *not* Bandura's social learning theory), because the individual is not passive, but actively attends to certain aspects of the environment, screens out other aspects, and reformulates incoming information (Endler, Boulter, & Osser, 1976). For Piaget, the developmental process encompassed biological growth, children's experiences, social transformation of information and attitudes from adults (especially parents) to children, and the inherent tendency for persons to seek equilibrium with the environment and within themselves (Salkind, 1981).

One of Piaget's significant contributions to developmental study was the notion of *stages*, that is, periods of time during which children's thinking and behavior reflect a certain type of underlying structure (Miller, 1983). Although other developmentalists before Piaget had used the concept of stages, Piaget envisioned stages based on qualitative, structural changes that (a) have a fixed order, and (b) cannot be skipped. Developmentalists today disagree on the definition of "stage" and its usage. Piaget's primary interest was the development of intelligence and the source of knowledge. However, because the performance of motor skills requires the processing of information, Piaget's theory has implications for motor development. Later in chapter 8, the ways in which motor developmentalists use Piagetian concepts to describe the processing demands of motor skills are more fully discussed.

The three theoretical approaches reviewed have very different basic assumptions: (a) Maturational theorists use assumptions that emphasize biological development; (b) behaviorists stress the importance of environment; and (c) cognitivists assume an incorporated biological and psychological influence on development. Behaviorists view an individual as reactive, whereas cognitivists see the individual as active. Behaviorists believe too, that development is a process of quantitative change wherein learning episodes accumulate with time, thus the description of stages is counterproductive (Miller, 1983). Maturationists, on the other hand, emphasize development as qualitative change by describing the sequence in which new skills merge. Cognitivists focus on qualitative changes that take place as one moves from stage to stage; further, cognitivists acknowledge that quantitative changes occur in the developmental process as behavior patterns and cognitive skills become stronger, more consistent, and more efficient (Miller, 1983). Diametrically opposed theories cannot be merged, but educators are free to select whichever view seems most appropriate to explain different aspects of development. It is important to remember that these theoretical viewpoints focus only on specific aspects of development. Thus, educators may need to combine aspects of several viewpoints to understand and explain motor behavior. In keeping with this line of reasoning, *basic concepts of motor development discussed in this text reflect a variety of theoretical perspectives.*

Contemporary Issues

As stated in Concept 1.3, some issues in motor development remain unresolved. In some cases, this has little affect on the study of specific aspects of motor development, but in others the impact on improving motor skill development may be dramatic. It is important, then, for students of motor development to be aware of these unsettled issues and be alerted to research findings that must be interpreted with caution.

Nature Versus Nurture

One of the longest standing issues in motor development is that of *nature* versus *nurture*, sometimes called heredity versus environment or nativism versus empiricism. The controversy centers on whether hereditary factors or environmental factors are the major influence on behavior. This issue has far-reaching implications for motor development. For example, if environmental factors are the chief determinants of motor behavior, a successful athletic career might be launched by structuring an infant's environment in a certain way. On the other hand, if genetic factors predominate and great athletes are "born," not "made," a parent or educator could do little to enhance the talents of a child beyond innate ability. Today, few theorists and teachers adopt the extreme position of one or the other, because neither position has been proven exclusively. The contemporary approach is far more reasonable in recognizing that heredity and environment are intertwined and that motor behavior is influenced by the interaction of heredity and environment. Thus, greater attention must shift toward the *mechanisms* that mediate development (Endler et al., 1976); that is, *how* do nature and nurture interact to produce development?

Critical Periods

A critical period is a time span during which an individual is most susceptible to the influence of an event or mitigating factor. This period may not be the *only* time when an event is influential, but rather the time when the individual is more likely to be affected by the event. In this sense, the term "critical" is a misnomer, and perhaps "sensitive" is a better descriptor of the concept. To illustrate the concept, suppose that a critical period exists between 4 and 8 months of age for the acquisition of reach-and-grasp skills. If the supposition is correct, an infant who does not have an opportunity to learn the skill during this age span may never be as proficient as if he or she had acquired it during the critical time.

Developmentalists disagree concerning the existence of critical periods. Although considerable evidence is available for the existence of critical periods in animals, the hypothesis remains difficult to test in humans for both ethical and moral reasons. Note that behaviorists strongly disagree that an individual is susceptible to influence during a biologically-based time period, because they argue in favor of developmental control by environmental factors. This controversy is especially relevant to the acquisition of basic motor skills. Consequently, more on this topic will be discussed in chapter 3.

Research Methodology

Longitudinal Research. The best research strategy for the study of human development is the longitudinal approach, in which measures on individual subjects are repeated periodically over the course of their development. Hence, development is observed directly, it is not implied. Unfortunately, the pluses of longitudinal research also create problems. One is that such research usually takes years, making it difficult for researchers to keep in contact with subjects and increasing the cost of the research. Also, it is many years before the study results are available. Repeated measures of the same subjects may become distorted because of a "practice effect" as the subjects become overly familiar with the assessment device. Too, a measurement tool appropriate for subjects at a young age may be inappropriate for them at an older age. Think how difficult it is to measure throwing accuracy of 2-year-old children compared with when they are 10 years old!

Cross-Sectional Research. As a result of these drawbacks to longitudinal research, many researchers adopt the cross-sectional research method. A cross-sectional study enables an experimenter to test subjects of different ages at the same time and *imply* developmental change if performance trends are shown across the different age-groups. Although this strategy shortcuts many of the problems associated with longitudinal research, the cross-sectional technique also has weaknesses; developmental change must be implied from group averages, which sacrifices attention at the individual level (Wohlwill, 1973). The subjects in a cross-sectional study also come from different *cohorts*, that is, different groups of individuals who share a common characteristic, such as age. Significant changes in nutrition, health care, education, play toys, and social attitudes occur over the years. If factors such as these affect the studied behavior, an improvement in behavior across age-groups could not be attributed to development to the exclusion of an intervening variable. For these reasons the traditional research methods in development—longitudinal and cross-sectional studies—require control or adjustment for time-of-measurement and cohort effects, respectively.

Sequential Research. A third type of research methodology, sequential research designs, has been suggested as a way to overcome longitudinal and cross-sectional problems. Sequential research is actually a combination of longitudinal and cross-sectional designs. One suggested sequential design includes three factors: cohort, time-of-measurement, and age (Schaie, 1965). A model sequential design is presented in Figure 1.1. In this example four cohorts are tested at three times, so that each row is a short longitudinal study and each column is a cross-sectional study. The advantage of the design is the time-lag component, wherein subjects from different cohorts can be compared at the same chronological age to identify any existing cohort differences. Nevertheless, this model has disadvantages as well. When the factors (age, cohort, time of measurement) are used as independent variables in a research study, they are not truly independent of one another, because setting two of

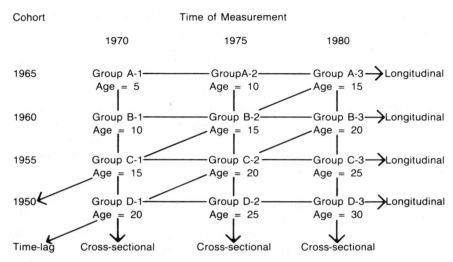

Figure 1.1 A model sequential research design. Note that each row is a short longitudinal study and that each column is a cross-sectional study. The time lag component, shown by the two diagonal lines, allows comparison of different cohorts at the same chronological age, thus identifying any cohort differences.

the factors automatically sets the third. Consequently, results of the study must be statistically analyzed three times, each using two of the three factors at a time. Questions remain as to the validity of comparing the results of the three analyses. A more thorough discussion on the analysis problem and others concerning sequential designs can be found in articles by Kausler (1982) and Wohlwill (1973). Despite the disadvantages of the sequential design, studies using this design make valuable contributions to the understanding of development.

Each research strategy has both strengths and weaknesses. The research strategy selected depends in part on the behavior to be studied and the factors expected to influence that behavior. Ideally, research results are ultimately confirmed by two or more research strategies.

Stages

Developmentalists have yet to adopt a standard definition and usage of the "stage" concept; hence, the concept has been used in different ways. Most developmentalists agree that stages should describe qualitative differences in overall behavior, yet some use the term to describe change in individual behaviors, for example, in grasping. Still others favor the term to describe change among two or more variables developing in parallel. In this sense, a stage unites a set of behaviors (Wohlwill, 1973). The imprecision in defining the stage concept is partly responsible for the skepticism of many developmentalists concerning its value. Although the term is used often and loosely in developmental literature, it is beneficial to define the concept more precisely and move toward a more accurate usage of the construct. Piaget outlined the most detailed set of criteria for defining the developmental process as stages (Miller, 1983; Salkind, 1981; Wohlwill, 1973). As a result, the term "stage" is most often used in the context described by Piaget, and we outline his criteria here.

Stages have several characteristics, but the major characteristic is *qualitative change*. That is, a stage contains new behavior previously unobserved, as opposed to more of an earlier behavior. Subsequent stages grow out of and incorporate previous stages, a characteristic that is termed *hierarchical integration*. Within a stage, behaviors emerge gradually and mix with the behaviors of the previous stage through a *consolidation process*. In this way the previous stage behaviors are reworked so that regression to the previous stage is impossible. Since stages lead to one another, they are *intransitive*, or unable to be reordered. Further, all individuals must progress through the stages in the same universal order, and stages cannot be skipped.

Movement to a new stage is stimulated by an imbalance between the individual's mental structures and the environment. This *equilibration process* is manifested in periods of relative stability at the end of each stage, followed by periods of instability during the transition between stages. The individual maintains *structural wholeness* as the patterns of behavior or operations within each stage are interconnected to form an organized whole. It is possible for individuals to acquire a given pattern of behavior or level of thought but not apply the new behavior to all the possible tasks or situations encountered. This time lag in the application of new behaviors within a stage is referred to as *horizontal decalage*. Sequential changes in behavior that conform to these characteristics, then, can be called "stages."

Behaviors that make qualitative transitions over time but do not meet the criteria for stages can be labeled in other ways. The terms "sequences," "patterns," "steps," and "phases" all might be used. On occasion, "steps" are used to describe changes within a stage. It is more appropriate, then, to use these terms unless behavioral transitions are known to meet the stage criteria. Students of motor development, however, should expect that these terms and the term stage will sometimes be interchanged in the literature.

Summary 1.3—Issues in Motor Development

It would be ideal if all the controversial issues in development were settled, but in fact, many remain unresolved. It is valuable to identify the differing perspectives and viewpoints taken in growth and development. To do so allows us to better understand the information gathered by researchers adopting one perspective, while recognizing the limitations of that knowledge. We can better untangle the controversies surrounding growth and development and sort through the various pieces of information to form a clearer total picture of the developing individual. In the next chapter, a biological approach is taken to discuss the concepts of physical growth that affect motor development.

Suggested Readings

Endler, N.S., Boulter, L.R., & Osser, H. (1976). *Contemporary issues in developmental psychology* (2nd ed.). New York: Holt, Rinehart and Winston.

Kausler, D.H. (1982). *Experimental psychology and human aging.* New York: John Wiley & Sons.

Miller, P.H. (1983). *Theories of developmental psychology.* San Francisco: W.H. Freeman.

Rogers, D. (1982). *Life-span human development.* Monterey, CA: Brooks/Cole.

Salkind, N.J. (1981). *Theories of human development.* New York: D. Van Nostrand.

Wohlwill, J.F. (1973). *The study of behavioral development.* New York: Academic Press.

2

Physical Growth, Maturation, and Aging

Should parents be concerned if a 12-month-old infant is not walking yet? Is a 6-year-old physically ready for youth league soccer? The answers to these questions are related in part to each child's physical maturity. To determine children's potential for motor skill performance at a given age, we must consider the status of their physical growth and maturation. Leg strength, for example, must develop to some minimal level before infants can support their weight and walk. The nervous system must mature sufficiently to permit voluntarily planned walking steps executed with coordination. Attempting to teach children skills before they are physically ready is often frustrating and can sometimes be harmful if the skeletal and muscular strength necessary for the skill is not yet developed. Growth and maturation are natural functions of increasing age, and developmentalists have determined the average ages for the acquisition of various motor skills.

All children are not the same. One 6-year-old cannot be measured to determine the growth status of all 6-year-olds. Children typically grow either faster or slower than "average-for-age" growth. Before an individual's potential for skill performance can be assessed, we must know the course of normal growth and the normal variations of growth for persons of a given age. We would then determine if the 6-year-old mentioned earlier is about the same height and weight as other 6-year-olds, or bigger, or smaller. This and other information should be considered when deciding if a child is ready for youth league soccer.

Assessment of physical growth and maturation requires a knowledge of normal growth patterns and an understanding of growth measures. Knowledge of normal growth includes not only the *average* extent of growth at a given age but also the normal *variations* of growth. These standards identify the range within which children's measurements should fall at a given age if their bodies are growing properly. Also, an examiner must understand the advantages and disadvantages of the many ways to measure growth. Some measures are useful for one age period but not another; some are influenced more by genetic inheritance than by the environment in which the child grows, and others are influenced more by the environment than by hereditary factors. An awareness of the strengths and weaknesses of each measure allows the examiner to appropriately use the information gained from the measure. The following discussion deals with the normal patterns of growth obtained with growth measures. This knowledge is helpful to those who teach skills because it allows individualization of both instruction and expectations of students based on the progress of physical growth. Additionally, children growing abnormally can be identified and referred to medical personnel for further evaluation.

Once an individual reaches adult size, you might think there is little reason to measure height, weight, and so on. But, the body is not static throughout adulthood. There may be many changes, especially in weight and in the composition of the body, such as the amount of fat weight. Many of the measures discussed are also useful for adults.

Concept 2.1   Physical growth and maturation can be assessed in many ways.

The branch of science involving human growth and body measurement is termed *anthropometry*. Anthropometric measures include height, weight, circumference, and breadth. Although most of us would consider these measures fairly routine, such measures must be precise if they are to provide us with reliable information about human growth (Boyd, 1929). Standard procedures for taking growth measures should be followed rigidly and are available from the International Biological Programme (Weiner & Lourie, 1969,

1981). Several common growth measures and maturation measures, including the accepted assessment procedure, are discussed next.

Growth Measures

Height

One of the most useful and common measures of growth is that of body height, or *stature*. Up to 3 years of age, height is measured with the child in a reclined position. Thereafter, measurements are taken with the person standing erect on a *stadiometer*. This instrument provides a rigid platform at right angles to an accurate linear scale (see Figure 2.1). A right triangle is placed flat against the scale and on the highest point (vertex) of the person's head

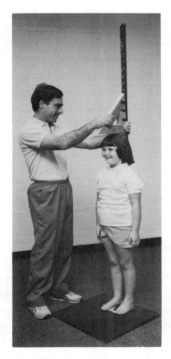

Figure 2.1   The measurement of standing height with inexpensive equipment. When the triangle is held against the measurement scale a level reading is assured.

to obtain a level reading. The person stands erect with heels together, shoulders relaxed, and arms at the side when the measure is taken. Anthropometrists have measured large groups of children and adolescents at various ages to determine average height-for-age. These averages and the range of height are often plotted against age, as in Figures 2.2a and 2.2b. The range of scores is expressed in percentiles which show relative position. For example, if a group of 100 8-year-olds were measured, a child whose height measured at the 50th percentile would be taller than 49 of the children and shorter than 50 of the children in the group.

Note that separate height charts are used for girls and boys. Height and weight differences for girls and boys are minimal during the prepubertal years. Girls begin their growth spurt about 9 years of age and experience peak height velocity (i.e., grow at a relatively faster rate) at 11 years of age. This growth spurt tapers off for girls at age 14, approximately. The boys' growth spurt typically begins at age 11, peaks at age 13, and does not taper off until age 17. In the 3 years between age 14 and 17, boys grow an average of 13 cm. Hence the longer growth period accounts for the greater total height achieved by boys compared with girls' height.

An individual's height can be measured and compared to the charted values for chronological age. Caution must be used in interpreting deviations from the average. For example, if the height of an 8-year-old boy falls at the 25th percentile, you may wonder if he is a late maturer, is growing abnormally, or if he will be a relatively short adult as dictated by his genetic inheritance. There is no way to answer this question from the height measure alone, so you must be careful not to jump to an incorrect conclusion. It is important to recognize, too, that some height charts are based on individuals of a particular race and socioeconomic background. Comparisons are best when made to data taken on a group similar to that of the measured individual. Despite the limitations outlined, measures of stature are helpful in assessing growth and are easily obtained.

Weight

Weight (body mass) is a common anthropometric measure that requires an accurate scale. The person to be weighed wears minimal (or no) clothing and stands in the center of the scale's platform. Both height and weight should be measured at the same time of day for consistency, particularly if the individual is measured repeatedly and compared to previous results. As with stature, weight-for-age is often plotted graphically, as in Figures 2.3a and 2.3b. Here, too, caution must be exercised in interpreting deviations from the average, because weight values (mass) give no information about body composi-

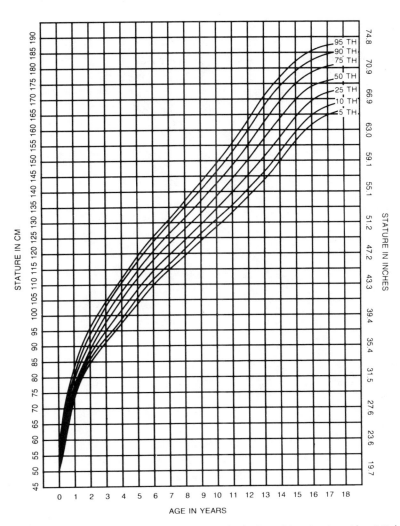

Figure 2.2(a) Stature (standing height) by age percentiles for boys. Note the sigmoid or "s" shape of the curves. From *NCHS Growth Curves for Children* by P.V.V. Hamill, 1977, Washington, DC: National Center for Health Statistics, DHEW Publication No. (PHS) 78-1650.

tion (leanness/fatness). Think for a moment about a 16-year-old boy whose weight measure coincides with the 85th percentile. This teenager might be overweight, heavily muscled, or he might have reached his adult size before most of his peers. Again, there is no way to tell from the weight measure alone.

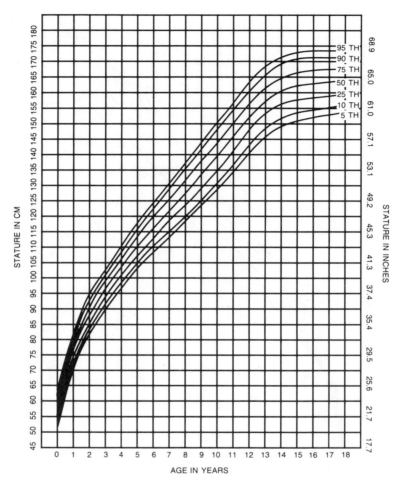

Figure 2.2(b) Stature (standing height) by age percentiles for girls. From *NCHS Growth Curves for Children* by P.V.V. Hamill, 1977, Washington, DC: National Center for Health Statistics, DHEW Publication No. (PHS) 78-1650.

To obtain more information about growth related to weight, estimates of leanness/fatness, or *body composition*, are made. The body weight is divided, for this purpose, into fat weight (adipose tissue) and lean body weight, which includes bone, muscle, organs, and tissues other than fat. The amount of body fat in a living individual cannot be measured directly but can be predicted by several methods. Underwater weighing is one method where

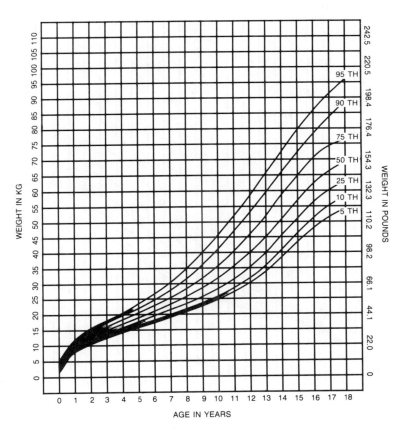

Figure 2.3(a) Weight by age percentiles for boys. From *NCHS Growth Curves for Children* by P.V.V. Hamill, 1977, Washington, DC: National Center for Health Statistics, DHEW Publication No. (PHS) 78-1650.

body denseness is estimated by contrasting body weight in air with body weight under water. It is difficult to submerge people and require them to expel the air in their lungs to obtain accurate underwater weight, so this method is rarely used with young children. Another body composition measure assesses the amount of potassium 40 naturally emitted from the body, because the amount is proportional to the lean body mass. It is easy to have persons lie in a whole-body counter that scans the body and records the potassium 40 radiation levels; however, the counters are expensive and often not available.

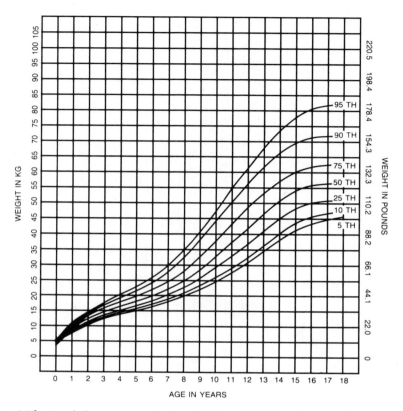

Figure 2.3(b) Weight by age percentiles for girls. From *NCHS Growth Curves for Children* by P.V.V. Hamill, 1977, Washington, DC: National Center for Health Statistics, DHEW Publication No. (PHS) 78-1650.

Estimates of body composition from skinfold thickness measures are the most practical in educational and recreational settings. Skinfold thickness is measured by placing a caliper over a fold of skin and the underlying fat tissue, lifted between the examiner's thumb and forefinger at clearly specified body sites (see Figure 2.4). The measures are then entered into mathematical equations that estimate body density and fat weight. These equations are, ideally, specific to age-group, race, fitness level, and after puberty, to gender. Although many equations are available for adults and some equations have been developed for preadolescents and adolescents (Shephard, Jones, & Ishii, 1969), further research is needed to identify the most accurate formulas for children.

Circumference

Head circumference is another body dimension of particular importance in the growth of infants and young children. It is taken just above the bony ridge over the eyes (see Figure 2.5). Normal head circumference measures fall within a fairly narrow range for any given age, so marked deviations might imply neurologic abnormalities. For example, an abnormally rapid increase in head measurements taken at frequent intervals might indicate that a child has hydrocephalus, an accumulation of intraventricular fluid. In some cases small head circumference for age has been associated with mental retardation, but there are notable exceptions and caution should be exercised in interpreting small head circumference measures. However, head circumference does serve as a valuable screening measure that may indicate medical examination is needed (Brandt, 1978).

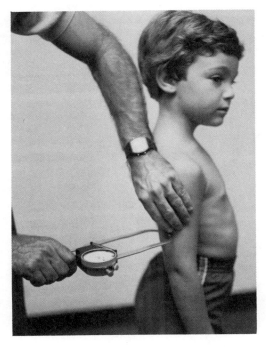

Figure 2.4   A skinfold measurement taken over the tricep muscle in the back of the upper arm.

Other common circumference measures include arm, calf, waist, and chest girth. In all of these measures it is important to measure at a specified site, making certain the tape measure is horizontal to the body segment. A steel, spring-loaded tape measure is preferable and assures consistent pressure on each measurement when the spring is stretched consistently. Due to variations in inspiration and in breast development, chest measures are often inaccurate; thus, chest girth is less desirable as a growth measure than other circumference measures.

Breadth and Length

Breadth measures are useful in assessing growth, particularly in body build, or physique. The most common measures are biacromial distance (shoulder

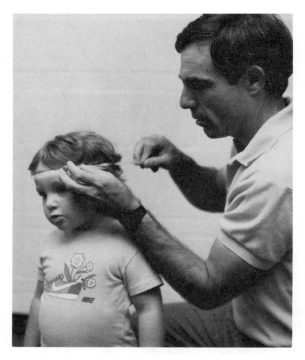

Figure 2.5 Measurement of head circumference with a spring-loaded steel tape measure.

width) and biiliac or bicristal distance (hip width). Biacromial width divided by the bicristal width provides a useful ratio to observe proportional changes in physique. Gender differences in growth at puberty are dramatically illustrated by this ratio, for which men tend to have a greater ratio than women, reflecting their relatively wider shoulders and narrower hips. The pelvis grows proportionately wider in women, of course, to accommodate childbirth, yielding a smaller shoulder-to-hip width ratio. Breadth measures are taken with a breadth caliper or blade anthropometer at specified bone locations, such as the acromion processes (shoulder) or the iliac crests (hip) (see Figure 2.6). It might be difficult to locate these bony sites in obese individuals.

Beside breadth measures, assessments of the length of various body parts can be taken, such as sitting height. The procedure for a sitting height measurement is identical to that for stature except the individual is seated with the feet hanging freely. Leg length can be estimated by subtracting the sitting

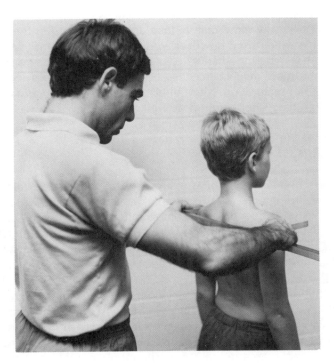

Figure 2.6 A breadth measurement taken at the shoulders, the biacromial breadth.

height from standing height, or it can be measured directly from the lateral malleolus (ankle bone) to the greater trochanter of the femur (thigh bone). Other length measurements are taken at definitive sites, usually a bony land-mark. A source such as Weiner and Lourie (1981) can be consulted for a complete description of each length measurement. These measures are useful in describing body proportions during growth, a topic discussed further in a later section.

Maturation Measures

Maturation, the progress toward maturity by qualitative rather than quantitative advancement, often must be implied from growth measures because direct measures of maturation are not easy to obtain. Suppose you measure a child's height, weight, biacromial breadth, and so on, and compare these values to those on standard growth charts for the child's age. If most of the body dimensions fall within the upper percentiles, you might conclude that the child is physically more mature than an average child of the same age. In making this conclusion, however, you may overlook other factors, such as the child's genetic inheritance, or perhaps excess fat weight that places the child in the upper weight percentiles. Hence, size alone does not accurately indicate level of maturation. More direct measures of maturation are available, but they have shortcomings as well.

Skeletal Age

The most useful method of assessing maturation is to determine *skeletal age* by taking radiographs (X rays), usually of the bones of the wrist, but occasionally of the long bones or teeth. Photographs of wrist and hand radiographs have been standardized to identify skeletal maturation at 6-month and 1-year intervals (Greulich & Pyle, 1959). To determine a child's skeletal age, for example, you must compare his or her radiograph to the standard radiographs of bone development. Figures 2.7 and 2.8 are wrist and hand radiographs that show the differences in bone development between a younger and an older child. Areas that appear as spaces in the wrist are actually cartilaginous bone not yet calcified and thus appear black or grayish in X rays. As each cartilaginous wrist bone begins to ossify, it becomes more dense and appears as a visible opaque area in the X ray. The number and size of the ossified area of each wrist bone increases as a child matures. Greater calcification in the long bones of the hand and forearm are also indicative of advanced development in a physically more mature child. If a wrist and hand X ray of a girl was analyzed and deemed closer in appearance to the X ray in Figure 2.8 than to any other photograph in the set of standards, the girl would be assigned a skeletal age of 128 months (10 years, 8 months). If her actual chronological age was 9 years old, she would be considered more mature

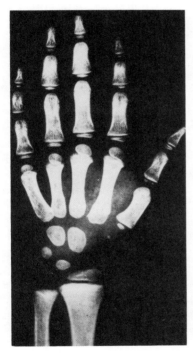
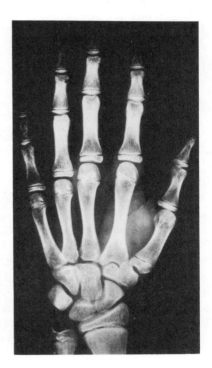

Figure 2.7 An X ray of the hand, skeletal age 48 months for boys and 37 months for girls. From *A Radiographic Standard of Reference for the Growing Hand and Wrist* (p. 53) by S.I. Pyle, 1971, Chicago, IL: Yearbook Medical Publishers. Copyright 1971 by Bolton-Brush Growth Center. Reprinted by permission.

Figure 2.8 An X ray of the hand, skeletal age 156 months for boys and 128 months for girls. From *A Radiographic Standard of Reference for the Growing Hand and Wrist* (p. 73) by S.I. Pyle, 1971, Chicago, IL: Yearbook Medical Publishers. Copyright 1971 by Bolton-Brush Growth Center. Reprinted by permission.

for her age; on the other hand, if she was 11½ years old, her skeletal age indicates she was maturing a little later than average for her age (i.e., she was less physically mature).

The difficulties in assessing skeletal age, aside from technical problems in x-raying and rater accuracy, include the expense of X rays and the doubtful advisability of repeated, unnecessary X ray exposure. Consequently, wrist and hand X rays are rarely available for large numbers of children. Hand and wrist radiographs of adults are used to measure not the degree of physical maturity, but rather the extent of osteoporosis (bone loss). A densiometric analysis may be done from the radiographs or the width of the bone cortex may be measured (Brewer, Meyer, Keele, Upton, & Hagan, 1983; Oyster, Morton, & Linnell, 1984). Hence, hand and wrist radiographs are informative at various times over the life span.

Other Maturational Measures

Several other direct measures of maturation can be used, but they have both advantages and disadvantages. One method assesses maturation by *dental eruption* (appearance of teeth), but it is restricted to the short age spans when deciduous (baby) teeth first appear and then are replaced by permanent teeth. Another simple, straightforward method of maturity assessment rates the *appearance of secondary sex characteristics*: genital and pubic hair development in boys, and breast and pubic hair development in girls. A rating from 1 to 5 is assigned for each measure by comparing development to standard photographs (Tanner, 1962; Weiner & Lourie, 1981). Axillary and facial hair development also may be rated. As with dental eruption, such ratings are useful only within a specific age period, in this case the adolescent years. Direct measures are preferred for maturation assessment purposes, but because they are not always available or applicable for use over wide age spans, maturation must sometimes be implied from anthropometric measures.

Plotting Growth

Anthropometric measures are often charted in relation to age, as illustrated earlier in Figures 2.2a, 2.2b, 2.3a, and 2.3b. The curve derived from this process is termed a *distance curve* because the absolute amount, or total accumulation of growth, is represented over regular time intervals, such as months or years. Several features of a distance curve are important: One is the rate, or speed, of growth. Where the curve is steep, growth is rapid; where it is relatively flat, growth is slow. The top curve in Figure 2.9 is a distance curve for height. Notice that the curve is particularly steep between 12 and 13 years, but it flattens out between 14 and 16 years. Another feature of the distance curve is the location of *inflection points*, that is, places where there is a transition from faster to slower growth, or vice versa. An inflection point in the distance curve of Figure 2.9 is at approximately 12.3 years. The rate of growth and the inflection points can be highlighted by plotting a *velocity curve*. The velocity curve is obtained by plotting the *rate* of incremental change in growth over time, rather than accumulated growth. For example, if a person grows 2 cm between ages 11 and 12, a point is plotted at 2 cm on the vertical, or "height gained," axis and at the midpoint of the growth interval, 11.5 years of age, on the horizontal axis. If the child grows 3 cm between ages 12 and 13, another point is plotted at 3 cm on the vertical axis and 12.5 years on the horizontal axis. The process is continued and the points are connected by a smoothed curve, the velocity curve. The middle curve in Figure 2.9 is the velocity curve for the distance curve at the top. Note that rapid growth is indicated by an upward trend in the velocity curve; slower growth is a downward trend; and the inflection point of the distance curve is a peak in the velocity curve. If you repeat this process by plotting the change in the velocity curve (instead of the distance curve), you obtain an *acceleration* curve that illustrates the rate of growth *change*. Figure 2.9 also shows an acceleration curve (bottom). An acceleration curve emphasizes the age periods when the rate of *change* in growth is constant, speeding up, or slowing down.

Summary 2.1—Assessing Physical Growth and Maturation

Physical growth is studied through careful and repeated measurement of body dimensions. Such growth measures are easily obtained, and standard growth curves can be derived from studies of large numbers of children. An individual child then can be measured and compared to the standard range for a given chronological age. Maturation level, the level of qualitative advancement of body tissues, can be implied from dimensional growth measures with caution. Direct measures of maturation are more desirable but are often impractical.

Growth assessment is a valuable tool for educators. Much of a child's progress in skill development is related to physical size and maturity. While

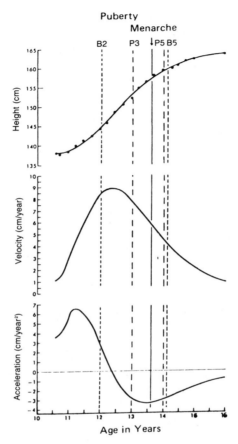

Figure 2.9 Height attained, height velocity, and height acceleration curves for a girl at adolescence. Note menarche came after peak height velocity. B2 marks beginning of breast development, B5, adult form. P3 marks intermediate stage of pubic hair development, P5, adult form. From *Advances in Reproductive Physiology* by A. Maclaren (Ed.), 1967, London: Elek Books. Copyright 1967 by Grafton Books division of Collins Publishing Group. Reprinted by permission.

size and maturity tend to increase with chronological age, they do so at a unique rate for each child. Any one child's capabilities can then be more realistically estimated with the level of physical maturity in mind so that expectations can be set and physical activities planned accordingly.

Concept 2.2   Embryonic and fetal growth are influenced by both genetic and environmental factors.

The instant an ovum (egg) and spermatozoan fuse in fertilization, the growth process begins. Early development is astonishingly precise, carried out under the control of genes. Genes, then, determine both the normal aspects of development and inherited abnormal development. At the same time, the growing embryo, and later, fetus is very sensitive to environmental factors. These include the environment in which the fetus is growing—the amniotic sac in the uterus—and the nutrients delivered to the fetus via the mother's circulation and the placenta. Some environmental factors, such as abnormal external pressure applied to the mother's abdomen or the presence of certain viruses and drugs in the mother's blood stream, are detrimental to the fetus. Other factors, such as delivery of all the proper nutrients, enhance the fetus' growth. So, environmental factors can positively or negatively affect growth and maturation.

That growth and development proceed normally, in an environment that maximizes genetic potential, is everyone's hope, but it is possible for the fetus to develop anomalies or be exposed to detrimental environmental influences. The individual's potential to function normally and participate fully in a wide range of physical activities can be affected. Factors that affect prenatal growth might later affect skill potential. Thus, an understanding of the normal developmental process is basic to a complete understanding of the active individual. Beyond this, an understanding of which environmental conditions can affect growth and development and how they do so is valuable because moving, active individuals are products of their genetic inheritance and the environmental factors present *throughout* their development. Such knowledge is valuable in reducing the risks to growing individuals and in prescribing activities for those whose potential for physical performance may be limited by genetic or environmental factors. These two aspects of prenatal growth, the normal process of development and environmental factors influencing it, are discussed next.

Normal Prenatal Development

Development begins with the fusion of two sex cells, an ovum from the female and a spermatozoan from the male. But how is the genetic inheritance of the new individual determined? The genetic information that determines hair and eye color, the potential for stature, skeletal structure, and many other characteristics is contained in genes in the form of DNA (deoxyribonucleic acid) molecules. The genes are located on chromosomes, filament-like bodies within the cell's nucleus. Human beings have 23 pairs of chromosomes. The sex cells are specialized cells formed by a type of cell reduction division termed *meiosis*. In meiosis, each "parent" sex cell divides into two "daughter" sex cells, during which one chromosome from each of the 23 pairs migrates to each daughter cell. Which one of the pair a daughter cell receives is a matter of chance; thus, there is a great deal of variability possible in the offspring of any set of parents. When an ovum and spermatozoan unite in fertilization, each donates the "chance" set of 23 chromosomes, reestablishing the total of 46 chromosomes (23 pairs). When we understand that each human chromosome has 30,000 or more pairs of genes, it is no wonder that each human being is unique!

The genes also direct the continuous development of the new organism, or embryo, in a precise and predictable pattern. The fertilized egg divides into two cells, then four, eight, and so on, all by *mitotic* cell division. In mitotic division, the parent cell passes the complete set of 46 chromosomes on to the daughter cell. After about 4 days, the embryo is transformed into a sphere termed a blastocyst (see Figures 2.10 and 2.11). By this time, the blastocyst contains about 60 cells, 5 of which form the inner cell mass. It implants itself in the uterus at about 5 to 6 days of age. The inner cell mass forms three

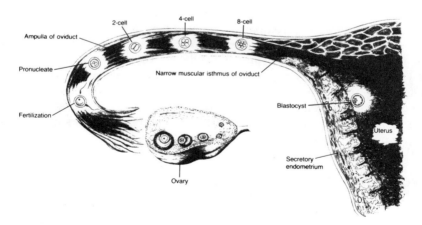

Figure 2.10 Movement of a human embryo through the oviduct and its implantation in the uterus. Reproduced with permission from *The Beginnings of Human Life* (p. 12) by R.G. Edwards, 1981, Burlington, NC: Carolina Biology Reader Series. Copyright 1981 by Finestride Ltd. and Carolina Biological Supply Co. Reprinted by permission.

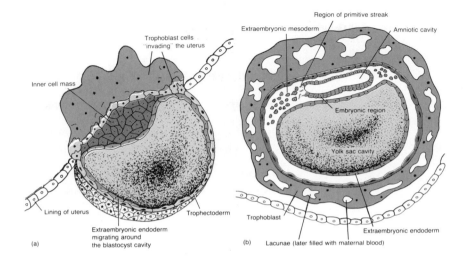

Figure 2.11   Diagrams of human embryos: (a) 9 days after fertilization, (b) 12 days after fertilization. The embryo by this time is embedded in the uterus. Reproduced with permission from *The Beginnings of Human Life* (p. 14) by R.G. Edwards, 1981, Burlington, NC: Carolina Biology Reader Series. Copyright 1981 by Finestride Ltd. and Carolina Biological Supply Co. Reprinted by permission.

layers of tissues through continued cell division and through the migration (movement) of cells to a new location. These three tissues, the ectoderm, the endoderm, and the mesoderm, give rise to all the various tissues and organs of the body. The ectoderm layer eventually becomes skin, tooth enamel, the nervous system, parts of different glands, and parts of the sensory receptors. The endoderm is the origin of the epithelial linings (avascular cellular layers) of many structures such as the auditory tube, larynx, urinary bladder, urethra, and prostate. The remaining body tissues and organs originate from the mesoderm. These include muscles, the blood, all connective tissues, the teeth, the adrenal cortex, and the skeleton (Timiras, 1972).

Formation of the tissues and organs proceeds in a predictable time line, summarized in Table 2.1. In general, the cells *differentiate* (become specialized) into the various body organs and form the human shape during the first 8 weeks after conception. This period is termed the embryonic stage. The period thereafter, the fetal stage, is characterized by further growth and cell differentiation leading to functional capacity. This continued growth of the organs and tissues occurs in two ways: by *hyperplasia*, an increase in the ab-

Table 2.1 Landmarks in Embryonic and Fetal Growth

Age (wks)	Length	Weight	Appearance	Internal Development
3	3 mm		Head, tail folds formed	Optic vesicles, head recognizable
4	4 mm	0.4 g	Limb rudiments formed	Heartbeat begins, organs recognizable
8	3.5 cm	2 g	Eyes, ears, nose, mouth, digits formed	Sensory organs developing, some bone ossification beginning
12	11.5 cm	19 g	Sex externally recognizable, head very large for body	Brain configuration nearly complete, blood forming in bone marow
16	19 cm	100 g	Motor activity; scalp hair present; trunk size gaining on head size	Heart muscle developed; sense organs formed
20	22 cm	300 g	Legs have grown appreciably	Myelination of spinal cord begins
24	32 cm	600 g	Respiratory-like movements begin	Cerebral cortex layers
28	36 cm	1,100 g	Increasing fat tissue development	Retina layered and light-receptive; cerebral convolutions appearing
32	41 cm	1,800 g	Weight increasing more than length	Taste sense operative
36	46 cm	2,200 g	Body more rounded	Ossification begins in distal femur
40	52 cm	3,200 g	Skin smooth and pink, at least moderate head hair	Proximal tibia begins ossification; myelination of brain begins; pulmonary branching ⅔ complete

Note. Adapted from *Developmental Physiology and Aging* (pp. 63-64) by P.S. Timiras, 1972, New York, NY: Macmillan. Copyright 1972 by Macmillan. Reprinted by permission.

solute number of cells, such as in blood, bone, or liver tissue; and by *hypertrophy*, an increase in the relative size of each individual cell, such as in the brain or lungs. If you examine the landmarks of growth carefully, you also see that growth tends to proceed in two directions. One direction is *cephalocaudal* (head-to-tail), meaning that the head and facial structures grow fastest, then the upper body, followed by the relatively slow-growing lower body. At the same time, growth is *proximodistal* (near-to-far) in direction, meaning the trunk tends to advance, then the nearest parts of the limbs, and finally the distal parts of the limbs. Although cells differentiate during growth to perform a specialized function, some cells have an amazing quality termed *plasticity*, the capability to take on a new function. If some of the cells in a system are injured, for example, the remaining cells might be stimulated to perform the role ordinarily carried out by the damaged cells. The cells of the central nervous system have a high degree of plasticity, and their structure, chemistry, and function can be modified pre- and postnatally (Timiras, 1972).

It is clear that normal prenatal growth occurs in a predictable pattern and on a predictable time line, under genetic control. But, it is also clear that the growth of some individuals does not proceed normally. Abnormal growth may arise from two sources: genetic factors and environmental factors. Genetic abnormalities may be inherited as dominant or recessive (including sex-linked) traits. Examples of dominant pathologic traits are hereditary multiple exostosis (formation of a tumor on a bony surface) and sickle-cell anemia. One recessive pathological trait is phenylketonuria (PKU), a condition in which phenylketonuric acid may accumulate, damaging the nervous system and resulting in mental retardation. Another recessive pathological trait is Down's syndrome (mongolism). In this trait, three chromosomes rather than two are present in one chromosome "pair," giving the individual a total of 47. Characteristics of Down's syndrome include mental retardation, cardiac abnormalities, and short stature. From these examples you can see that genetic abnormalities vary considerably in both appearance and severity.

Environmental Factors Influencing Prenatal Growth

Many characteristics of the fetus' environment have the potential to affect growth, and the impact is experienced most through the nourishment system. It is helpful to first examine how the fetus is nourished.

Fetal Nourishment

The structure involved in fetal nourishment is the *placenta*, a network of blood capillaries that is formed in early development from a part of the egg's outer membrane. The placenta actually consists of two parallel "plates" separated by a maternal blood-filled space (see Figure 2.12). *Villi* (vascular finger-like projections) extend into the space, thereby increasing the surface area for fetal-maternal exchanges. Fetal blood flows through capillaries that

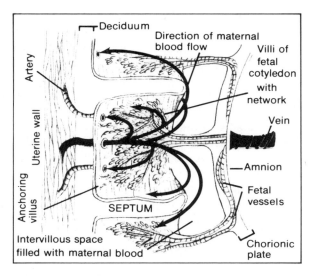

Figure 2.12 A diagram of the placenta showing the two circulations (mother and fetus) which are intimate but never mingle. From *Reproductive Physiology for Medical Students* (p. 191) by P. Rhodes, 1969, London: J. & A. Churchill Ltd. Copyright 1969 by Churchill Livingstone. Reprinted by permission.

lie intermingled with the villi. Respiratory and nutritive exchanges take place via diffusion between fetal blood in the capillaries and maternal blood in the space without direct mixing of the two blood supplies. One of the most important exchanges is that of oxygen to the fetus and carbon dioxide to the mother for elimination by her respiratory system. Nutrients transferred to the fetus via the placenta include proteins, amino acids, polypeptides, carbohydrates, water, inorganic ions (sodium, potassium, iron, etc.), and vitamins. Excretory by-products of fetal metabolism are removed from the fetus via this process as well.

Teratogens

In addition to oxygen and nutrients necessary for the life and growth of the fetus, viral infections, drugs, and inappropriate amounts of nutrients and hormones also can be delivered through the placenta. Some of these substances act as a malformation-producing agent, or *teratogen*. The effect they have on the fetus depends on the fetus' stage of development when the substance is introduced as well as the amount of the substance. The fetus is particularly vulnerable in the early stages of development (the first 16 weeks) when organs and limbs are forming. Any tissues undergoing rapid development at the time a teratogen is introduced are especially susceptible to malformation. Some teratogens have a specific action on certain tissues or cells, affecting one kind of tissue at a certain stage of development, and another tissue at another time. In other words, there are *critical periods*, periods of particular vulnerability to change, for the growth and development of body tissues and organs. Teratogens often have little or no effect on the mother. For this reason, they have been difficult to identify sometimes and, therefore, difficult to guard against. Some of the known teratogens and their possible effects on growth and development are listed in Table 2.2. Some malformation-producing or growth-retarding conditions arise because the amount of a nutrient normally delivered to the embryo/fetus through the placenta is insufficient. Other abnormal conditions arise because a substance is present in excess amounts. Vitamins are an excellent example: A *deficiency* of vitamin A can be dangerous, and an *excess* of vitamin D may cause abnormalities.

Still other congenital defects are traced to the presence of a substance in the maternal blood. For example, small virus particles, such as rubella, present in maternal blood can cross the placenta and harm the fetus. Drugs with molecular weights under 1,000 also cross the placenta easily; a tragic example is that of thalidomide. This drug was tested extensively on adult animals and humans with no toxic effects, and subsequently sold without prescription as a sleeping pill, tranquilizer, or sedative. Only after the births of many infants with limb deformities did medical personnel realize that thalidomide acted as a teratogen, especially when ingested, even in small doses, by the mother between the 3rd and 8th weeks after conception. After the thalidomide experience, medical personnel recognized more and more that adult data could not be extrapolated safely to the fetus (Timiras, 1972). The growth and development of the fetus is maximized when the mother avoids ingesting substances that might be teratogenic and maintains a diet adequate, but not excessive, in nutrients. Otherwise, the fetus might develop a specific malformation or be generally retarded in growth and small-for-date at birth. It is important to recognize that these conditions, including low birth weight, can affect postnatal growth and development.

Other Prenatal Environmental Factors

Not all harmful conditions arise through the fetal nourishment system. Malformation, retarded growth, or life-threatening conditions can result, too, from factors affecting the fetus' environment. Examples include: (a) external or internal pressure on the infant, including pressure from another fetus in utero; (b) extreme internal environmental temperature, as when the mother suffers from high fever or hypothermia; (c) exposure to X rays or gamma rays;

Table 2.2 A Partial List of Teratogens and Their Possible Effects

Teratogen	Possible Effect on Fetus

Nutritional deficiencies
  Vitamin A, vitamin E,
  riboflavin, fatty acids,
  glucose
	General influence on all aspects of growth
	and development, including low birth
	weight; possible effect on placental
	function; possible malformations

Hypervitaminosis Excess vitamin D	Cardiac defects, mental retardation, sensory abnormalities
Drugs	
Morphine/heroine addiction	Addiction in infant
Barbiturates	Depression of central nervous system
Antibiotics	Sensory disorders, deafness
Tetracycline	Impaired growth
Antithyroid medications	Thyroid gland enlargement, mental retardation
Alcohol	Fetal Alcohol Syndrome; in extreme alcoholism, low birth weight, suppressed growth, mental retardation, physical deformities
Thalidomide	Various malformations (limbs, heart, viscera)
LSD	Chromosomal damage
Nicotine/heavy smoking	Growth retardation, low birth weight, spontaneous abortion, premature birth
Infections	
Rubella	Cardiac defects, impaired growth, mental retardation, cataracts, deafness
Cytomegalic inclusion disease	Mental retardation, microcephaly
Excess hormones	
Androgens	Masculinization of female fetus
ACTN	Cleft palate
Hormonal deficiencies	
Alloxan diabetes	Suppressed growth

Note. Information summarized from *Developmental Physiology and Aging* (p. 382) by P.S. Timiras, 1972, New York, NY: Macmillan. Copyright 1972 by Macmillan. Reprinted by permission.

and (d) changes in atmospheric pressure, especially those leading to hypoxia (oxygen deficiency) in the fetus. The precise effects of these factors also depend upon the fetus' stage of development. They, like the teratogens, have the potential to affect both pre- and postnatal growth and development.

Summary 2.2—Factors Influencing Prenatal Growth

Fertilization begins a process of growth and development that is under both genetic control and environmental influence. Early in embryonic life the pattern and timing of organ and tissue formation are remarkably precise and predictable, but abnormalities can arise from two sources. The fetus might inherit a trait that retards growth and development, or a characteristic of the environment might do the same. Some abnormal conditions are a product of both genetic inheritance and the environment. That is, a tendency for a disease might be inherited and subsequently the disease will appear *only* if certain environmental conditions occur (Timiras, 1972). A healthy environment maximizes the fetus' chance of reaching its full genetic potential. Individuals involved in the care of the fetus can attempt to control environmental factors known to be influential. A proper diet is important, as is avoidance of smoking, alcohol, and harmful drugs.

Physical growth and development, then, should be viewed as a continuous process that begins at conception. Individuals are in part products of the factors that affected their prenatal growth and development. The fetus has either grown in an environment maximizing its chances of survival and of reaching full growth potential, or it may already have been harmed or placed at risk during birth and the days thereafter. Next on the growth continuum, birth and postnatal growth and development are examined.

Concept 2.3   Postnatal growth proceeds in precise and orderly patterns that differ among the body systems.

What is the capacity of an 11-year-old for long distance running? Or of a 60-year-old? Of course, there is no one answer for all 11-year-olds or all 60-year-olds. Educators often find themselves in the position of evaluating the status and potential of individuals to help them set reasonable goals. As discussed in concept 2.1, part of this evaluation is an assessment of physical maturity. The educator must be aware of several important aspects of growth and development or aging. The average pattern of postnatal growth and the typical pattern of aging in adults are important. An individual may be compared with the "average" and expectations for performance adjusted accordingly. Educators must also know the growth rates and maturation patterns of various body tissues and systems. Does muscle growth keep pace with whole body growth? Do the muscles and skeletal framework maintain their young-adult levels of strength with aging? Or, does one weaken while the other does not? In order to plan appropriate activities, educators must know what body systems are changing and when they are changing.

Normal Postnatal Growth

Overall Growth

The pattern of body growth after birth is a continuation of prenatal life. It is predictable and consistent but not linear. This seems to be true no matter which measure of overall growth is chosen. For example, look back at the growth curves for height and weight in Figures 2.2 and 2.3. They are characterized by a period of rapid growth after birth, followed by a period of gradual but steady growth, a second period of rapid growth during early adolescence, and then a leveling off. Thus, the curves are roughly s-shaped, so that we call the pattern of overall body growth a sigmoid curve. Although a normal individual's growth curve is always the sigmoid shape, the timing of spurts and steady growth periods is likely to vary from the average. That is, a child might be in the gradual growth phase or enter the adolescent growth spurt at a slightly different age than that indicated by the average curve. The timing and rate of growth are genetically controlled, but environmental factors also can have a great impact on growth, especially those factors influencing body metabolism. The periods of most rapid growth, the one following birth and the other in early adolescence, are particularly sensitive to alteration by environmental factors.

The susceptibility of body growth to environmental influence is best illustrated by the phenomenon of "catch-up" growth. A child might experience catch-up growth after a period of severe malnutrition or perhaps after a bout with a severe disease such as chronic renal failure. During such a period, body growth is retarded. After improvement of the diet or recovery from the disease (i.e., restoration of a positive environment for growth), the growth rate increases until the child approaches or "catches-up" to what otherwise would have been the extent of growth during that period (Prader, Tanner, & von Harnack, 1963) (see Figure 2.13). Whether some or all of the growth is "recovered" depends on the timing, duration, and severity of the negative environmental condition. So you can see from this example that negative environmental influences can retard growth, while positive influences maximize growth within genetic limits.

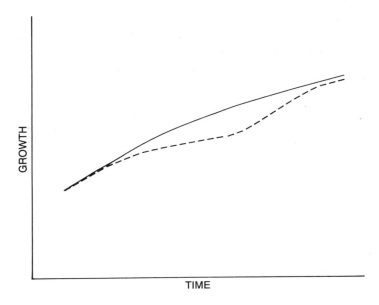

GROWTH

TIME

Figure 2.13 A hypothetical illustration of catch-up growth. The solid line represents the course of normal growth, the dotted line actual growth. A negative environmental influence can cause a retardation of growth compared to the "normal" course growth would have taken. If the negative factor is removed, catch-up growth (bracket) might occur to restore eventual growth to its normal or near-normal level.

Gender Differences. Gender is a major factor in the timing of growth as well as the extent of growth. There are important gender differences in growth and development, which are especially pronounced at adolescence. The differences are minimal in early childhood, with boys being slightly taller and heavier. Throughout childhood, though, girls tend to mature at a faster rate than boys so that at any given age, girls, as a group, are biologically more mature than boys. At approximately 9 years of age the average girl begins to pass the average boy in height and weight. She then enters her adolescent growth spurt at about 10½, nearly 2 years ahead of the average boy.

During the adolescent growth spurt, secondary sex characteristics appear. In girls, the breasts enlarge, pubic hair appears, and *menarche*, the first menstrual cycle, occurs. In boys, the testes and scrotum grow in size and pubic hair appears. Regardless of the exact chronological age when a girl begins her growth spurt, the peak of her gain in height is typically followed by menarche (see Figure 2.9). It is suggested that menarche occurs at a critical body weight (Frisch, 1972). While this view is still controversial, if a relationship between age at menarche and critical body weight exists, it is clear that menarche might be influenced by environmental factors such as nutrition. Boys have no landmark comparable to girls' menarche for puberty: The production of viable sperm is a gradual process. Young women, having begun their growth spurt earlier than young men, also end their growth at an earlier age, which accounts for much of the average absolute height difference between the sexes. That is, men have a longer period in which to grow in height. Height increases taper off at about age 16 for women and age 18 for men, although some investigators have measured slight increases in trunk length into the mid-40s. Generally, height is stable through adulthood.

It is common for stature to decrease slightly in older adulthood. Some of this decrease is due to compression and flattening of the body's connective tissues, especially the cartilage pads between the vertebrae in the spinal column. The result is a compression of the spinal column and a decrease in trunk length. The bones also lose density as a consequence of progressive modifications in the protein matrix of the skeleton (Timiras, 1972). This breakdown is more severe in persons with osteoporosis and can result in collapse of one or more vertebrae. In this case, the loss of stature is pronounced.

Regular Growth Assessment. A regular program of assessing growth in children and comparing the results with average values can help detect abnormal growth. Medical or environmental factors influencing abnormal growth can then be identified and corrected. Of course, the individual's genetic potential for height and body build (often "hinted" by the parents' height and build) as well as the individual's personal "timing" of growth are reflected in such growth measures. Those children and teens who are above the 90th percentile for age or below the 10th percentile, especially those whose parents are not exceptionally tall or short, respectively, should be referred to medical personnel for examination (Lowrey, 1973).

Teachers are in a particularly good position to regularly assess height and weight. Besides the potential for detecting growth problems, height and weight data can be used to teach children basic concepts of hereditary and environmental influence. Knowledge of the growth process can alleviate children's anxieties about their body size. These anxieties often come about because of the timing differences in maturation rate. For example, a late-maturing 13-year-old boy could be 20 cm (approximately 8 in) shorter than his early-maturing friends and not yet possess any of the secondary sex characteristics such as a deepened voice. These differences often leave the late-maturer feeling inadequate or inferior. Teachers can make children aware of the changes likely to take place in their bodies and help them set reasonable goals for their physical endeavors in the interim before they reach adult size.

Relative Growth

While the body as a whole consistently follows the sigmoid pattern of growth, specific body parts, tissues, and organs have differential rates of growth. In other words, each part of the growing individual has its own precise and orderly growth rate. These differential growth rates can result in notable changes in form. Observe how the body proportions illustrated in Figure 2.14 change rather dramatically throughout the life span. The head is one fourth of the height at birth but only one eighth of the adult height. The legs are about three eighths of the height at birth but almost half of adult height. Body proportions at birth reflect the cephalocaudal and proximodistal directions of prenatal growth. Hence, the newborn has a form quite different from an adult's form. To achieve adult proportions, body parts such as the legs must grow faster than other body areas during postnatal growth. At very young ages the form of the body might have implications for skill performance.

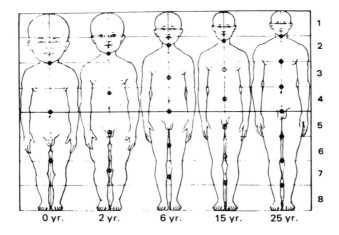

Figure 2.14 Postnatal body proportion changes. From *Developmental Physiology and Aging* (p. 283) by P.S. Timiras, 1972, New York, NY: Macmillan. Copyright 1972 by Macmillan. Reprinted by permission.

For example, even if the newborn were neurologically ready to walk, it is unlikely that such a top heavy body could be balanced easily on small legs and feet! Notice in Figure 2.14 that a 6-year-old still does not have adult form, although the differences are decreasing. It is possible that form differences account for some of the child-adult performance differences in skill. The varying limb lengths and weights can affect momentum and potential speed in ballistic skills such as throwing, balance, and so on. No research studies, however, have quantified a performance difference attributable to the proportional differences in form at the childhood ages (Haywood & Patryla, 1978).

Specific tissues and organs also grow differentially. While their prenatal growth tends to follow the increase in body weight, the postnatal growth of some tissues and systems follows unique patterns, as we see in Figure 2.15. The brain, for example, achieves over 80% of its adult weight by age 4, but adrenal weight is minimal until it increases rapidly during the teens. Because various tissues of the body grow differentially after birth, postnatal growth is best examined by considering the body systems individually. In planning vigorous activities for children it is important to know if some systems such as the skeleton or heart keep pace with whole-body growth. A discussion of the normal pattern of growth in individual systems—the skeletal, muscle, adipose tissue, endocrine, and nervous systems—is in order before we can deal with the environmental influences that can alter this growth.

Skeletal Growth

Early in embryonic life the skeletal system exists as a "cartilage model" of the bones. At a fetal age of 2 months, *ossification centers* appear in the midportion of the long bones such as the humerus (upper arm) and femur (thigh) to begin forming bone cells (see Figure 2.16). The bone shafts ossify outwardly in both directions from these primary centers until at birth the entire shaft is ossified. Thereafter, postnatal bone growth in length occurs at a secondary center at each end of the shaft, termed the "epiphyseal plate" or "growth plate" (see Figure 2.17). The epiphyseal plate has four cellular layers. The outermost layer is the *zone of resting cells*, which serves as a reservoir for future cartilage cells and is nourished by a blood supply from the epiphysis. In the next layer, the *proliferative zone*, cartilage cells increase in size and an extracellular cartilage matrix is formed. The third layer, or *hypertrophic zone*, is an area where cartilage cells arrange themselves in vertical columns. In the *calcified cartilage zone* cartilage cells erode and bone is deposited by osteoblasts (cells engaged in making new bone) on the walls of cavities in the cartilage. Bone is thus laid down at the epiphyseal plates. This process depends on nourishment through the blood supply, shown as the capillary invasion zone in Figure 2.17.

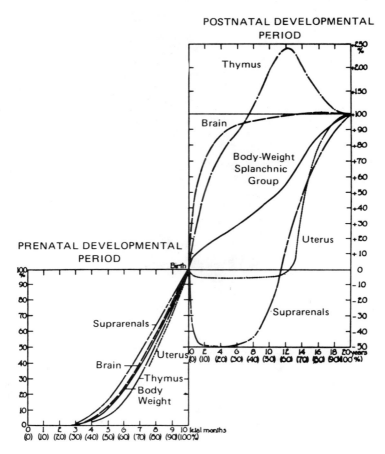

Figure 2.15 Growth in weight of the body and selected tissues during prenatal and postnatal growth. The ordinate indicates size attained in percentage of final weight (100%). From *Developmental Physiology and Aging* (p. 284) by P.S. Timiras, 1972, New York, NY: Macmillan. Copyright 1972 by Macmillan. Reprinted by permission.

Small round bones, like those in the wrist, ossify from the center outward. At birth about 400 ossification centers exist. Another 400 appear after birth. The various centers appear at earlier chronological ages in girls than in boys. Growth at the ossification centers ceases at different times in various bones. At the epiphyseal plates the cartilage zone eventually disappears and the shaft or diaphysis of the bone fuses with the end or epiphysis; this, too, usually occurs at an earlier age in girls than in boys. Once the epiphyseal plates of a long bone fuse, the length of the bone is fixed. Almost all epiphyseal plates are closed by 18 to 19 years of age. While bones are growing in length, they

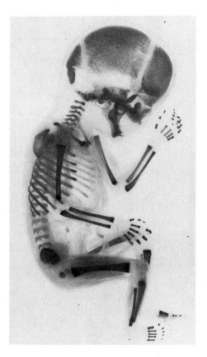

Figure 2.16 A human fetal skeleton at about 18 weeks of age. Dark areas are the ossified portions of the developing skeleton. Spaces between dark areas are occupied by cartilage models. Photo provided by Carolina Biological Supply Company of Burlington, North Carolina, from their Human Development slide series.

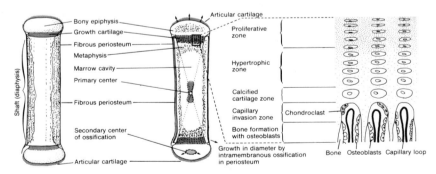

Figure 2.17 Development of a long bone in childhood. The epiphyseal growth plate, between the epiphysis and shaft, is enlarged on the right to show the zones wherein new cells ossify. Reproduced with permission from *Bones* (2nd ed.) by J.J. Pritchard, 1979, Burlington, NC: Carolina Biology Reader Series. Copyright 1979 by Carolina Biological Supply Co. Reprinted by permission.

also increase in girth, called *appositional* growth. This is achieved by the addition of new tissue layers under the *periosteum*, a very thin outer covering of the bone, much like a tree adds to its girth under its bark.

As discussed earlier, it is this process of bone growth that is used to assess skeletal age. Skeletal age can easily be a year or more ahead or behind chronological age, meaning that within a group of children who are the same chronological age, there could be a span of 3 years or more in skeletal maturation. This certainly emphasizes the need to assess children's physical maturity individually. Since linear growth is almost completely the result of skeletal growth, measures of stature reflect the linear growth of bone. In the absence of a direct measure of maturation, height can imply maturation within the limits discussed in concept 2.1.

Skeletal Injuries.   Injuries to the growing skeleton rarely have a lifelong impact. Broken bones, for example, are typically repaired quickly and efficiently by the young body. There is the potential, though, for severe injury to the epiphyseal plate. An injury to the epiphyseal plate that cuts off the blood supply in the capillary invasion zone can result in the early cessation of growth at the site. A significant difference in the eventual length of the right and left limbs is possible if the injury occurs early in the growth period. Fortunately, epiphyseal injuries are not common and of those that occur, only a few involve the blood supply. But, even the rare occurrence of epiphyseal injuries gives educators reason to question the wisdom of programming some activities, such as contact sports, for young children.

In addition to the epiphyseal plates, there are epiphyses at the muscle tendon attachment sites of the bones. These *traction epiphyses* are also subject to irritation and injury. For example, the traction epiphysis at the attachment site of the flexor-pronator muscles of the forearm (the *medial epicondyle* of the *humerus*) can be injured or irritated in throwing (see Figure 2.18). A study of 162 male baseball players, 9 to 14 years old, showed that all 80 of those who pitched had some irritation of this epiphysis (Adams, 1965). Of those who played baseball but did not pitch, and those who did not play, few showed inflammation. Findings such as this have led to the establishment of guidelines for the frequency and length of pitching in many youth baseball programs. Another familiar example of epiphyseal irritation is the tenderness of the *tibial tubercle* (below the knee) at the *patellar* tendon attachment. Known as *Osgood-Schlatter* disease, its occurrence might result in a recommendation of rest from vigorous, especially weight-bearing, activities.

Osteoporosis.   There is little change in the skeletal structure in young adulthood, although at any age poor posture can lead to skeletal misalignment. Researchers who have studied aging believe that some bone loss will naturally occur in the aging process (Smith, Sempos, & Purvis, 1981). Beyond this,

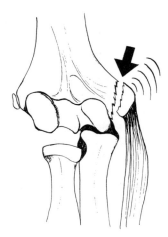

Figure 2.18 A drawing of an elbow joint. An injury to growth plate of the medial epiphysis (a traction epiphysis) has occurred from a violent contraction of the flexor-pronator muscle group in the act of throwing. From *Physical Activity: Human Growth and Development* (p. 44) by G.L. Rarick (Ed.), 1973, New York, NY: Academic Press. Copyright 1973 by Academic Press. Reprinted by permission.

many older adults suffer from a major bone mineral disorder, *osteoporosis*, that is characterized by a loss of bone mass, and consequently, bone strength. The bone becomes abnormally porous through enlargement of the canals in bone or the formation of spaces. This condition increases the risk of fractures, especially at the hip, and adds to the difficulty of fracture repair (Timiras, 1972). Prolonged deficiency of calcium in the diet is a major factor in osteoporosis, although many factors can contribute to its occurrence, either alone or in combination. Deficient osteoblastic activity might be involved. In postmenopausal women, decreased levels of estrogen are implicated because estrogen hormones stimulate osteoblastic activity. Osteoporosis has been treated by dietary supplements of calcium, vitamin D, and fluoride with some success. Estrogen supplements are sometimes prescribed to postmenopausal women, but estrogen therapy is associated with increased risk of endometrial cancer. Concurrent use of progestogens can reduce this risk. Evidence also indicates that physically active women of both premenopausal and postmenopausal age have significantly less osteoporosis and bone loss than sedentary women (Brewer et al., 1983; Oyster et al., 1984).

Muscle Growth

Muscle fibers grow during prenatal life by *hyperplasia*, an increase in the *number* of muscle cells, and *hypertrophy*, an increase in muscle cell *size*.

An increase in the number of fiber nuclei accompanies this growth. Hyperplasia continues for a short time after birth, but thereafter muscle growth is predominantly achieved by hypertrophy (Malina, 1978). In adult muscle there are several types of fibers: *Type I* (slow twitch) fibers that are suited to endurance activities, and *Type II*, *a* and *b*, (fast twitch) fibers that are suited to short-duration, intense activity (see Figure 2.19). In this context, a twitch is a brief period of contraction followed by relaxation of the muscle fiber. At birth, 15% to 20% of the muscle fibers have yet to differentiate into Type I, Type IIa, or Type IIb fibers (Baldwin, 1984; Colling-Saltin, 1980). This has led to speculation that the ultimate proportion of Type I, Type IIa, and Type IIb fibers might be influenced by the infant's early activities, but this issue remains unresolved. Differentiation of muscle cells is controlled genetically, yet the process might respond to interventions during early development, such as activity-induced transformations of fiber type. Questions about the alteration of fiber type proportions will be answered by future research on the biochemical factors involved in muscle development (Baldwin, 1984).

Naturally, muscles must increase in length as the skeleton grows, and this is achieved by the addition of *sarcomeres* (contractile units) at the muscle-tendon junction (see Figure 2.20). Increases in diameter come with age and increased body size but are related also to the intensity of activity to which the muscle is subjected. Gender differences in muscle mass are minimal during childhood, with muscle mass constituting a slightly greater proportion of the body weight in boys. During and after adolescence, gender differences are

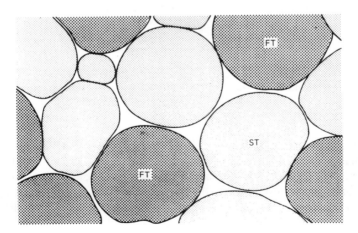

Figure 2.19 A cross-section of muscle showing that fast twitch (FT) and slow twitch (ST fibers are intermingled. From *Physiology of Fitness* (2nd ed.) (p. 238) by B.J. Sharkey, 1984, Champaign, IL: Human Kinetics. Copyright 1984 by B.J. Sharkey. Reprinted by permission.

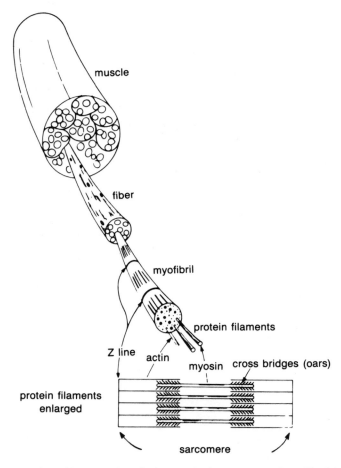

Figure 2.20 Muscle architecture. Note the basic unit, the sarcomere. From *Physiology of Fitness* (2nd ed.) (p. 237) by B.J. Sharkey, 1984, Champaign, IL: Human Kinetics. Copyright 1984 by B.J. Sharkey. Reprinted by permission.

marked. Muscle mass increases in boys up to about age 17 and ultimately accounts for 54% of their body weight. In sharp contrast, girls add muscle mass only until age 13, on the average, and this muscle mass is only 45% of their body weight (Malina, 1978). These gender differences in the addition of muscle mass are the result of hormonal influences, which are discussed later in this chapter.

In young adulthood the percentage of body weight that is muscle decreases in the average person, reflecting not a loss of muscle, but an increase in fat weight. Changes in diet and physical activity level are probably responsible for this shift. In old age, both the number of muscle fibers and their diameter (size) appear to gradually decrease. There is a greater loss of Type II than Type I fibers. By very old age, the loss of muscle mass can be as high as 50% of that possessed in young adulthood. While these trends describe the average growth and decline of muscle, remember that muscle mass is influenced by a variety of factors including genetic inheritance, insulin level, growth hormone and sex hormone level, nutrition, and activity or training level.

The heart is muscle tissue, too. Like skeletal muscle it grows by hyperplasia and hypertrophy with an accompanying increase in fiber nuclei. The right ventricle (lower chamber) is larger than the left ventricle at birth, but the left ventricle catches up after birth by growing more rapidly than the right so that adult proportions are soon achieved (see Figure 2.21). The heart generally follows the sigmoid pattern of whole-body growth, including a spurt of growth in adolescence. For several decades of this century it was thought that the large blood vessels around the heart developed more slowly than the heart itself. Later it was shown that this myth had resulted from a misinterpretation of measurements taken in the late 1800s; in fact, blood vessel growth is proportional to that of the heart. Yet, even until recent years, at least one researcher cited the original mistaken data as a reason to limit the vigorous activity of

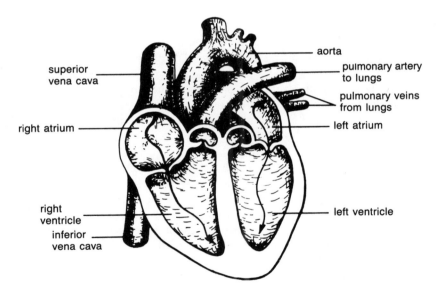

Figure 2.21 The human heart. From *Physiology of Fitness* (2nd ed.) (p. 249) by B.J. Sharkey, 1984, Champaign, IL: Human Kinetics. Copyright 1984 by B.J. Sharkey. Reprinted by permission.

children (Karpovich, 1937). In older age, the heart's ability to adapt to increased work load declines. This might be related in part to degeneration of the heart muscle, a decrease in elasticity, and changes in the fibers of the heart valves (Shephard, 1981). There is also a loss of elasticity in the major blood vessels. With all of these changes, however, it has been difficult for researchers to distinguish the changes that come inevitably with age from those that reflect a lack of fitness in the average older adult.

Adipose Tissue

With the recent popularity of fitness, some enthusiasts consider the presence of *adipose* tissue (fat tissue) in any amount to be undesirable. Yet, adipose tissue plays a vital role in energy storage, insulation, and protection, and the amount of adipose tissue necessarily increases in early life. Adipose tissue appears in the fetus around the 7th prenatal month and by birth the distribution of fat tissue is well defined. The body's fat weight continues to increase during the first 6 postnatal months before tapering off to a plateau that spans ages 1 to 7. At this time the proportion of body fat again increases (Knittle, 1978). This preadolescent gain later ceases (and may reverse for a time) in boys but tends to continue throughout adolescence in girls. Both sexes tend to gain fat weight during the adult years, reflecting changes in nutrition and the activity levels of most adults. Total body weight begins to decline after 50 years of age, but this may reflect loss of bone and muscle rather than fat. It is difficult to identify the typical pattern of adipose tissue gain or loss in older adulthood. Because obese individuals have a higher mortality rate, lighter individuals might either survive to be included in studies of older adults whereas obese individuals do not, or thinner adults might be more eager to participate in research studies. It appears that an increase in fat weight with aging is *not* inevitable; for example, persons from undernourished parts of the world and Masters'-class athletes do not demonstrate such gains (Shephard, 1978b).

Many aspects of adipose tissue development are undergoing further study. Maternal weight gain during pregnancy, early infant feeding, and genetic factors in adipose tissue development are among the topics being examined. Of particular interest is the possible existence of critical periods for fat tissue development, because there is some indication that both adipose cell size and number increase during the periods of rapid development. Increases in cell number are significant because, once formed, adipose cells can persist, even with malnutrition; that is, the cells may be "empty" of fat, but the cell is still there. Hence, cell size, but not cell number, can be changed in adulthood. Weight control in later life may be more difficult for those persons who have more adipose cells.

The Endocrine System

Growth and development are under the influence of three major types of hormones: pituitary *growth hormone* (GH), the *thyroid hormones* (*T3, T4, thyroxine, triiodothyronine*), and the *gonadal hormones* (*androgen, estrogen*) (Timiras, 1972). Either an excess or a deficiency of these hormones may disturb the normal process of growth and development. Although different in their chemical structure, all three promote growth in the same way: They stimulate protein *anabolism* (constructive metabolism) resulting in the retention of substances needed to build tissues. Each hormone plays a unique role in growth at a unique time.

Growth Hormone. Growth hormone (GH) influences growth during childhood and adolescence. It is secreted by the pituitary gland, under the control of the central nervous system, via a substance called the GH-releasing factor. To emphasize its importance, you should realize that a deficiency or absence of GH results in growth abnormalities, and in some cases the cessation of linear growth.

Thyroid Hormones. The thyroid hormones also influence postnatal whole body growth, but are particularly influential in the development of certain organs and tissues, including the brain and liver. Note the relative increase in the weight of the thymus during adolescence, as shown earlier in Figure 2.15. The size of this organ, which is necessary for the development of immunological function, is increased by growth and thyroid hormones. The thymus then involutes (decreases in relative size) during late adolescence when these hormones subside and growth slows. Secretion of the thyroid hormones is regulated by the level of pituitary *thyrotropic hormone* (TSH). TSH excretion is, in turn, increased by a releasing factor found in the brain's *hypothalamus*. Thus, two systems appear to be acting in concert: a pituitary-thyroid system, and a nervous system-thyroid system. You can see that the endocrine system is delicately balanced. In fact, there is also a GH-thyroid relationship, because thyroxine must be present for GH to be effective.

Gonadal Hormones. The gonadal hormones affect growth and sexual maturation, particularly during adolescence, by stimulating the development of the respective sex organs. The androgens, specifically *testosterone* from the testes and *androgens* (*dehydroepiandrosterone, androstenedione,* and *11β-hydroxyandrostenedione*) from the cortex of the adrenal glands, hasten fusion of the epiphyseal growth plates in the bones. Thus, skeletal maturation (fusion) is promoted by these hormones at the expense of linear growth; this explains why early maturers tend to be shorter in stature than later maturers. Androgens also play a role in the adolescent growth spurt of muscle mass by increasing nitrogen retention and protein synthesis. This spurt is more significant in young men than young women because men secrete both testosterone and adrenal androgens, but women produce only the adrenal androgens. *Estrogens* are secreted in women by the ovaries and the adrenal cortex. Increased estrogen secretion during adolescence, as with androgens, speeds epiphyseal closure, but estrogen also promotes fat accumulation, primarily in the breasts and hips.

Other Hormones Affecting Growth.   The hormones discussed up to this point all play a major, direct role in growth and development. Another familiar hormone, *insulin*, has an indirect role in growth. Produced in the pancreas, insulin is vital to carbohydrate metabolism rather than protein metabolism; but a deficiency of insulin can decrease protein synthesis, too. This is detrimental at any time of life, but especially during the growth period.

Hormonal Activity During Older Adulthood.   In adulthood, hormones play a role in three areas that are related to physical activity: regulation of cardiovascular performance, mobilization of fuel, and synthesis of new protein (Shephard, 1978). Information about age-related hormonal changes is limited, but several features of hormonal function in aging are known. Basal levels of GH seem to be stable throughout the life span, but during exercise, older adults can have a more pronounced increase in GH levels than younger exercisers. This increase may be an attempt by the body's metabolism to conserve *glycogen* (the form in which glucose, a sugar, is stored in the body) and reduce protein breakdown through the release of stored fat. Thyroid hormone levels also increase with aging; this can have a negative effect on liver *cholesterol* utilization, *free fatty acid* (from adipose tissue) mobilization, and body heat production. A long-term increase can be related to congestive heart failure. *Gonadal* hormone levels decrease with age. While information on this aspect of aging is lacking, androgen supplements have been prescribed successfully to counter muscle wasting and osteoporosis. It is known that the secretion level of insulin is maintained in older adults, but the incidence of clinical *diabetes* (caused by insulin deficiency) increases markedly with age. Even though insulin level is maintained, it is possible that older adults do not utilize insulin to promote glycogen storage as effectively as younger adults. Thus, the mobilization of fuel for exercise could be retarded.

The Nervous System

Growth and development of the nervous system provides a prime example of the interplay of genetic and environmental factors. The precise and predictable course of early nervous system development appears to be under genetic regulation. Immature neurons are generated, differentiate in their general type, and migrate to a final position. Formation of cell processes (*dendrites* and *axons*) occurs next with arborization (branching) of the processes and further differentiation. Finally, *myelination* of the processes (an insulating process) takes place (Williams, 1983) (see Figure 2.22). For the most part, proliferation and migration of cells occur prenatally, and most of cell arborization and myelination takes place postnatally.

Throughout its growth and development, the nervous system is vulnerable to environmental factors, despite its plasticity. This is particularly true during several critical periods of rapid development. These critical periods occur early in life—prenatally and the first year postnatally—but nervous system development continues through puberty (some myelination may occur as late as young adulthood) and is susceptible to environmental influence until this time. To understand how and when the nervous system development is subject to genetic and environmental influence, its structural development must be outlined briefly.

Early Development. Since neurons of the brain are formed prenatally, the rapid gains in brain weight during the 1st postnatal year (when half of the adult weight of the brain is achieved) primarily reflect two processes. The *glial* cells and myelin increase, and the neurons increase in size and undergo arborization. The glial cells support and nourish the neurons. The arborization, or branching of neurons, includes the establishment for each neuron of 1,000 to 100,000 connections with other neurons during the 1st year after birth. The two large lobes of the brain, the right and left cerebral hemispheres, are formed but not fully functional at birth (see Figure 2.23). The *cortex*, or outer layer, of these hemispheres is involved in purposeful movement and goal-directed behavior.

The first clear evidence of successful, *intentional* movement occurs at 4 to 5 postnatal months (Bushnell, 1982; McDonnell, 1979) and probably signals the functioning of the cortex. The cells of the cortex continue to differentiate in the early postnatal years, as do the cortical cells of the *cerebellum*, the two smaller lobes at the base of the brain. Some of the lower brain areas, which are relatively small at birth, grow rapidly in the 1st year. Exceptions to this are the areas involved in vital tasks, such as respiration and food intake, that are already relatively mature at birth. These lower brain centers also mediate many reactions and reflexes in the late prenatal and early postnatal months. In general, then, the ontogenetically and phylogenetically older parts of the brain are the most mature at birth, and the 1st year after birth is an important period of brain maturation.

Myelin. The development of myelin in the nervous system is of particular interest because it contributes to speedy conduction of nerve impulses. Myelin is formed by *Schwann cells*, which wrap themselves around the out-

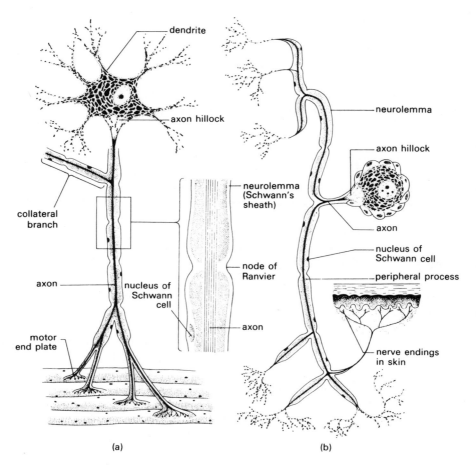

Figure 2.22 A myelinated (a) motor neuron and (b) sensory neuron. From *Functional Human Anatomy* (4th ed.) (p. 274) by J.E. Crouch, 1985, Philadelphia: Lea & Febiger. Copyright 1985 by Lea & Febiger. Reprinted by permission.

going neuron cell process, or axon (see Figure 2.24). The myelin sheath is interrupted periodically by nodes (called *nodes of Ranvier*). The neuron cell membrane is involved in nerve impulse conduction only at the nodes, so the impulse jumps from node to node. This type of nerve impulse conduction is known as *saltatory* conduction, and it is much faster than conduction in nonmyelinated axons. Saltatory conduction also requires less metabolic energy

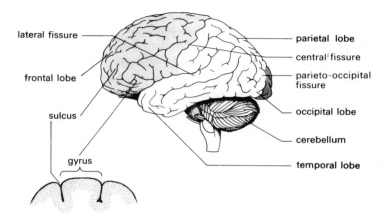

Figure 2.23 The cerebrum and a cross-section of the cerebral cortex. From *Dynamic Anatomy and Physiology* (3rd ed.) (p. 244) by L.L. Langley, I.R. Telford, & J.B. Christensen, 1969, New York, NY: McGraw-Hill. Reprinted by permission.

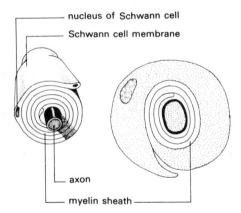

Figure 2.24 A myelinated axon. Adapted from *The Human Oranism* (5th ed.) (p. 260) by R.M. DeCoursey and J.L. Renfro, 1980, New York, NY: McGraw-Hill. Copyright 1980 by McGraw-Hill. Reprinted by permission.

so that myelinated axons can fire nerve impulses at higher frequencies for longer periods of time (Kuffler, Nicholls, & Martin, 1984). Axons that are as yet unmyelinated in the newborn are probably functional, but myelination improves the speed and frequency of firing. The function of the nervous system in movements requiring or benefiting from speedy conduction of nerve impulses, such as a series of rapid movements, might be related to the myelination process during development. Note that *multiple sclerosis*, a disease that strikes young adults and breaks down the myelin sheath, results in tremor, loss of coordination, or even paralysis.

Spinal Cord. The spinal cord is relatively small and short at birth. The myelination pattern that the spinal cord and nerve pathways undergo might have implications for motor development. Myelination proceeds in two directions in the cord: first in the cervical portion, followed by the progressively lower portions; and then in the motor (*ventral*) horns, followed by the sensory (*dorsal*) horns. The *horns* are areas of the center portion of the spinal cord. This center, H-shaped area contains tightly-packed neuron cell bodies (see Figure 2.25). Two major *motor pathways*, or nerve tracts, carry impulses from the brain down the spinal cord to various parts of the body. One pathway, the *extrapyramidal tract*, probably is involved in delivering the commands for both random and postural movements made by the infant in the first days after birth (see Figure 2.26). The other, the *pyramidal tract*, myelinates after birth and is probably functional by 4 to 5 months, when intentional behavior can be observed in the infant (see Figure 2.27). In studies where the pyramidal tracts of monkeys have been severed (Lawrence & Hopkins, 1972; Lawrence & Kuypers, 1968), the effect has been a loss of individual finger movement with an accompanying decrease in the speed and agility of movement. The direction of myelination tends to be *away* from the brain in both of these motor tracts. In contrast, the direction of myelination is *toward* the brain in sensory tracts, occurring first in the tactile and olfactory pathways, then in the visual, and finally in the auditory pathways. Sensory pathways mature slightly faster than motor pathways, except in the *motor roots* and cerebral hemispheres. The roots are areas just outside the cord that contain the axons of the cord's neurons and, in the case of the sensory roots, nerve cell bodies as well. Fibers from the dorsal and ventral roots merge to form the peripheral (spinal) nerves outside the cord. A marked increase in the myelination of these peripheral nerves occurs 2 to 3 weeks after birth, but this process continues through the 2nd or 3rd year of life.

The Older Brain. With aging there is a decrease in the number of neurons in the nervous system, including the cerebral cortex, but an increase in the number of glial cells. Overall, this results in decreased brain weight by old age. This decrease might be related to a gradual reduction in circulation and in oxygen utilization by the brain after adolescence. The electrophysiologic effects of aging seem to be a lower nerve signal strength, an increase in "neural noise" (random background activity in the central nervous system), a lesser number of neural connections to "smooth" signals, and longer-lasting after-

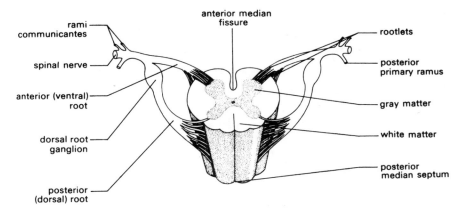

Figure 2.25 A cross-section of the spinal cord. From *Dynamic Anatomy and Physiology* (3rd ed.) (p. 256) by L.L. Langley, I.R. Telford, & J.B. Christensen, 1969, New York, NY: McGraw-Hill. Copyright 1969 by McGraw-Hill. Reprinted by permission.

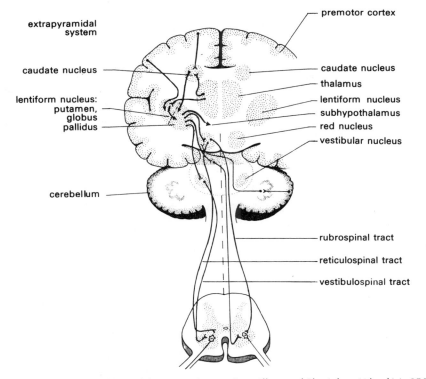

Figure 2.26 The extrapyramidal motor pathways. From *Illustrated Physiology* (4th ed.) (p 256) by A.B. McNaught & R. Callander, 1983, Ediburgh, Scotland: Churchill Livingstone. Copyright 1983 by Churchill Livingstone. Reprinted by permission.

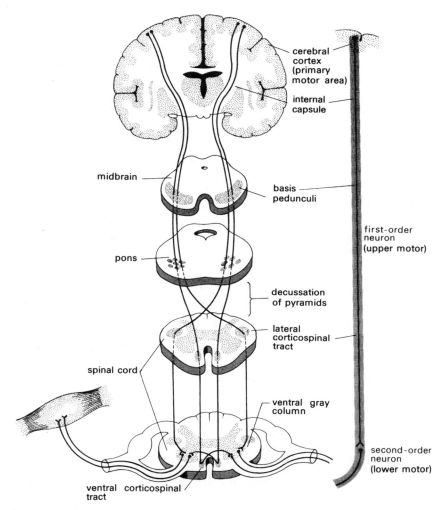

Figure 2.27 The pyramidal motor pathways. From *Dynamic Anatomy and Physiology* (3rd ed.) (p. 301) by L.L. Langley, I.R. Telford, & J.B. Christensen, 1969, New York, NY: McGraw-Hill. Copyright 1969 by McGraw-Hill. Reprinted by permission.

effects (prolonged electrical activity after stimulus cessation). These effects can be manifested behaviorily in a general slowing of sensory and motor function.

Summary 2.3—Postnatal Growth Patterns

In working with individual persons it is important to understand normal growth and maturation of the body and its tissues. Whole-body growth proceeds in a characteristic pattern known as the sigmoid growth pattern, but the rate of maturation varies between the sexes and among individuals. Allowing for these individual differences, abnormal or retarded growth can be detected by comparing an individual child to "average" growth curves. The various body tissues and systems can have unique growth patterns. Awareness of these patterns is important because growth is more susceptible to external influence during periods of rapid change. Some of these external or environmental influences can be positive and help persons attain their full growth potential. Others can retard growth or permanently affect growth and maturation. A review of many of the environmental factors that can affect growth, development, and maturation follows.

Concept 2.4   Environmental factors become more important in post-natal growth and maturation.

Educators must recognize the influence of environmental factors on postnatal growth, development, and aging. These environmental influences become increasingly more important, relative to genetic factors, as one matures. In fact, critical periods might exist for some aspects of postnatal growth because vulnerability to environmental influence is greatest during periods of rapid development. The presence or absence of an environmental factor at a given time might affect an individual's potential for skilled performance for the remainder of his or her lifetime. What are these environmental factors, and how might they affect the physical growth and development of individuals throughout their life spans?

Environmental Factors Influencing Postnatal Growth

Birth Process

First, consider that the *birth* process, as the transition from a prenatal, internal environment to a postnatal, external environment, has the potential to affect growth and development. The birth process is somewhat traumatic for the fetus even under normal circumstances. Abnormal labor or delivery can be harmful to the infant (see Figure 2.28). Recall from our earlier discussion of prenatal growth that the fetus' oxygen supply passes through the placenta via the umbilical cord, and that hypoxia (oxygen deficiency) can im-

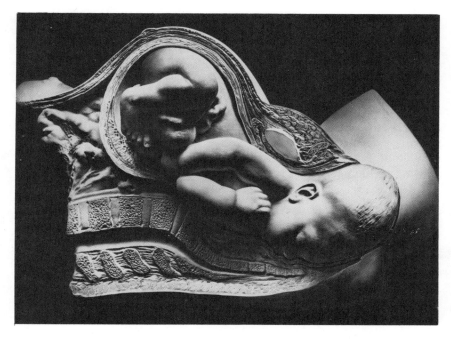

Figure 2.28 The second stage of labor. The baby's head is now showing. From the *Birth Atlas*, New York, NY: The Maternity Center Assn. Copyright by the Maternity Center Association. Reprinted by permission.

pair normal brain development. Circumstances that put pressure on the cord, such as breech birth, are of concern because they can reduce or block the infant's oxygen and blood supply, causing brain damage. Also of concern for brain development is abnormal pressure on the head of the infant as might occur in breech birth or with the use of forceps during delivery. The use of forceps can cause other injuries, too, notably those to the epiphyseal growth plates of the bones.

Low birth weight (under 2,500 gm) is associated with increased health risks during early postnatal growth and development (Brandt, 1978). It is important to distinguish between low birth weight infants who are born prematurely and those born after full term. A premature infant is expected to be small at birth and small-for-age when compared with average growth charts. In fact, many premature children compare favorably to growth charts if their age is adjusted downward for their early birth date. In contrast, the small but full-term infant has grown slowly during the prenatal period, probably as the result of a negative prenatal environmental factor. In such cases, normal postnatal growth is jeopardized by the presence of certain environmental factors during prenatal growth. A mother's cigarette smoking during pregnancy is a common example of an adverse prenatal factor strongly associated with low birth weight. Maternal malnutrition is another. Fortunately, improvement of environmental factors in the early postnatal months can bring about a period of "catch-up" growth, so it is difficult to predict the effect of low birth weight on adult size. The long-term effect of low birth weight depends on the timing, duration, and severity of the adverse factor as well as postnatal nutrition and care (Brandt, 1978).

Postnatal Nutrition

A major environmental factor affecting growth and development is *nutrition*. The body needs the energy provided by food to grow and to maintain normal bodily functions. The need is greatest during periods of rapid growth, but good nutrition is important for the maintenance and repair of body tissues throughout life. The three basic foodstuffs—proteins, carbohydrates, and fats—each play a role in growth and development. *Amino acids* from proteins provide the building material for different tissues and are needed for protein synthesis. Carbohydrates are the chief source of fuel to meet the body's energy requirements, and fats provide energy storage and insulation against heat loss. Water, minerals, and vitamins are the other essential nutrients that support growth and development.

Adequate nutrition is necessary for an individual to attain growth potential, but under- or overnutrition can affect growth adversely. These conditions can result from an inadequate quantity or quality of nutrients, or both. The effects of *chronic* malnutrition on stature alone are so severe that children suffering from prolonged malnutrition often do not attain their potential growth level. Puberty also may be delayed. The effects of protein malnutrition are dramatically illustrated by two diseases, *kwashiorkor* and *marasmus*, that cause not only growth retardation but muscle wasting. Malnutrition can affect the body systems differentially; remember that the nervous system develops rapidly in early life, thus malnutrition during this time period can limit nervous system development *irreversibly*. Similarly, any system developing rapidly during malnutritious conditions can be affected greatly.

Malnutrition is not limited to underdeveloped nations. Persons living in affluent countries can be malnourished. Even affluent nations have homeless and jobless people who cannot afford to eat properly. It is also possible for individuals to suffer from intestinal diseases that limit the assimilation of nutrients. Psychologic conditions can also affect diet. An example of such a condition is anorexia nervosa, an eating disorder characterized by aversion to food for fear of weight gain. Excessive physical activity can cause undernourishment when the diet cannot keep pace with the energy demands of the activity. The consumption of "empty" calories from junk food is also problematic: One can eat an adequate number of calories but not obtain sufficient vitamins and minerals. The typical problem of affluent areas is overnutrition. Childhood obesity is associated with accelerated growth and development but also exhibits unusually high levels of cholesterol and *triglycerides*. The result can be a young child already at risk of coronary disease. At the same time, many overweight persons adopt popular fad diets in an attempt to lose excess fat weight. Many of these diets are unbalanced in nutrients and result in malnourishment for the dieter.

The influence of an environmental factor like nutrition is clearly illustrated by a *secular trend* in body size and maturity (Van Wieringen, 1978). The effect of this trend is a tendency for people living today to be taller and heavier and to reach puberty sooner than those generations ago. Whether nutrition contributes to this secular trend through an increase in total calories or in protein is unclear. Adequate nutrition is also associated with increased life span, because malnutrition predisposes an individual to disease. At the other extreme, obesity is correlated with a higher death rate in middle and old age.

Physical Environment Characteristics

Several characteristics of the *physical environment* in which children grow can potentially affect growth patterns: climate, seasons of the year, and altitude. A relationship between climate and body physique has been observed. Tall/thin physiques are more common in hot climates and short/stocky physiques in cold. Nutrition and exercise patterns might be involved in these climatic/physique relationships, and genetic factors cannot be ruled out. Yet, these physique trends are not entirely dependent upon exercise, nutrition, and genetic inheritance. American children reared in tropical areas tend to a more linear physique than Americans raised in temperate zones (Malina, 1975). These American children are of a different genetic make-up than native children and probably have adequate nutrition provided to them. Eskimo children living in extremely cold zones grow over a prolonged period and attain their adult height at an older age than average. This suggests that some energy is diverted from growth to heat production and body temperature maintenance in these children (Little & Hochner, 1973). Patterns of growth might also be influenced by seasonal cycles. Greater weight gains have been recorded in the fall than in the spring, and greater height gains in the spring than in fall, in at least one early study (Tanner, 1961). Nutrition and exercise patterns could be other environmental factors acting in concert to produce this pattern of growth.

Living at high altitude can affect growth, too. Children growing up high in the Andes and Himalayas have a smaller body size and slower growth rate than those living at lower altitudes. Adequate oxygen is important for normal growth and development. Since less environmental oxygen is present in the air at high altitudes compared with lower altitudes, children living at very high altitudes over a long period can suffer hypoxia. This could result in retarded growth and development. It is possible, too, that the cold climate of high altitudes and the nutritional status of these children simultaneously affect growth patterns. The adaptability of the body to environmental factors is also demonstrated by another aspect of growth: Children living at high altitude develop greater lung capacities than their peers at sea level. This allows individuals living at high altitudes to offset hypoxia, at least in part, by extracting oxygen from a larger quantity of air in the lungs.

Radiation can have a harmful effect on growth. Children can be exposed to radiation from natural sources, such as cosmic rays, or from artificial sources, such as therapeutic radiation or nuclear testing. High dosages of radiation have a variety of devastating effects on any growing organism, especially early in life. Among these effects are cell mutations, nervous system damage, growth retardation, and leukemia.

Physical Activity and Exercise

Of particular interest to educators is the effect of physical activity on growth, development, and aging. It is generally agreed that a certain amount of physical activity is needed to support normal growth. That amount, however, is not easily determined; neither is the effect of excessive activity. Because the benefits of an active lifestyle have received widespread attention in recent years, it is important to know the effects of exercise on growth and aging. These effects will now be examined more closely, but a discussion of fitness development will be reserved for a later chapter.

Does physical activity affect skeletal growth? To answer this question, let's consider the various aspects of bone growth—length, width, and density—separately. The effect of physical activity on bone length is unclear except that strenuous labor, such as carrying heavy loads on the shoulders, is known to be detrimental (Kato & Ishiko, 1966, cited by Rarick, 1973). It is difficult to assess the effect of sport participation on stature. Some studies indicate that athletes as a group are taller than nonathletes, but this can be attributed to self-selection or screening for tall athletes by coaches. On the other hand, Ivanitsky (cited by Rarick, 1973) found that the diameter of the long bones was larger in athletes than nonathletes. He cites larger femurs (thigh bones) in soccer players and larger radius bones (in the forearm) in tennis players.

Bone *diameter*, then, might be increased by activity during the growing years. Bone *density* increases with exercise and decreases with inactivity at any age (Nilsson & Westlin, 1971). Exercise plays a role in preventing osteoporosis in adults. In summary, long-term physical activity, short of strenuous labor, promotes bone density and might increase the diameter of involved bones. Bone adapts favorably to the stimulation of physical activity.

It is well established that activity brings about an increase in muscle mass, but our knowledge of the exact mechanism by which this happens is incomplete. As noted earlier, the majority of muscle increase occurs by hypertrophy rather than hyperplasia. During growth it is sometimes difficult to distinguish an increase in muscle mass brought about by overload exercise (high resistance, low repetition) from that due to normal growth. Also, sex hormones play a role in increased muscle mass such that women and prepubescent boys, neither of whom have large amounts of testosterone, do not experience significant gains in muscle mass typical of postpubescent boys who engage in overload exercise. Regular physical activity is also associated with a decrease in body fat. The intensity and duration of exercise undoubtedly influences the extent of this decrease. Both increases in muscle mass and decreases in body fat are associated with activity programs of some duration. Parizkova (1972) found that a regularly trained (6 hr/wk) group of boys had significantly less fat at 18 years than an untrained (2.5 hr/wk or less) group of the same age, even though the groups were similar in fat level at age 11. This study and other changes in body composition with growth and aging are discussed more fully in chapter 7.

The capacity for exercise decreases with aging, but there is increasing evidence that appropriate amounts of regular activity throughout life lessen this decline. Extreme levels of activity harm adults: Both immobility and extremely strenuous work without rest are associated with shortened life span. Excessive training in sport, dance, and exercise can bring injury. Modest anatomical imperfections and misalignments can be tolerated in daily activities and moderate exercise. But overuse causes injury when bones, tendons, and muscles cannot withstand the repetitive forces to which they are subjected (Stanish, 1984).

Summary 2.4—Postnatal Environmental Factors

During postnatal growth the environment in which the child grows becomes increasingly important to the attainment of growth potential. Body tissues and systems are more susceptible to negative environmental factors during periods of rapid growth. Exposure to a negative environmental influence, then, can have an irreversible effect at one point in life but a minimal effect at another. In working with children it is important to understand the environmental factors that can affect growth and development. Maintenance of a healthy environment is critical to full attainment of the growth potential.

In working with adults it is important to understand those factors that affected growth and development in earlier years as well as those that can still affect good health. As we now turn to consider the acquisition and performance of motor skills, it is important to keep in mind the physical growth status of children and the extent of variability in physical status among persons of any age as they enter a performance situation.

Suggested Readings

Edwards, R.G. (1981). *The beginnings of human life.* Burlington, NC: Carolina Biological Supply.

Falkner, F., & Tanner, J.M. (Eds.). (1978). *Human growth* (Vols. 1-2). New York: Plenum Press.

Lowrey, G.H. (1973). *Growth and development of children.* Chicago: Year Book Medical.

Malina, R.M. (1975). *Growth and development: The first twenty years in man.* Minneapolis: Burgess.

Rarick, G.L. (1973). *Physical activity: Human growth and development.* New York: Academic Press.

Rhodes, P. (1981). *Childbirth.* Burlington, NC: Carolina Biological Supply.

Shephard, R.J. (1982). *Physical activity and growth.* Chicago: Year Book Medical.

Smith, E.L., Sempos, C.T., & Purvis, R.W. (1981). Bone mass and strength decline with age. In E.L. Smith & R.C. Serfass (Eds.), *Exercise and aging: The scientific basis.* Hillside, NJ: Enslow Publishers.

Timiras, P.S. (1972). *Developmental physiology and aging.* New York: Macmillan.

3

Early Motor Behavior

If you watch a newborn move, you will notice that some of his or her movements are undirected and without purpose and that some of them are reflexive or automatic. An example of the latter is the sucking motion elicited by stroking the upper lip. At a later age the infant acquires the skills to control posture, to grasp objects, and to move about by sitting up, reaching, crawling, standing, and walking. The process whereby the newborn's undirected movements are replaced years later with a mature athlete's graceful and coordinated skills is intriguing. At what age are children capable of the skilled movements adults take for granted? And how do children refine their skills? This chapter will first examine the sequence of motor development, beginning with a discussion of the ways motor development is assessed, and then will consider reflexive movements, followed by the voluntary, basic skills acquired during the first 2 years of life.

Concept 3.1   Motor development is reflected in the appearance of new skills and their refinement in movement process and product.

The first 3 to 4 months of an infant's life are characterized by involuntary, reflexive movements and by undirected movements of the arms and legs. During the next year or two, many of the reflexes gradually disappear while the infant acquires the basic rudimentary, but voluntary movements leading to grasping by the hands (prehension), upright posture, and locomotion. Motor development, then, could be described in terms of the new skills learned by the infant. These skills appear, after all, in a sequence that is consistent from child to child, even though the *time* of their appearance is variable. But consider motor development in early childhood. Children acquire new skills, additional locomotor skills such as running and skipping, stationary movements such as turning and twisting, and manipulative skills such as throwing, catching, and kicking. Yet, when children attempt any of these skills for the first time, the result is only an approximation of the perfected skill seen in elite performances. Children must repeat these skills again and again to perfect them. Therefore, motor development in early childhood is not just the acquisition of new skills but the refinement of new skills as well.

Skill Refinement

Skill refinement can be gauged in two ways. One way is the *movement form* or *process* used by the child. For example, a right-handed boy who steps forward with his right foot, lifts his elbow up by his ear, and throws by extending his forearm has not mastered the skill of throwing! He could refine his throw by performing it in a more mechanically efficient manner. It is this gradual transition that is termed skill refinement by movement process. The second way to gauge skill refinement is by *movement outcome* or *product*. For example, as children refine their throwing skills, they throw faster, more accurately, and for longer distances. Process and product are not independent of one another. Refinements in the skill process tend to yield improvements in the product because energy is used more efficiently. Once an advanced form is mastered, improvement in the movement product is still possible. Some of this improvement is attributable to physical growth and maturation and some to increased strength and endurance. The preadolescent and adolescent years are characterized by improvements in the product of a skill. Continued refinement in the process of skill performance can still occur in this age period, as can improvements in the ability to combine single skills into complex sequences and improvements in matching a movement to environmental demands.

Thus, we see that progress in motor development can be gauged in several ways: (a) the appearance of new skills, (b) refinements in the movement process, (c) increases in the movement product, (d) acquisition of skill combinations, and (e) improved environmental-response match. Often an age period can be characterized by advancement in one of these areas (new skills, refinement, etc.), but improvement can be simultaneously ongoing in several ways. That does not mean that all children and adolescents automatically make improvements characteristic of a particular age period and thus reach the optimal level of motor performance. Motor development can be slowed or arrested in individual children during the growing years. On the other hand, motor development can be accelerated in some children. The improvements described as characteristic of a given age range are made by *most*, but not necessarily *all*, children. Often a wide range of skill levels is exhibited among children of the same chronological age.

In chapter 2 the importance of physical maturity to motor development was stressed. Because children mature physically at different rates, they acquire new skills at different rates and achieve specific levels of movement outcomes (such as the distance of a throw) at different rates. Some of the variability in skill level at a given chronological age is attributable to the variability in physical maturity. Experience influences motor development, also. A child is likely to refine a skill at an earlier age if practice opportunities are plentiful. This means individual children might be relatively advanced in some skills but unskilled in others. We can expect, then, skill acquisition and refinement to be variable among different children as well as with each individual child.

Summary 3.1—Acquisition and Refinement of New Skills

Motor development can be described in terms of the appearance of new skills, in refinement in the form used to execute a skill, or in the outcome of a movement. During infancy, motor development is often gauged by the appearance of new basic skills. In childhood, it is often measured by refinements in the skill process and product. All of these processes are ongoing throughout infancy and childhood, although the rate of skill acquisition and refinement is variable. This variability is attributable in large part to differing rates of physical growth and maturation among children and movement experiences unique to each child. With the extent of this variability in mind, the motor development process characteristic of the various age periods is examined next, beginning with infancy.

Concept 3.2   Many reflexive movements are evident in the first months of life, but their role in motor development is unclear.

You may have placed your finger in the palm of an infant and felt the baby grasp your finger. This involuntary, reflexive act is known as the *palmar grasping reflex*. Many of the movements of the fetus in the womb and some of an infant's movements in the early postnatal months are reflexive. Later, other reflexes appear, which help an infant to maintain posture in changing environmental conditions. The exact role of reflexive movements in motor development is not known, and considerable controversy exists regarding the relationship of reflexes to later voluntary responses. For example, can you accelerate the learning of voluntary skills by repeatedly stimulating reflexes in early life? Several theories have been proposed and are reviewed in detail in our discussion.

Infantile Reflexes

Primitive Reflexes

Many of the infantile reflexes and reactions are listed in Table 3.1 under one of three categories: primitive reflexes, postural reactions, and locomotor reflexes (see also Figure 3.1). The first group, the *primitive* reflexes, are involuntary responses, many of which are mediated by the lower brain centers (Peiper, 1963). Many of these reflexes are functional prenatally and can be elicited in utero or in premature infants. One of their prenatal functions might be to help the fetus move around in the uterine cavity to position itself for birth (Milani Comparetti, 1981). At birth and in the first postnatal days some primitive reflexes are necessary for survival. For example, the Moro reflex assists with the first inspiration, and the sucking and rooting reflexes are needed for feeding (Milani Comparetti, 1981). The high level of reflex activity in prenatal and early postnatal life might be an indication of cerebral cortex (higher brain) immaturity. As the cortex matures, it assumes control of the lower brain centers at about 3 to 4 postnatal months, which is also a time when many primitive reflexes either disappear (that is, they are inhibited) or become localized (specific to a particular part of the nervous system) (Peiper, 1963). This transition occurs in a fairly predictable but gradual time sequence.

Typically, the reflexive response is at first rather strong and then gradually weakens with advancing maturity until it can no longer be stimulated. In fact, deviation from the typical pattern of reflex disappearance can indicate an abnormality in neurologic maturation. Persistence of a reflex in an infant well after the average age of disappearance might indicate that the infant has a pathological cerebral condition (Peiper, 1963). Remember that individuals develop on their own time schedule and can be ahead or behind these aver-

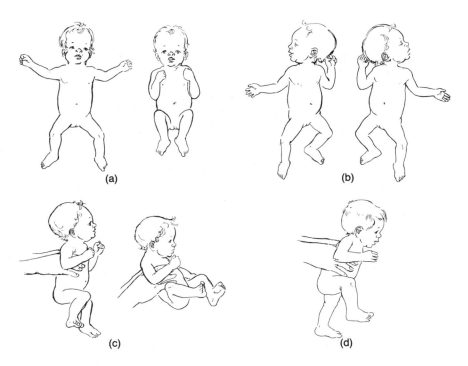

Figure 3.1 Selected reflexes. (a) The Moro reflex. Arms and legs extend then flex. (b) The asymmetrical tonic neck reflex. Note the "fencer's" position. (c) The labyrinthine righting reflex. The infant rights the head when tipped backward. (d) The walking reflex.

age ages. Too, the exact time of a reflex's disappearance is often difficult to establish. Only when the reflex persists for several months past average might it constitute a warning signal of a pathological condition. A reflex should be of comparable strength when stimulated on the right and left sides of the body: A weak response on one side could also reflect a pathological condition.

Postural Reactions

As their name implies, the *postural* reactions (or gravity reflexes) help the infant to automatically maintain posture with a changing environment (Peiper, 1963). Some of these responses keep the head upright and therefore breathing passages open. Others help the infant roll over and eventually attain a vertical position. They generally appear after the second postnatal month. By late in the 1st year or early in the 2nd year of life, the postural reactions drop

Table 3.1 The Reflexes

Reflex/Reaction	Starting Position (If Important)	Stimulus	Response	Time	Warning Signs
Primitive reflexes					
Asymmetrical tonic neck reflex	Supine	Turn head to one side	Same-side arm and leg extends	Prenatal to 4 mo	Persistence after 6 mo
Symmetrical tonic neck reflex	Supported sitting	Extend head and neck / Flex head and neck	Arms extend, legs flex / Arms flex, legs extend	Prenatal to 4 mo	Persistence after 6 mo
Doll-eye		Flex head / Extend head	Eyes look up / Eyes look down	Prenatal to 2 wk	Persistence after first days of life
Palmar grasping		Touch palm with finger or object	Hand closes tightly around object	Prenatal to 4 mo	Persistence after 1 yr; asymmetrical reflex
Moro	Supine	Shake head, as by tapping pillow	Arms and legs extend, fingers spread; then arms and legs flex	Prenatal to 3 mo	Presence after 6 mo; asymmetrical reflex
Sucking		Touch face above or below lips	Sucking motion begins	B to 3 mo	
Babinski		Stroke sole of foot	Toes extend	B to 4 mo	Persistence after 6 mo
Searching or rooting		Touch cheek with smooth object	Head turns to side stimulated	B to 1 yr	Absence of reflex; persistence after 1 yr
Palmar-mandibular (Babkin)		Apply pressure to both palms	Mouth opens; eyes close; head flexes	1 to 3 mo	
Plantar grasping		Stroke sole of foot	Toes contract around object stroking foot	B to 12 mo	
Startle	Supine	Tap abdomen or startle infant	Arms and legs flex	7 to 12 mo	

Table 3.1 (Cont.)

Reflex/Reaction	Starting Position (If Important)	Stimulus	Response	Time	Warning Signs
Postural reactions					
Body righting		Turn legs and pelvis to other side	Trunk and head follow rotation	2 to 6 mo	
Neck righting	Supine	Turn head sideward	Body follows head in rotation	2 to 6 mo	
Labyrinthine righting reflex	Supported upright	Tilt infant	Head moves to stay upright	2 to 12 mo	
Pull-up	Sitting upright, held by 1 or 2 hands	Tip infant backward or forward	Arms flex	3 to 12 mo	
Parachute	Held upright	Lower infant toward ground rapidly or tilt forward to prone position	Legs and arms extend and abduct	4 mo into 2nd yr	
Locomotor reflexes					
Crawling	Prone	Apply pressure to sole of one foot or both feet alternately	Crawling pattern in arms and legs	B to 4 mo	
Walking	Held upright	Place infant on flat surface	Walking pattern in legs	B to 5 mo	
Swimming	Prone	Place infant in or over water	Swimming movement of arms and legs	11 days to 5 mo	

out of the infant's repertoire of movements as isolated reactions and are replaced by voluntary movements.

Locomotor Reflexes

The last category of reflexes is that of the *locomotor* reflexes. These appear to be actions related to the voluntary behaviors from which they take their individual names, such as the "walking" reflex. The locomotor reflexes, though, appear much earlier than the voluntary behaviors for which they are named and typically disappear weeks before the infant attempts the voluntary locomotor skill.

Views on the Role of Reflexes

The role of reflexes in motor development is unclear. Some theorists believe that the reflexes merely reflect the structure of the nervous system, in other words, the way we are "wired." Others take the view that reflexive movements lead to coordinated limb movements (Peiper, 1963). They give the infant the opportunity to practice coordinated movements before the higher brain centers are ready to mediate such movements. We will consider some of the various views on reflexes in more detail.

An interesting controversy has surrounded the theory that systematic stimulation of a locomotor reflex could enhance acquisition of the related locomotor skill. Hence, repeated stimulation of the swimming reflex during the early months after birth would lead to advanced swimming skills. Zelazo and his co-workers (Zelazo, Konner, Kolb, & Zelazo, 1974; Zelazo, Zelazo, & Kolb, 1972a, b) proposed this view after an investigation in which they elicited the walking reflex in a small number of children during their first 8 weeks. These children later tended to be early walkers. The investigators concluded that the walking reflex could be transformed to an instrumental action (see also Zelazo, 1983).

The established view of reflexes has been that the locomotor reflexes *must* disappear several months before the onset of the voluntary behavior, so the Zelazo view was heavily criticized. Pontius (1973), for example, pointed out that there was no evidence for the notion that the reflex underwent a transformation to a voluntary response. He argued first that without intervention there is a natural gap of at least several months between the disappearance of the reflex and the onset of the voluntary skill, rather than a smooth transition from one to the other. Second, the reflex and the voluntary skill are mediated by different brain centers. The 1st year is a period of ongoing maturation in the higher brain centers and the pyramidal tracts (motor nerve pathways). Thus, it is likely that this maturation process brings the higher brain centers to a point at which they can first inhibit lower brain centers and then mediate voluntary skills. Further, little is known about the effect of overstimulation of the reflexes on normal neurologic development. Since the prolonged presence of a reflex is often linked to pathological conditions (Peiper, 1963), it might be suspected that prolonged overstimulation is, if not useless, perhaps detrimental to the normal course of neurologic development (McGraw, 1943; Gotts, 1972).

Recently, Thelen (1983) argued that the Zelazo studies do, in fact, demonstrate continuity between reflexive walking and voluntary walking. The locomotor reflexes need not disappear; they can be maintained with practice, and a period of reflex inhibition before voluntary locomotion is unnecessary. However, she proposes an alternative explanation to Zelazo's view that a reflex is transformed to a learned, instrumental response by practice. Thelen hypothesizes that the walking reflex disappears because the infant's leg mass increases. Practice of the reflex improves lower body strength and allows an infant to continue the reflexive response by lifting the legs alternately. Thelen did note that 4- to 6-week-old infants reduced their reflexive walking responses when weight was added to their legs, but increased them when their legs were submerged in and consequently buoyed by water. Hence, we see from these various views that interrelationships between neural, physical, and mechanical factors remain cloudy in accounting for the role of the locomotor reflexes in motor development.

A slightly different viewpoint has been taken for the role of the primitive reflexes and the postural reactions in the development of voluntary movement. Molnar (1978) suggests that certain primitive reflexes *must* disappear and postural reactions appear before an infant can undertake some of the basic voluntary motor skills such as rolling, sitting, and walking. For example, the asymmetrical tonic neck reflex, a primitive reflex, must be inhibited so that the infant can perform the body and neck righting reactions without an extended arm preventing the roll. The body and neck righting reactions are necessary for voluntary rolling because the upper and lower trunk must turn sequentially (Roberton, 1984). Similar transitions can be followed for other voluntary skills.

Another established view of reflexive movements holds that they lead up to coordinated movements of the limbs (Peiper, 1963). That is, before the higher brain centers are mature enough to prepare instructions for a coordinated movement such as stepping, a reflexive movement allows practice of the pattern. Recent work with animals, however, has led to speculation that locomotion is not even controlled by the higher brain centers, but rather by "(movement) pattern generators" in the spinal cord (Grillner, 1975). Even more recent research on the control of movement has caused theorists (Kelso, Holt, Kugler, & Turvey, 1980; Kugler, Kelso, & Turvey, 1980) to argue that a movement pattern such as a reach or step results from a systematic relationship among the muscles that is established at the spinal cord. This view implies that many of the detailed specifications for a movement do not have to be controlled at the higher brain centers for a movement to occur. Biodynamic theory is a young but promising theory. It is partially supported by experimental work but critical questions (e.g., whether the musculoskeletal structure controls the movement based on time or force) remain. If this theory is correct, early motor development would involve more than maturation of the nervous system. Physical changes, such as those in limb length and limb mass with growth, would be important. Obviously, the role of reflexive movement in motor development will be further clarified as research continues on both neurologic development and control of movement.

Summary 3.2—Reflexive Movement

Some of an infant's movements in the early months are primitive, involuntary reflexes presumably mediated by lower brain centers. With rapid maturation of the cerebral cortex and myelination of the pyramidal tracts during the 1st year, these reflexes disappear and postural reactions appear. Locomotor reflexes also appear during the 1st year. They tend to disappear weeks before voluntary locomotion, but whether this is a necessary consequence of neurologic maturation is not clear. In fact, recent research on the biodynamics of movement leads to speculation that a patterned limb response such as a walking step reflects construction of the musculoskeletal system, rather than neurological maturation alone. If so, we can see that this phase of motor development is a result of the maturation of several systems that are in turn interrelated. As the reflexes disappear during infancy, voluntary motor skills are acquired. It is this phase of motor development that will be discussed next.

Concept 3.3   Infants achieve control of their environment by acquiring rudimentary motor skills in an identified sequence.

In the 1st year of life children acquire locomotion and visually guided reaching through a series of "motor milestones." For example, the infant first learns to hold the head erect, then to sit, then to stand, and then to walk. Individual infants vary in the time they reach a motor milestone, but they acquire these different rudimentary skills in a relatively consistent sequence. The average ages at which these various skills appear in infants are well documented (Bayley, 1935; Shirley, 1963). This progressive pattern of skill acquisition is related in large part to physical maturation, especially maturation of the central nervous system, the development of muscular strength and endurance, and improvement in sensory processing. Thus, diversity in the rate of physical development among infants is partly responsible for variations in the rate of appearance of the motor milestones. Environmental factors also play a role in individual variability. The orderly, sequential acquisition of the rudimentary skills is the beginning of the process that leads to the amazingly complex movements of mature performers. This process will be examined in more detail to better understand the development of motor skills, by considering first the acquisition of locomotor skills, and then the achievement of visually guided reaching.

Motor Milestones

Locomotion

Five classic studies of infants provide us with information about the appearance of the motor milestones. These studies are the descriptive works of Shirley (1931, 1933), Bayley (1935), Ames (1937), Gesell and Ames (1940), and McGraw (1940, 1943). The authors basically agree on the sequential appearance of the motor milestones but show minor variations in the age of onset of some milestone skills. The variations are probably due to several factors that could affect the infant groups studied by each author: differences in growth and maturation rate, differences in environmental factors (such as climate, the number of siblings, and child-rearing practices), and differences in the author's scoring criteria. The researchers also approach motor development from slightly different viewpoints. By considering each viewpoint, we add to our understanding of locomotive motor development in early postnatal life.

Shirley and Bayley. The studies by Shirley and Bayley are largely descriptive. The sequence and average age at onset of the motor milestones were determined by careful observation of groups of infants. Selected milestone skills from Shirley's early work and from the Bayley Scale of Infant Development (Bayley, 1969), based on Bayley's 1935 work, are displayed in Table 3.2. Infants generally achieve postural control of the upper body by about 5 months of age, then control of the entire trunk during the next 3 months. By about the 9th month they attempt locomotion through a sequence of achievements leading to creeping. In everyday terms we often call moving on hands and knees "crawling." In the developmental literature, "crawling" usually indicates movement with the abdomen still on the floor. "Creeping" describes the movement on hands and knees with the stomach off the floor.

The milestone skills identified by Bayley and Shirley in Table 3.2 (see also Figure 3.2) also point out that coordination for walking is achieved at approximately 11 to 15 months. The child initially learns to stand with help or the support of furniture, then to walk along the furniture or when led by an adult. Eventually the infant is able to stand and then walk alone. In the next few months the child masters walking in different directions and on steps. Children usually begin negotiating steps with a "mark time" pattern: One foot is placed on a step followed by the other foot on the same step rather than the next higher one. Eventually the mature, alternate stepping pattern is mastered. These classic studies of Bayley and Shirley identify the sequence of locomotor skill acquisition in the first 2 years.

Ames.   The work of Ames (1937) focused on the sequential pattern of development leading to creeping. This progression begins with infants drawing the knee and thigh forward beside the body at about 7 months. Within a few weeks they can assume a low creeping position and several weeks later creep about the floor. Once infants can assume the high creep position, they may rock back and forth on hands and knees or creep backward before learning to creep forward.

Gesell and Ames.   The work of Gesell and Ames (1940) emphasizes the changes between *extension* (straightening) and *flexion* (bending) movements of the limbs as children achieve upright locomotion. *Unilateral* (one side of the body), *bilateral* (both sides), and *cross-lateral* (opposite hand and foot) transitional movements are identified as well. For example, the newborn's dominant pattern of limb movement is bilateral flexion, as in bending both arms. Over the first 7 months bilateral flexion is gradually replaced by unilateral flexion of the limbs.

But the infant reverts to bilateral flexion when first attempting locomotor skills (crawling, rocking, creeping) around the 8th month. As the infant becomes more skilled, bilateral arm extension and bilateral leg flexion-and-extension are adopted. The infant is on the way to proficient creeping when he or she learns to move the opposite limbs alternately, that is, to use cross-lateral patterns of movement. This process is repeated with standing and walking. The infant again reverts to bilateral extension when learning to stand at 10 to 14 months, but he or she eventually masters alternate arm and leg movements in order to walk proficiently.

This type of analysis of early motor development highlights an interesting facet of skill development: *reversion* or *regression*. Infants revert to a pattern of movement previously "outgrown" when faced with learning a new skill in a new posture. After all, this new skill requires a higher center of gravity

Table 3.2 Selected Motor Milestones

Average Age (mo)	Age Range (mo)	Milestone (Bayley Scale of Infant Development)	Milestone (Shirley Sequence)
0.1		Lifts head when held at shoulder	
0.1		Lateral head movements	
0.8	0.3- 3.0	Retains red ring	
0.8	0.3- 2.0	Arm thrusts in play	
0.8	0.3- 2.0	Leg thrusts in play	Chin up
1.6	0.7- 4.0	Head erect and steady	
1.8	0.7- 5.0	Turns from side to back	
2.0			Chest up
2.3	1.0- 5.0	Sits with slight support	
4.0			Sits with support
4.4	2.0- 7.0	Turns from back to side	
4.9	4.0- 8.0	Partial thumb opposition	
5.0			Sits on lap
			Grasps object
5.3	4.0- 8.0	Sits alone momentarily	
5.4	4.0- 8.0	Unilateral reaching	
5.7	4.0- 8.0	Rotates wrist	
6.0			Sits in chair
			Grasps dangling object
6.4	4.0-10.0	Rolls from back to front	
6.6	5.0- 9.0	Sits alone steadily	
6.9	5.0- 9.0	Complete thumb opposition	
7.0			Sits alone
7.1	5.0-11.0	Prewalking progression	
7.4	6.0-10.0	Partial finger prehension	
8.0			Stands with help
8.1	5.0-12.0	Pulls to standing	
8.6	6.0-12.0	Stands up by furniture	
8.8	6.0-12.0	Stepping movements	
9.0			Stands holding furniture
9.6	7.0-12.0	Walks with help	
10.0			Creeps
11.0	9.0-16.0	Stands alone	Walks when led
11.7	9.0-17.0	Walks alone	
12.0			Pulls to stand
14.0			Stands alone
14.6	11.0-20.0	Walks backward	
15.0			Walks alone
16.1	12.0-23.0	Walks up stairs with help	
16.4	13.0-23.0	Walks down stairs with help	
23.4	17.0-30.0 +	Jumps off floor, both feet	
24.8	19.0-30.0 +	Jumps from bottom step	

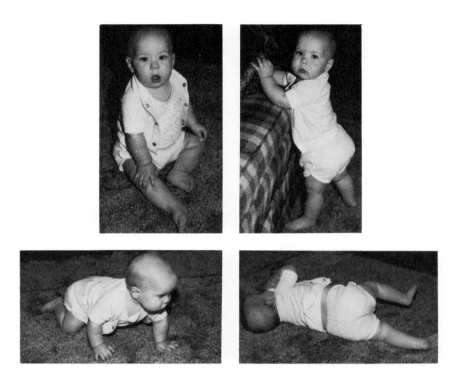

Figure 3.2 Some of the motor "milestone skills."

and smaller base of support than previously-learned skills. An infant initially meets the challenge of this more difficult skill by using a simple bilateral limb movement to assume a stationary position. As skill and confidence are gained, the infant progresses to the mature, alternate-limb actions. Gesell and Ames note that the direction of progress in locomotion is cephalocaudal and proximodistal, the pattern reflecting advancement in neuromotor coordination.

McGraw. McGraw (1940, 1943) describes prone progression (to creeping) and erect locomotion from yet another viewpoint. She emphasizes that achievement of the motor milestones reflects the development of cortical (cerebral cortex) control over muscle function. This acquisition of muscle function control occurs in a cephalocaudal direction. McGraw uses seven phases to describe the progression to erect locomotion. The first phase, the *Walking Reflex* (from birth to 5 months of age), indicates that the lower brain centers control the movement. In the next phase, *Inhibition* (at 4 to 5 months of age), higher brain centers may inhibit this subcortical control and control of head movement is achieved. Advancing cortical maturation is evident in the *Tran-

sition phase, which is characterized by better trunk control (4 to 7.5 months). The *Deliberate Stepping* phase follows with the infant showing better foot control (7.5 to 9 months). During the *Independent Stepping* phase (9 to 15 months), less cortical attention is demanded as walking movements become more and more automatic. This trend toward automaticity continues in the *Heel-Toe Progression* phase (after 18 months). Finally, the most mature level of muscular control is reached (at approximately 2.5 years) wherein little attention is required to execute walking steps. Hence, cortical control is achieved, leading to the establishment of muscle action patterns that can be carried out without conscious control.

The early descriptive studies were instrumental in identifying the sequence and direction of locomotor development. They were also helpful in establishing the average rate of skill development during the early months. While this regular progress toward locomotion was traditionally accepted as evidence of development by maturation alone (rather than environmental experience), recent research has countered this one-sided view. There is still little agreement on the origin of the motor milestone skills. Nevertheless, these early works are used today as the basis for assessments of normal motor development in infancy.

Motor Scales. The scales developed by Shirley (1931, 1933, 1963), Bayley (1935), and others can be used to assess an individual's rate of motor development through comparison of the individual's age at acquisition of a given skill to the average age provided by the scale. This process is particularly valuable in identifying infants who lag behind the majority of children in the acquisition of locomotor skills. It is possible that some of these infants are growing and maturing normally but a bit more slowly than other children. They may eventually catch up with the average scores. However, it is also possible that the developmental lag indicates a neurologic impairment. In this case comparison of a child's performance to a motor scale may provide early detection of the problem. Remember that the average age for appearance of a motor skill is really the middle of an *age span* during which most children acquire the skill. This age span typically widens as we deal with skills acquired at an older age and is evident in Table 3.2. The increasing variation in age at onset is related in part to the environment in which the child develops and in part to individual maturation rates. The longer an environmental factor influences both the growth of a child and his or her experiences with motor skills, the greater the effect on age of acquisition. Lags in motor development that may indicate a neurologic impairment are only the ones that are so large as to fall outside the normal age span for acquisition of a skill. Caution must also be used in evaluating individual children because it is not unusual for infants to "skip" a milestone skill. For example, some infants never crawl. They do, though, acquire subsequent skills in the normal time frame, whereas a slowly developing child might acquire the skill, but at a relatively late age, and subsequent skills would also be remarkably delayed.

Visually Guided Reaching and Grasping

The mature skill of reaching for and grasping an object is achieved through a progression of reaching and grasping skills learned during the 1st year or so of life. Prehension (grasping) and manipulation are very important to mature skill performance. We can appreciate this quickly by thinking of fielding a baseball, rebounding a basketball, or using a racquet. Further, grasping and manipulative skills are necessary for a variety of everyday and artistic endeavors such as typing and piano playing.

H.M. Halverson published a classic description of grasping development in 1931. He identified 10 phases of prehension development, which are summarized in Figure 3.3. In early grasping the infant squeezes objects against the palm. Soon he or she can place the object in the thumb-side of the palm and eventually use the thumb in a pincer movement opposing the forefinger. Early arm reaches are imprecise and tend to be a thrusting forward, then lowering of the hand onto the object. Later the infant might reach for even a small object with both hands, because an error with one hand still pushes the object into the other hand so it can be squeezed between the two. At about 10 months the infant begins to master a continuous, direct reach and grasp with one hand.

More recent research has focused on the extent of visually guided reaching in the newborn. This research was prompted by contradictory hypotheses that newborn motor activity is limited to excited thrashing of the limbs (White, Castle, & Held, 1964) versus the view that newborn movements demonstrate advanced eye-hand coordination (Bower, 1972; Bower, Broughton, & Moore, 1970). The latter view was developed when Bower noted that newborns could make more grasping motions when their bodies were supported and their hands free to move. Newborns are typically not positioned such that this is possible. Newborns also make frequent contact with objects that are dangled near them, whereas freestanding objects are often knocked out of reach within the first few hand movements (Bower, 1977). It is obvious that newborns cannot catch or voluntarily grasp objects. But newborns can reach in the general direction of an object placed in front of them. The function of these arm extensions is probably more attentional, that is, pointing, than manipulative (McDonnell, 1979; Von Hofsten, 1982).

Visually guided reaching has been observed at about 4 to 5 months of age. Infants at about this age will adapt their reach when their view of an object is distorted by prisms (McDonnell, 1975), and their reaching is disrupted when they cannot see their hand (Lasky, 1977). Later in the 1st year,

Type of Grasp	Weeks of Age	
No Contact	16	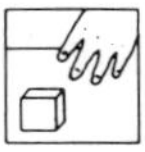
Contact Only	20	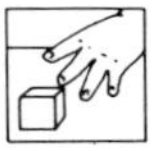
Primitive Squeeze	20	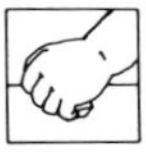
Squeeze Grasp	24	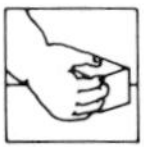
Hand Grasp	28	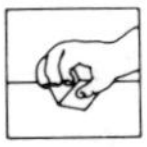
Palm Grasp	28	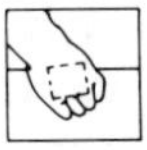
Superior-Palm Grasp	32	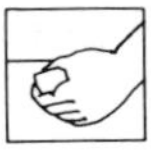
Inferior-Forefinger Grasp	36	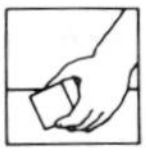
Forefinger Grasp	52	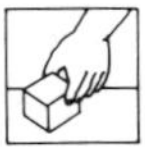
Superior-Forefinger Grasp	52	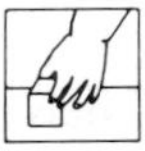

Figure 3.3 A developmental grasping progression. From "An experimental study of prehension in infants by means of systematic cinema records" by H.M. Halverson, 1931, *Genetic Psychology Monographs*, **10**, pp. 212-215. Copyright 1931 by Helen Dwight Reid Educational Foundation. Reprinted by permission.

infants demonstrate ballistic reaches, that is, complete and fast arm movements planned on initial information of an object's position rather than the slower method of comparing arm and object position (McDonnell, 1979). Very little research is available on the reaching of children older than 1 year of age. Hay (1978, 1979) has noted that reaching accuracy is refined between 4 and 6 years of age but then declines around 7 years before progressively improving through at least 11 years of age. Hay suggests that younger children perform reaching tasks ballistically, but children around 7 years of age begin to rely heavily on feedback from the arm reach. By 9 or so years, children are better able to integrate the ballistic and feedback systems to reach accurately.

Just as in locomotion, these reaching and grasping developments reflect neurologic development. The area of the motor cortex associated with the hand undergoes rapid maturation in early postnatal life. At about 3 months of age the cerebral cortex begins to develop rapidly, and soon thereafter the infant demonstrates visually guided reaching. The eye-hand coordination of accurate reaching achieves an adult pattern around 9 years of age, while continued maturation of the cerebral cortex is noted over the first decade (Woollacott, 1983).

Although reaching and grasping developments can be associated with neurologic development, it might also be associated with changing mechanical factors. The biodynamic hypothesis of Kugler, Kelso, and Turvey (1982) (mentioned in concept 3.2) would predict that continuous change of a factor such as arm length and weight that occurs with physical growth could bring about sudden qualitative changes in the control of arm reaches. More research is needed on the transitions in these motor behaviors and their associations with mechanical and neurologic factors (Woollacott, 1983).

Gender Differences

None of the motor milestone charts gives separate ages of skill acquisition for boys and girls, simply because there are no significant gender differences in the sequence of skill acquisition or in the average ages for skill onset. As we noted in chapter 2, girls mature physically a bit faster than boys on the average, so the average girl may acquire the milestones slightly earlier than the average boy. But for all practical purposes, individual differences in the rate of development overshadow these small average gender differences.

Critical Periods

We have identified the sequence of motor skill acquisition in infancy and the normal age span during which each skill is acquired. Can this normal progression be altered by environmental factors? Might a deprived environment retard motor development and an enriched environment accelerate it? These questions could be answered if it were known whether *critical periods* exist for motor skills. Remember that critical periods are defined as a finite time period during which a child is most sensitive to learning a particular skill. These periods are critical because a child who does not learn a skill during its critical period might find it difficult or even impossible to learn the skill at an older age.

There is strong evidence for the existence of critical periods in the development of many animals. It also appears that critical periods exist for certain aspects of human development, such as language acquisition (Dennis, 1963). Unfortunately, the information on critical periods of motor development is not as clear. Let us review the evidence available on this topic, first with regard to deprived environments, then enriched environments.

Deprived Environments. For obvious ethical reasons researchers cannot place human infants in deprived living conditions. Some information about humans is available, though, from studies of institutionalized infants. The institutional environment typically cannot provide the same degree of parental care and interaction as is possible in the home. Infants may not be given an adequate amount of space in an institution or the freedom to attempt and practice motor skills, because one adult must supervise many babies. Hence, some institutions may be considered a deprived environment for development. In fact, lags in physical, intellectual, emotional, and social development have been documented in some institutions (Bowlby, 1978).

Dennis (1963) reported that institutionalized children in Iran demonstrated retarded locomotor development: Sitting alone, creeping, standing, and walking alone were all delayed. In one institution, only 15% of the children could walk alone when tested between their 3rd and 4th birthdays. Dennis noted that infants at the institution spent most of their time supine. They were rarely placed in sitting and prone positions from which they could more easily attempt locomotion. Bowlby (1978) concluded from a review of four studies that institutionalized children do develop more slowly than those raised in homes, although locomotor skills and manual dexterity are not as severely affected as social responsiveness and speech.

On the other hand, a study of motor development among Hopi Indians indicates that some degree of physical restriction may be tolerated within normal motor development. The Hopi practice at the time of the study, 1940, was to bind infants to a cradle board worn on the mother's back for all but a few hours of the day until the age of 9 months. The average age for the onset of walking among these cradle-bound infants was only ½ month later than that of a group of Hopi infants not cradle-bound (Dennis, 1940). It seems that early deprivation has a negative effect on motor development only if it is long and severe enough. Shorter and milder instances of deprivation may be tolerated and normal progress still made. In this case even the few hours of freedom each day and the time between 9 months of age and the onset of walking probably gave Hopi infants time to explore and practice moving. We must realize, though, that the assessment criteria used in this study make it difficult to ascertain all the effects of deprivation on early motor development. Recording the acquisition of a motor milestone such as walking is a quantitative assessment. This process may be somewhat resilient to mild deprivation. Very little is known about the effect of deprivation on performance *quality*, that is, the movement *process*, yet this could have tremendous impact on later motor development. For example, a skill might never be performed with the smoothness and precision otherwise possible. More information is needed before we can definitively assess the effect of mild deprivation.

Enriched Environments. The existence of critical periods for motor development could also be demonstrated by lasting beneficial effects of enriching the environment. Several programs for maximizing motor development exist, but they have undergone little objective assessment. Ridenour (1978) reviewed these programs and categorized them as "Programming Plan" or "No Programming Plan." Advocates of the Programming Plan approach suggest that prepractice of the motor skills soon to be acquired is beneficial. For example, the Prudden Infant Fitness Program calls for a daily 20-minute period of mother-infant activities during the infant's 1st year. The activities include manipulation of the limbs and trunk. The use of infant walkers and baby bouncers is encouraged. In contrast, advocates of the No Programming Plan discourage prepractice of skills, manipulation of the infant, and use of special equipment. Instead, infants are allowed to achieve new postural positions (upright sitting, standing) on their own. Toys are placed near the infant, to be obtained on the infant's own initiative. They are never placed in the infant's hand by an adult. The Pikler Program at the National Methodological Institute for Infant Care in Budapest is an example of the No Programming Plan (Pikler, 1968). Pikler reports that the age at onset of the motor milestones is not appreciably delayed in the program's infants and that their quality of movement is better than that of instructed children. However, very little independent research has been conducted on the merits of such programs, and no reported studies have assessed programs from both categories simultaneously. It is difficult, then, to judge the value of programs attempting to optimize motor development. In the absence of research information it seems sensible for parents to provide an environment that facilitates the infant's natural motor development but to avoid activities the infant is obviously not ready to perform. Parents should also avoid programs that promise unrealistic acceleration of motor development.

The McGraw Twin Study—Jimmy and Johnny. McGraw (1935) conducted a well-known motor development study that dealt with the issue of critical periods and enrichment activities. She used a co-twin method, realizing that twins of identical genetic background could be raised in different environments. Any differences in behavior could be attributed to environmental rather than genetic factors. Unfortunately, McGraw's set of twins were later determined to be fraternal rather than identical twins and therefore their heredity was not identical.

Several aspects of the study, however, are still noteworthy. The twins were observed from 21 days of age to 22 months. One twin, Johnny, was exercised in motor activities while the other, Jimmy, spent most of his time in a crib. Their ages at the onset of the important motor skills were recorded and compared. From this comparison McGraw concluded that the basic behaviors every child acquires to function biologically are not appreciably modified by practice. In contrast, those activities variably acquired by individuals, that is, not necessarily learned by everyone, are enhanced with practice, depending upon the age when they are introduced. McGraw felt strongly that critical periods exist for the modification of performance. Johnny actually learned skills such as roller skating at a younger age than most children who are probably not encouraged to attempt them, much less practice them, as Johnny did. After the enrichment program McGraw (1939) observed Johnny and Jimmy for several years. While both boys scored similarly on objective tests of skill, Johnny appeared to have superior motor coordination and confidence in his movements.

The latter finding emphasizes, like the Hopi Indian study, the importance of using several criteria to evaluate early practice of motor skills. The sequence and timing of motor skill acquisition in early life may not be greatly modified by early practice experiences. Undoubtedly, the emergence of rudimentary motor skills is related to the ongoing development of other body systems, such as the neurologic and muscular systems. Children may not be capable of some skills until these systems mature, no matter how much "practice" they are given by adults. For example, children confined to a crib in an institution cannot develop much leg strength and therefore are not well prepared for locomotor skills even if suddenly given the opportunity to move about. Also, passive movements (as with adults manipulating infants) are not neurologically controlled in the same manner as movement actively undertaken by the infant. On the other hand, early but appropriately-timed practice experiences may improve the quality of movement and the confidence of the child. More study is needed of these aspects of early motor development, especially of the interrelationships between neurologic and musculoskeletal development and of environment-induced opportunities to undertake and practice motor skills.

Summary 3.3—Locomotion and Reaching

Upright locomotion and visually guided reaching are acquired through a relatively consistent set of steps or "motor milestones." The average age spans for acquisition of these milestones are known and seem to reflect ongoing neurologic development, although there are suggestions that they also reflect mechanical changes accompanying growth. This process appears somewhat resilient to mild deprivation. Likewise, it seems that enrichment programs do not have a great impact on skill acquisition in the first 18 months of life. Yet, the quality of skill performance may be affected by environmental factors. Children may be more or less confident of their movement abilities depending upon the extent of their early experience with motor activities. Continued research will tell us which, if any, skills can be enhanced by early practice and which methods of early practice are best.

Infants enter the early childhood period well on their way to mastering basic locomotion and grasping. Their challenge then is to acquire various more complex locomotor and manipulative skills, such as jumping, hopping, running, skipping, catching, throwing, and striking. The next chapter begins by discussing the acquisition and refinement of these basic motor skills.

Suggested Readings

McGraw, M.B. (1939). Later development of children specially trained during infancy. *Child Development*, **10**, 1-19.

Peiper, A. (1963). *Cerebral function in infancy and childhood*. New York, NY: Consultants Bureau.

Ridenour, M.V. (1978). Programs to optimize infant motor development. In M.V. Ridenour (Ed.), *Motor development: Issues and applications* (pp. 39-61). Princeton, NJ: Princeton Book Company.

4

Motor Behavior During Childhood

Infants begin to walk around 1 year of age, and soon after this they attempt other basic skills. Running and jumping are learned during the 2nd year, and other forms of locomotion follow in early childhood. Children might try throwing and kicking as early as the 2nd year, depending upon opportunity and encouragement from family members, but the initial attempts at these basic skills typically are crude and inconsistent, that is, mechanically inefficient. With experience, instruction, and imitation of others, children become more efficient in their performance of the basic skills. This improvement happens gradually, with the child continually refining the skills to more closely approximate a form consistent with mechanical principles of movement. Increases in body size and strength account for many of the improvements achieved during childhood. Yet size and strength alone do not account for the progression of a mechanically inefficient 2-year-old to the level of elite performance. A good example is the skill of overhand throwing. The 2-year-old usually performs this skill by pointing the elbow toward the target, extending the lower arm, and releasing the ball for the throw; there is no leg or trunk action. Using such inefficient mechanical movements, even a full-size adult could not execute a maximal throw in this way! To maximize performance, a form that takes advantage of mechanical principles, size, and strength is needed. Because the development of the basic skills generally follows a trend toward increased mechanical efficiency, motor development during childhood will be considered by first examining the pertinent mechanical laws, and then the process whereby children gain motor efficiency.

Concept 4.1   Children improve their basic skill performance by increasing their mechanical efficiency.

An understanding of applicable mechanical principles involved in motor skills is important in order to focus on the critical aspects of performance, that is, what makes a movement skilled or unskilled. Once understood, the improvements needed to make unskilled performance more proficient can be identified. Biomechanics, the mechanics of muscular activity, is an area of study in itself and beyond the scope of this text. The purpose here is to discuss the application of established mechanical principles relative to basic skill performance. Of primary concern in motor development are the principles that apply to human motion and stability. A more detailed explanation of these principles is available in any biomechanics text (cf. Hay & Reid, 1982; Kreighbaum & Barthels, 1985).

Laws of Motion and Stability

Application of Force

Newton's First Law of Motion states that an external force must act on a resting object to cause it to move or to change an object already moving. Hence, to throw a ball, one applies force to it. Performance can be maximized by applying this force over the greatest distance possible. In executing motor skills performance is increased by taking a step forward when projecting an object; this motion increases the *linear (straight-line)* distance over which force is applied. Using a full range of body motion to increase the *rotary* distance over which force is applied also increases performance. A preparatory crouch or wind-up puts the performer in a position to maximize both the linear and rotary distance of force application. The preparatory positioning also stretches the muscles to be used, thus readying them for maximal contraction. These actions permit projection of the object at greater velocity than would be accomplished without a wind-up and a full range of motion. So, mature skill performance is characterized in part by a preparatory phase as well as a force application phase of movement through a full range of motion.

Action and Reaction

Another of Newton's Laws, the Third, states that for every force one body exerts on another body, the second body exerts an equal force on the first in the opposite direction. For example, when sprinters round the curve on a track, they push backward and to the right so they are projected forward and to the left. On the straightaway, they push directly backward. Any forces exerted in a plane other than that of the desired movement direction detract from the performance. If athletes are attempting a maximal performance, such as long jumping for the greatest distance possible, they want to exert as much force on the ground as possible to get the biggest return push possible. This maximal effort is characterized by full extension (straightening) of the push-off limbs, in this case the legs. Application of this action-reaction law is also seen among parts of the body. For example, in locomotor skills such as running, one leg swings forward and the arm on the opposite side of the body swings forward in reaction. This familiar pattern is termed the *opposition* of arm and leg movement and is a characteristic of skilled locomotor movements.

Straightening of the Projecting Limb

When athletes perform ballistic tasks, their limbs trace part of a circle; the arm travels in an arc in throwing, the leg in an arc in kicking. Releasing or striking an object causes it to fly away from this curved path in a straight line from the release or impact point. The velocity an object has when it leaves this path is a product of its rotational velocity (speed along a curved path) and the radius of the circular path it is tracing. In other words, the object's straight line velocity is determined by the length of an athlete's limb and the speed it is moving. If athletes are already moving their limbs as fast as possible when attempting a maximal performance such as pitching a baseball, the only other way to increase the projecting velocity of the object is to increase the length of the limb. This increase is achieved by straightening the limb just before release in a throw or impact in a kick or strike. So, skilled performers giving a maximal effort begin with their limbs bent or cocked and then straighten them. Why not keep the limb straight throughout the throw, strike, or kick? It takes more effort to move the weight of an extended limb (and any held object) than a flexed limb. This conservation of effort is seen in skilled sprinting when the recovering (returning) leg is brought forward bent. To conserve energy in maximal efforts, athletes move their limbs in a bent position, but they maximize the velocity of a projection by straightening their limbs just before release or impact.

The Open Kinetic Chain

Tossing or kicking an object a short distance can be done easily with a small movement of the arm or leg. But for a maximal ballistic effort, more body parts must be involved, and they must be moved in a series of movements rather than one movement. The movement series must be "timed" so that each succeeding movement applies its force just after the previous movement has applied its greatest force to accelerate the object. As a brief example, recall that in a throw the thrower steps forward and rotates the pelvis, then rotates the upper trunk as the throwing arm comes forward, extends and rotates inwardly, all in a sequence of movements. A sequence such as this is termed the *open kinetic chain* of movements. One of the most significant changes seen in the skill development of children is the transition from mechanically inefficient skill performance by using a single action, to skills executed via a pattern of efficient, properly timed sequential movements.

Force Absorption

Earlier, the benefit of maximizing force application over distance was identified. The natural reverse of this principle is that force can be minimized by dissipating it over distance. In addition, force can be dissipated over *area*. The greater the distance and larger the area, the more gradually force is absorbed. In catching, then, one meets the ball well in front of the body and lets the hands and arms "give" to absorb the force. In landing from a jump, the legs are flexed after touchdown to increase the distance over which the force is absorbed. To decrease the force of a fall, one rolls to spread the impact of the fall over a larger area of the body.

Base of Support

The stability of any object is related in part to the size of its support base. A refrigerator on its side is more difficult to tip over than one standing up! If one wants to become more stable, the body's support base can be increased by spreading the feet apart if in a standing position, or spreading the hands apart if doing a handstand. The reverse is true if one wants to lose stability. In locomotor skills, one sacrifices stability (two-feet base of support) momentarily, in order to move by alternately losing and gaining balance (one-foot support base). The body's weight is pushed forward, ahead of the support base, and the leg is moved forward to regain balance. When young children first learn locomotor skills they attempt to control their stability by keeping a wide base of support. For example, they walk with their toes out and plant their feet out to the side. As they gain greater muscular control, experience, and confidence, they narrow their base of support. Skilled performers use a base of support just wide enough to achieve stability.

Summary 4.1—Applying Mechanical Principles

Motor performance is improved throughout childhood by a gradual increase in motor efficiency, resulting from better application of the mechanical principles of movement combined with increases in body size and strength. The major mechanical principles involved in efficient, skilled movement include the application and absorption of force, action and reaction, linear and rotational velocity, sequentially timed movements, and stability in the base of support. Children's progress toward skilled motor performance is demonstrated by increasingly consistent motor patterns that effectively utilize mechanical principles.

Concept 4.2   Children's skill development includes qualitative changes that mark steps in a developmental sequence.

Basic skill development in children is a gradual process of refining skills so that they are executed in a more mechanically efficient way. Often this process includes a qualitative change in the skill, such as beginning to take a step forward with a throw. Some authors have described development of a particular skill through stages or levels. These stages are based on the qualitative change in a critical feature of the skill, which is indicative of how closely a child follows efficient mechanical principles. Examples of critical changes that mark the achievement of a new level are use of the swing leg in hopping or use of leg-and-arm opposition in a run. In other words, the stages are based on a qualitative change in how the child performs, rather than a quantitative performance change such as hopping longer distances or running faster.

Qualitative Changes in Motor Skills

In chapter 1, labeling the qualitative changes in motor skills as stages was discussed. Recall that a precise usage of the term stage is desirable and that the developmental process should exhibit behavior that meets certain criteria before identification as stages of development. The criteria included (a) a universal sequence, (b) intransitive order, and (c) hierarchical integration of the preceding stage. While many authors have *labeled* changes in the basic motor skills as stages, only a few researchers have *tested* these stages for conformity to the stage criteria. For example, Roberton (1978b, 1978c) tested her hypothesized stages of the forceful overarm throw for the criteria of universal sequence and intransitivity. She found that only some of the stages for change in specific body areas met these two criteria (see also Clarke, Phillips, Peterson, & Welker, 1982; Haubenstricker, Seefeldt, & Branta, 1983). Until more of the hypothesized stages are tested, it is best to label these developmental changes as *steps* and keep in mind that they may not meet the criteria of stages. However, the proposed steps are useful ways to study the continuous process of skill development because they attempt to delineate qualitative changes in performance. As basic motor skills are discussed in this chapter, the proposed steps that appear to facilitate better understanding of skill development are noted. In motor skills where steps have not been formalized for the development of a particular skill, the qualitative changes between a child's initial attempts at a skill and proficient performance are stressed.

Developmental steps can be applied to skill development in two different ways. In one method, all the characteristic positions or movements of the various body components are described for the initial step, or "Step 1"; then they are described for a more advanced level, "Step 2," and so on, to the most advanced level (Seefeldt & Haubenstricker, 1982). A description of Step 1 performance would outline, perhaps, the leg action, the trunk action, and the arm action (c.f. Table 4.3, p. 109).

The alternative method, proposed by Roberton (1977, 1978b, 1978c), is a *component* model. Each separate body component is followed through whatever number of steps accounts for the qualitative changes observed in that component over time. The basic unit of description, then, is the body component, rather than the step. For example, the leg action for jumping might be described in terms of three steps, and the arm action for jumping in terms of five steps, and so on (c.f. Table 4.4, p. 110). This can result in a different number of steps for each component, rather than a fixed number of steps as in the previously described method. Further, the transition from one step to the next can occur at different times (ages) for the various body segments. An individual child's leg action in hopping could be classified as Step 2, but arm action could be classified as Step 3. This means that individual children can reach mature performance levels in different ways: Sally's leg action might be more efficient than her arm action as she learns to throw, but Tommy's arm action in throwing might be ahead of his leg action. The component model is the model used in this text. Observation of one body component at a time is well-suited to the novice observer, and categorization by body component of the behavior follows more easily.

As a final point, remember that at times, children will be in transition between steps. If their skill performance is observed during a transition period, they might use inefficient movements on some motor skill attempts but more advanced movements on others. In this case, the children would be categorized into a step based on the developmental level most often shown, that is, their *modal* level (Roberton & Halverson, 1984). If neither level is predominant in a certain child, his or her level can be noted as "in transition" between Step 2 and Step 3, for example, or perhaps as 2½.

Locomotor Skills

Walking

As noted earlier, walking solo typically begins between 9 and 17 months of age. Figure 4.1a shows a child who has just learned to walk. The infant's leg action is inefficient. He takes short steps with limited leg and hip extension and contacts the ground flat-footed with a bent knee, thus accentuating vertical leg lift. His toes point out, and his feet are spread wide apart when planted as he attempts to maintain his lateral balance (see Figure 4.1b). There is little (if any) trunk rotation, which is consistent with the short stride. His hands and arms are carried high in a bent position often termed the "high guard" position. They are fixed and do not swing on each stride. The high guard position is seen often in beginning walkers because it assists their unsteady balance and provides some protection in case of a fall. With continued development, the arms will drop to about waist level (middle guard position), and later to an extended position at the sides (low guard position), but they still will not swing (see Figure 4.1c). When children begin to use arm swing, it frequently is not equal and regular; both hands might swing forward together (Roberton, 1984).

An infant's initial attempts to walk are mechanically inefficient. Achievement of an efficient walking pattern is dependent upon certain developmental changes:

- Absolute *stride length* must increase, reflecting greater application of force and greater leg extension at push-off. Also, as children grow, increased leg length contributes to a longer stride.

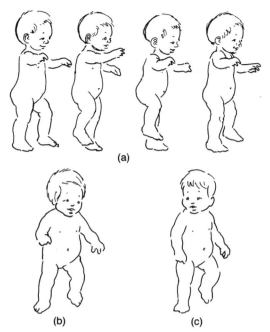

(a)

(b)   (c)

Figure 4.1 (a) A beginning walker. Note the short stride and high guard arm position. (b) To maintain balance beginning walkers often plant the feet wide apart and with the toes out. (c) Rather than swinging the arms in time with the legs, beginning walkers often hold the arms in a middle or low guard position. (a) and (c) Redrawn from film tracings provided by the Motor Development and Child Study Laboratory, Department of Physical Education and Dance, University of Wisconsin-Madison. (b) Redrawn from *Fundamental Motor Patterns* (3rd ed.) (p. 29) by R.L. Wickstrom, 1983, Philadelphia, PA: Lea & Febiger.

- Foot plant on the ground must change to the *heel-then-forefoot* pattern which results from increased range of leg motion.
- *Outtoeing* must be reduced and the base of support narrowed laterally to keep the forces exerted in the forward-backward plane.
- The *double knee-lock* pattern must be adopted to assist full range of leg motion. In this pattern the knee extends at heel strike, flexes slightly as the body weight moves forward over this supporting leg, then extends once more at foot push-off.
- Pelvic rotation must occur to allow full range of leg motion and oppositional movement of the upper and lower body segments. Improvement in balance occurs; forward trunk inclination is reduced.
- Oppositional arm swing, with the arms extended at the sides, must be coordinated with the legs. This is consistent with the principle of action and reaction; that is, the opposite arm and leg move forward and back-

ward in unison. The arm swing must become relaxed and move from the shoulders with slight accompanying movement at the elbow.

An advanced walker is pictured in Figure 4.2. The heel contacts the ground first, and the knee locks in extension before flexing as the weight of the body comes over the foot. The knee extends again in midstance. Pelvic rotation accompanies leg swing, and the arms swing in opposition to the legs.

Developmental Changes in Walking.   Developmental changes in walking are usually achieved at an early age, so that by 2 years of age most children have the essential ingredients of an advanced walk. For example, pelvic rotation is seen on the average at 13.8 months, knee flexion at midsupport at 16.3 months, foot contact within a trunk-width base of support at 17.0 months, synchronous arm swing at 18.0 months, and heel-then-forefoot strike at 18.5 months (Burnett & Johnson, 1971). Stride length increases through mid-adolescence, partly because of fuller range of motion at the hips, knees, and ankles (especially at the younger ages) and partly because of the increase in leg length resulting from growth. Rhythm and coordination of the walk improve observably until age 5 or so, but beyond this age, pattern improvements are subtle and probably not detectable to the unpracticed observer.

Observing Movement Patterns.   It is easier to understand the characteristics of walking if time is spent watching infants and young children walk. Critical

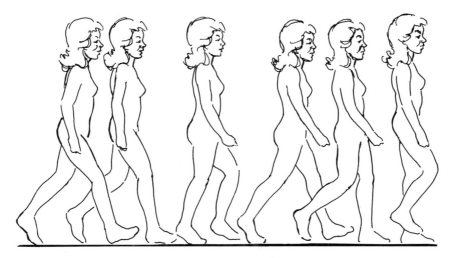

Figure 4.2 An advanced walker. Note the double knee lock pattern, trunk rotation, and oppositional arm swing.

observation of movement is a skill that must be practiced. It is necessary to focus on specific body components to assess the quality of the movement pattern. Attention must be focused on one body segment at a time, such as the legs; it is also important to position oneself where these body segments can be seen clearly. For example, when watching walking from the side, an observer can check first for the heel-strike pattern, then full extension at push-off, knee flexion at midsupport, and the range of leg motion. It is difficult to see the several aspects of leg action all at once. Focusing on one body part (such as the knee) over time (several steps) is the best observation strategy. Next, attention can be directed toward arm position and opposition to leg action, which are also easily observed from the side. From the front or rear position, foot angle (to check for outtoeing or intoeing), the width of the support base, and degree of trunk rotation can be observed. It is reasonable for beginning observers to select one body area or joint to observe at one time. Experienced observers can see several aspects of the pattern at once, but most focus only on a limited number of critical features at any one time. Videotaping the action of a quickly-performed skill is particularly helpful in initial attempts to analyze the skill. Movements can be viewed several times at normal speed, in slow motion, and in stop action.

Running

Running is a more advanced motor skill than walking, but many of the critical features of the two movement patterns are similar. By definition, running has a period of "flight" when neither foot is touching the ground, in contrast to walking, where one foot is always in contact with the ground. Children typically achieve this flight phase around 2 years of age. Earlier running attempts are probably a very fast walk. Sometimes attempts at more complex skills exhibit less mature movement patterns than other less complex skills. Despite the fact that these less mature patterns were previously "outgrown" in walking, one often sees examples of regression to less mature movement patterns in very early running attempts (Burnett & Johnson, 1971). That is, when first learning to run, the child may adopt a wide base of support, a flat-footed landing, leg extension at midsupport, and the high guard arm position. With practice, more mature movement patterns are quickly adopted.

Characteristics of Early Running. Some of the characteristics of early running are pictured in Figure 4.3a. Focusing first on the leg action, a period of flight is seen but the legs still have a limited range of motion. The rear leg does not extend fully at push-off. The recovering thigh comes forward with enough acceleration that the knee bends, but not with enough acceleration to carry the thigh to a level parallel with the ground at the end of leg

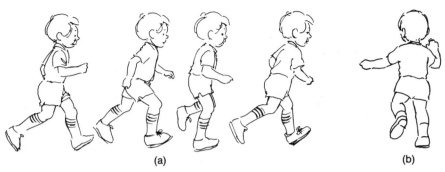

(a)   (b)

Figure 4.3 (a) A beginning runner. The legs have a limited range of motion. The arms extend at the elbow and swing slightly to the side rather than driving forward and back. (b) The thigh and arms swing out rather than forward and back. (a) Redrawn from film tracings provided by the Motor Development and Child Study Laboratory, Department of Physical Education and Dance, University of Wisconsin-Madison. (b) Redrawn from *Fundamental Motor Patterns* (3rd ed.) (p. 50) by R.L. Wickstrom, 1983, Philadelphia, PA: Lea & Febiger.

swing. Thus the range of motion is limited and the stride length short. Looking next at the arm swing, opposition of the arms to the legs is seen. The arms swing to accompany trunk rotation, though, rather than driving forward and back as in an advanced sprint. The elbows extend and the arms rotate when they swing back, which are unnecessary movements; the arms even swing out slightly to the side, wasting energy. Beginning runners sometimes swing their arms more horizontally, across their body, rather than forward and back, probably to aid unsteady balance.

Figure 4.3b pictures some characteristics of early running that can be seen from the rear. As the recovering thigh is swung forward, it inefficiently rotates to the side rather than moving straight forward. The arm swings to the side, away from the body, probably to assist with balance, but again wasting energy that could be directed toward running forward.

Developmental Changes in More Advanced Running. As with early walking, the movement patterns used in early running are mechanically inefficient. Applying the mechanical principles discussed earlier, the developmental changes needed for beginning runners to reach a more advanced run, as pictured in Figure 4.4, can be identified as follows:

* Stride length must increase, indicating that greater force is being applied. As greater force is used, several characteristics of mature running emerge: The rear leg is fully extended at push-off, the heel is tucked close to the buttocks as the thigh swings forward with greater acceleration, and before foot strike the thigh has come to a level parallel to the ground. When

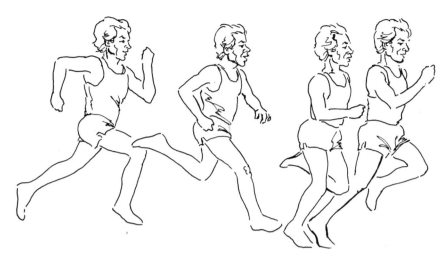

Figure 4.4 An advanced runner. Note the fuller range of leg motion.

the recovery leg is swung forward in a tucked position, the runner's effort is conserved.

- Lateral leg movements must be eliminated so that forces are kept in the forward-backward plane.
- Foot strike must be in a heel-then-forefoot or approximately flat pattern for extended running. Outtoeing must be eliminated and the base of support narrowed.
- The support leg must be allowed to flex at the knee as the body weight comes over the leg.
- Trunk rotation must increase to allow for a longer stride and better arm-leg opposition. Forward trunk lean should be slight.
- Arm swing must be forward and back, with the elbows at approximately right angles and in opposition to the legs.

Most of these advanced characteristics can be identified in the running form pictured in Figure 4.4. These qualitative changes, together with growth in body size and strength and improved coordination, typically result in improved quantitative measures of time in flight and running speed. Such changes have been well documented in several University of Wisconsin studies covering the age span of 1.5 to 10.0 years (Beck, 1966; Clouse, 1959; Dittmer, 1962). Hence, improvement can be expected in both the process and the product of running performance in childhood. Improvements in the product of running performance, increased speed for example, certainly may continue through adolescence. It is not the case, however, that every individual achieves all of the improvements in running pattern during childhood. Most teenagers continue to make refinements in their running form, and it is not uncommon to observe inefficient characteristics in adults' running, especially the characteristics of outtoeing, lateral leg movements, and limited stride. So, age alone does not guarantee mature running form; adolescents and adults alike may have inefficient running patterns.

As with walking, it is necessary to observe running patterns in people of all ages to better understand the critical features of running. Running should also be observed from both the side and the front or back, focusing on one particular aspect of the running pattern at one time, as outlined for walking.

Jumping

Typically, jumping tasks are attempted by children at a young age, with the simplest forms often achieved before age 2. Jumping includes tasks wherein the body is propelled from a surface with either one foot or both feet and lands on both feet (see Table 4.1). Specialized forms of jumping, such as hopping and leaping, also are acquired during childhood. Hopping requires a take-off and landing on the same leg, often repeatedly. Leaping is described as a run with a projection forward from one foot to a landing on the other. Several examples of hopping and leaping are included in Table 4.1. Jumping is considered first.

Assessing Jumping. Jumping by young children can be assessed in several ways: the age at which certain *kinds* of jumps can be performed (age norms), the distance or height of a jump (the *product*), or the maturity of the jumping pattern (the *process*). Age norms for jumping achievements of preschool children (Wickstrom, 1983) are shown in Table 4.2. The table indicates that children learn to step down off a higher surface from one foot to the other before jumping off the floor with both feet. Children then learn to jump down from progressively greater heights onto both feet. Later, forward jumps and jumps over objects are mastered, as is hopping a few times on one foot. These tasks are achieved before age 4. By the time a child reaches school age, all of these jumps usually can be performed. Product assessments, that is, measuring the *distance* jumped horizontally or vertically, are frequently used to assess jumping skill once the movement process has been refined. We will focus here on the movement process, because the measurement of distance jumped is rather self-explanatory and straightforward.

A process assessment of jumping improvement emphasizes the increased efficiency children obtain by gradually adopting movement patterns consistent with sound mechanical principles. These improvements can be seen in both the vertical and the horizontal (standing long) jump, although several

Table 4.1 Types of Jumps Arranged by Progressive Difficulty

Jump down from one foot to the other foot.
Jump up from two feet to two feet.
Jump down from one foot to two feet.
Jump down from two feet to two feet.
Run and jump forward from one foot to the other.
Jump forward from two feet to two feet.
Run and jump forward from one foot to two feet.
Jump over object from two feet to two feet.
Jump from one foot to same foot rhythmically.

Note. From *Fundamental Motor Patterns* (3rd ed.) (p. 69) by R.L. Wickstrom, 1983, Philadelphia, PA: Lea & Febiger. Copyright 1983 by Lea & Febiger. Reprinted by permission.

Table 4.2 Jumping Achievements of Young Children

Achievement	Motor Age (mo)	Source
Jump from 12 in. height; one foot	24	M&W
Jump off floor; both feet	28	B
Jump from 18 in. height; one foot	31	M&W
Jump from chair 26 cm high; both feet	32	B
Jump from 8 in. height; both feet	33	M&W
Jump from 12 in. height; both feet	34	M&W
Jump from 18 in. height; both feet	37	M&W
Jump from 30 cm height; both feet	37.1	B
Jump forward 10 to 35 cm from 30 cm height; both feet	37.3	B
Hop on two feet 1 to 3 times	38	M&W
Jump over rope 20 cm high; both feet	41.5	B
Hop on one foot 1 to 3 times	43	B

Note. Adapted from information in studies by Bayley (1935) (B) and McCaskill & Wellman (1938) (M&W). From *Fundamental Motor Patterns* (3rd ed.) (p. 68) by R.L. Wickstrom, 1983, Philadelphia: Lea & Febiger. Copyright 1983 by Lea & Febiger. Reprinted by permission.

Table 4.3 Developmental Sequence of the Standing Long Jump for the Whole Body by Step

Step 1 Vertical component of force may be greater than horizontal, resulting jump is then upward rather than forward. Arms move backward, acting as brakes to stop the momentum of the trunk as the legs extend in front of the center of mass.

Step 2 The arms move in an anterior-posterior direction during the preparatory phase, but move sideward (winging action) during the "in-flight" phase. The knees and hips flex and extend more fully than in step one. The angle of take-off is still markedly above 45°. The landing is made with the center of gravity above the base of support, with the thighs perpendicular to the surface rather than parallel as in the reaching position of step four.

Step 3 The arms swing backward and then forward during the preparatory phase. The knees and hips flex fully prior to take-off. Upon take-off the arms extend and move forward but do not exceed the height of the head. The knee extension may be complete, but the take-off angle is still greater than 45°. Upon landing, the thigh is still less than parallel to the surface, and the center of gravity is near the base of support when viewed from the frontal plane.

Step 4 The arms extend vigorously forward and upward upon take-off, reaching full extension above the head at "lift-off." The hips and knees are extended fully with the take-off angle at 45° or less. In preparation for landing the arms are brought downward and the legs are thrust forward until the thigh is parallel to the surface. The center of gravity is far behind the base of support upon foot contact, but at the moment of contact the knees are flexed and the arms are thrust forward in order to maintain the momentum to carry the center of gravity beyond the feet.

Note. Degrees are measured from horizontal. Adapted from "Sequencing Motor Skills Within the Physical Education Curriculum" by V. Seefeldt, S. Reuschlein, & P. Vogel, 1972. Paper presented to the annual conference of the American Association for Health, Physical Education and Recreation.

developmental sequences of the improvement typically made during childhood in the standing long jump have been outlined. Developmental changes for all body components at one time are shown in Table 4.3, while in Table 4.4, the developmental sequence using the body component approach is displayed. The component approach is used for discussion here.

Table 4.4 Developmental Sequences for the Standing Long Jump

Take-off: Leg action component

Step 1   One foot leads in asymmetrical take-off.
Step 2   Both feet leave ground symmetrically, but hips or knees or both do not reach full extension by take-off.
Step 3   Take-off is symmetrical, with hips and knees fully extended.

Take-off: Trunk action

Step 1   Trunk is inclined forward less than 30° from vertical. Neck is hyperextended.
Step 2   Trunk leans forward less than 30°, with neck flexed or aligned with trunk at take-off.
Step 3   Trunk is inclined forward 30° or more at take-off, with neck flexed.
Step 4   Trunk is inclined forward 30° or more. Neck is aligned with trunk, or slightly extended.

Take-off: Arm action component

Step 1   Arms move in opposition to legs or are held at side, with elbows flexed.
Step 2   Shoulders retract, arms extend backward in winging posture at take-off.
Step 3   Arms are abducted about 90°, with elbows frequently flexed, in high or middle guard position.
Step 4   Arms flex forward and upward with minimal abduction, reaching incomplete extension overhead by take-off.
Step 5   Arms flex forward, reaching full extension overhead by take-off.

Flight and landing: Leg action component

Step 1   Legs assume asymmetrical run pattern in flight, with one-footed landing.
Step 2   Legs assume asymmetrical run pattern, but swing to two-footed landing.
Step 3   During flight, hips and knees flex in a synchronous fashion. Knees then extend for two-footed landing.
Step 4   During flight, flexion of both knees precedes hip flexion. As hips flex, knees extend, reaching forward to two-footed landing.

Flight and landing: Trunk action component

Step 1   Trunk maintains forward inclination of less than 30° in flight, then flexes for landing.
Step 2   Trunk corrects forward lean of 30° or more by hyperextending. It then flexes for landing.
Step 3   Trunk maintains forward lean of 30° or more from take-off to midflight, then flexes forward for landing.

Flight and landing: Arm action component

Step 1   Arms move in opposition to legs as if child were running in flight and on landing.
Step 2   Shoulders retract and arms extend backward (winging) during flight and move forward (parachuting) during landing.

Table 4.4 (cont.)

Step 3   During flight, arms assume high or middle guard positions and may move backward in windmill fashion. They parachute for landing.

Step 4   Arms lower or extend from flexed position overhead, reaching forward at landing.

Note. Trunk angle is measured from vertical. Validation of these sequences is in progress (VanSant, in progress). From *Motor development during childhood and adolescence* (p. 69) by J.R. Thomas (Ed.), 1984, Minneapolis, MN: Burgess. Copyright 1984 by Burgess. Reprinted by permission.

Characteristics of Inefficient and Efficient Jumpers.   It is helpful to first identify some of the characteristics of inefficient beginning jumpers in both the vertical jump and the standing long jump. Most young children begin jumping by executing a vertical jump, even if their intention is to jump horizontally. Several beginning jumpers are shown in Figures 4.5, 4.6, and 4.7. Note that their preparatory crouch is slight, and their legs are not fully extended at lift-off. In fact, the vertical jumper in Figure 4.5 tucks her legs to leave the ground, rather than extending her legs at take-off to project her body off the ground. Notice that in this example her head is no higher at the peak of her jump than at take-off. Another characteristic of inefficient jumpers is lack of a two-foot (symmetrical) take-off or landing, as shown in Figure 4.5, when one is intended. The legs may also be in an asymmetrical position during flight. The improvements needed in leg action are first, a symmetrical take-off, flight, and landing, and second, a full extension of the ankles, knees, and hips at take-off, following a deep preparatory crouch. Notice that the jumper pictured in Figure 4.7 has begun to flex the knees and hips together in the flight phase of her standing long jump.

In a standing long jump the trunk must be inclined forward at least 30° from vertical to achieve a long-distance jump. Inefficient jumpers often keep the trunk too erect and hyperextend their necks at take-off. Their trunk action must improve by having the trunk inclined more than 30° during take-off and early flight and by aligning their head and neck with their trunk. The trunk must flex forward for the landing.

Lack of coordinated arm action also is characteristic of inefficient vertical and horizontal jumpers. Rather than assisting the jumping action, the arms may be used asymmetrically, held in a stationary position at the sides, or held in a high guard position as a precaution against falling. Arms may ''wing'' (extend backward) ineffectively during flight (see Figure 4.5) or ''parachute'' (extend down and out to the side) during landing (see Figure 4.6). To achieve

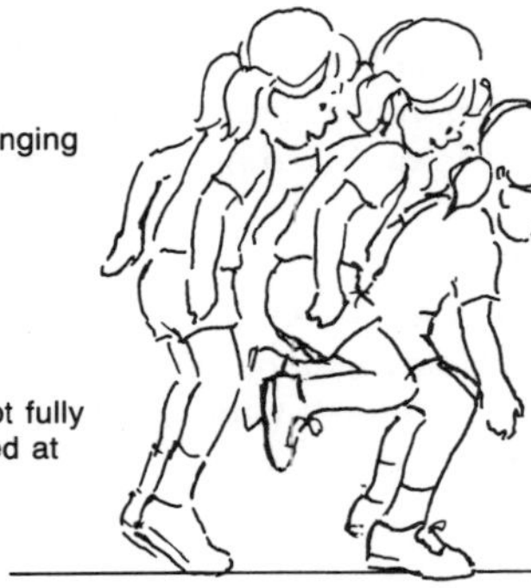

Head is flexed

Arms in winging
posture

Legs not fully
extended at
take-off

One foot touches
first

Legs tucked
under body

Figure 4.5 Sequential views of a vertical jump. The form here is immature. The legs are tucked up under the body rather than fully extending to project the body off the ground. Notice that one foot touches down first. The arms do not assist the jump. They are simply held in the winging posture. Redrawn from *Fundamental Motor Patterns* (p. 74) by R.L. Wickstrom, 1983, Philadelphia, PA: Lea & Febiger.

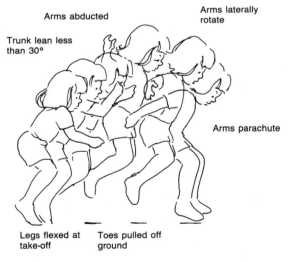

Arms abducted

Arms laterally
rotate

Trunk lean less
than 30°

Arms parachute

Legs flexed at
take-off

Toes pulled off
ground

Figure 4.6 A beginning long jumper with Step 1 leg action (see Table 4.4) in both the take-off and in flight. As the weight is shifted forward the toes are pulled off the floor to "catch" the body at landing. The trunk lean at take-off is less than 30° from vertical but the head is aligned so that this jump is in Step 2 trunk action at take-off. During flight the trunk action is only at Step 1 because of small forward lean. The arms are used at take-off but are in an abducted position, Step 3, laterally rotate in flight and "parachute" for the landing, a Step 2 arm action. Redrawn from the longitudinal film collection, Motor Development and Child Study Laboratory, Department of Physical Education and Dance, University of Wisconsin-Madison.

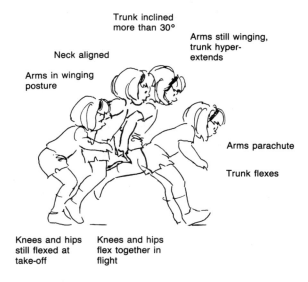

Trunk inclined more than 30°

Arms still winging, trunk hyper-extends

Neck aligned

Arms in winging posture

Arms parachute

Trunk flexes

Knees and hips still flexed at take-off

Knees and hips flex together in flight

Figure 4.7 A beginning jumper. The leg action is in Step 2 at take-off because the feet leave the ground together but the legs and hips are still flexed. The knees and hips flex together during flight and knees then extend before landing, Step 3 leg action. The trunk action is at Step 4 during take-off because the trunk is inclined more than 30°. The trunk hyperextends in flight, then flexes for landing, Step 2. The arm action is Step 2 throughout. They are held in winging at take-off and in flight before "parachuting" for the landing.

an efficient jump, the jumper must use the arms symmetrically to lead the jump from a preparatory extended position to an overhead swing.

Through these developmental changes, performers can develop a mechanically efficient jumping pattern. The efficient jumpers pictured in Figure 4.8 and 4.9 demonstrate sound technique. To execute efficient jumps they

- get into a preparatory crouch that will put the muscles on stretch and allow a maximal force to be applied as indicated by full leg extension at the moment of lift-off. Both feet leave the ground at the same time.
- begin the jump with a vigorous arm swing upward and forward from an extended preparatory position.
- direct force downward and extend the body throughout flight in a jump for height. If an object is to be struck or touched overhead, the dominant arm reaches upward and the opposite arm swings downward to gain height by lateral tilt of the shoulders. The trunk remains relatively upright throughout. The ankles, knees, and hips flex upon touchdown to allow the force of landing to be absorbed.
- direct force down and back in a jump for horizontal distance, resulting in a forward lean body angle at take-off of 30° or more from vertical. Dur-

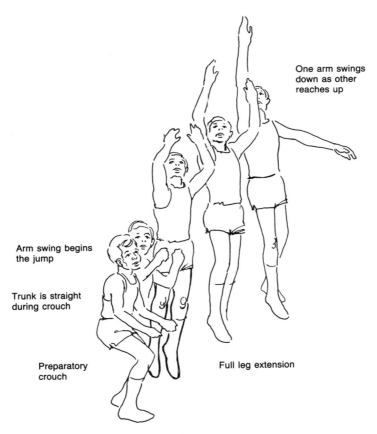

One arm swings
down as other
reaches up

Arm swing begins
the jump

Trunk is straight
during crouch

Preparatory
crouch

Full leg extension

Figure 4.8 An advanced vertical jump for the purpose of reaching high. From a preparatory crouch this basketball player swings his arms forward and up to lead the jump. There is complete hip, knee, and ankle extension at take-off. Near the peak of the jump, one hand continues up while the other comes down, tilting the shoulder girdle to assist the high reach. Notice that the trunk tends to remain upright throughout. Redrawn from *Fundamental Motor Patterns* (p. 77) by R.L. Wickstrom, 1983, Philadelphia, PA: Lea & Febiger.

ing flight the knees flex, then the thighs come forward to a position parallel with the ground. The lower legs swing forward for a two-foot landing. The trunk comes forward in reaction to the thighs flexing, putting the body in a "jackknife" position. When the heels touch the ground, ankles and knees flex to absorb the momentum of the body over distance as the body continues to move forward.

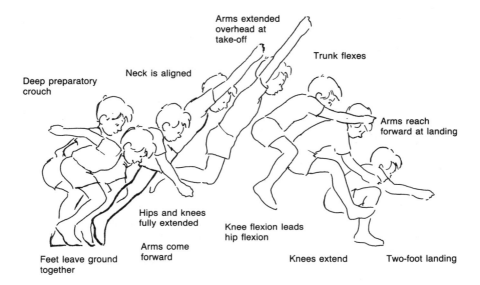

Arms extended overhead at take-off

Trunk flexes

Neck is aligned

Deep preparatory crouch

Arms reach forward at landing

Hips and knees fully extended

Knee flexion leads hip flexion

Arms come forward

Feet leave ground together

Knees extend

Two-foot landing

Figure 4.9 An advanced long jump. The feet leave the ground together and touch down together. The legs are fully extended at take-off, the knees then flex in flight followed by hip flexion and finally knee extension to reach forward for landing. The trunk is inclined more than 30° at take-off and this lean is maintained in flight until the trunk flexes for landing. The arms lead the jump and reach overhead at take-off. They then lower to reach forward at landing.

Efficient jumpers, after a preparatory crouch, direct force in the proper direction for a vertical or a horizontal jump by extending fully at take-off. Their arms are used extensively and initiate the chain of movements in the jump. With practice, these refinements in jumping pattern can be made during childhood. Continuous growth in body size and strength also contributes to quantitative improvements in the maximal distance jumped. During the elementary school years, children average increases of 3 to 5 in. per year in distance jumped horizontally and approximately 2 in. per year in height jumped vertically (DeOreo & Keogh, 1980). The qualitative improvements in jumping during childhood are variable among children. For example, compare the jumper in Figure 4.7 to the developmental steps in Table 4.4 (p. 110). Her trunk action is Step 4 at take-off, but her leg and arm action patterns are only Step 2.

It is clear that all persons do not master jumping in childhood or even in adolescence. Zimmerman (1956) found many inefficient jumping characteristics among college women, including limited arm swing and incomplete leg extension at take-off. In order for children and teens to receive assistance from their instructors in perfecting an advanced jumping pattern, instructors must be able to critically observe and analyze jumping performance. As with the previous skills discussed it is necessary to practice this observation process. Most aspects of jumping are easily observed from the side: arm swing, leg extension at take-off, body angle, leg action in flight, and leg action in landing. Sideward movements of the arms, though, can be seen best from the front or back.

Hopping

Many of the mechanical principles applicable to jumping are involved in hopping as well. Roberton and Halverson (1984) present suggested developmental levels for hopping in Table 4.5. This sequence has been modified and validated by Halverson and Williams (1985). The authors used a component approach, so levels are identified for leg action and for arm action separately. Four levels of leg action and five levels of arm action are suggested.

Table 4.5   Developmental Sequence for Hopping

Leg action

Step 1   **Momentary flight.** The support knee and hip quickly flex, pulling (instead of projecting) the foot from the floor. The flight is momentary. Only one or two hops can be achieved. The swing leg is lifted high and held in an inactive position to the side or in front of the body.

Step 2   **Fall and catch; swing leg inactive.** Body lean forward allows the minimal knee and ankle extension to help the body "fall" forward of the support foot and, then, quickly catch itself again. The swing leg is inactive. Repeat hops are now possible.

Step 3   **Projected takeoff; swing leg assists.** Perceptible pretakeoff extension occurs in the hip, knee, and ankle in the support leg. There is little or no delay in changing from knee and ankle flexion on landing to extension prior to takeoff. The swing leg now pumps up and down to assist in projection. The range of the swing is insufficient to carry it behind the support leg when viewed from the side.

Step 4   **Projection delay; swing leg leads.** The weight of the child on landing is now smoothly transferred along the foot to the ball before the knee and ankle extend to takeoff. The support leg nearly reaches full extension on the takeoff. The swing leg now leads the upward-forward movement of the takeoff phase, while the support leg is still rotating over the ball of the foot. The range of the pumping action in the swing leg increases so that it passes behind the support leg when viewed from the side.

Table 4.5 (cont.)

Arm action

Step 1 **Bilateral inactive.** The arms are held bilaterally, usually high and out to the side, although other positions behind or in front of the body may occur. Any arm action is usually slight and not consistent.

Step 2 **Bilateral reactive.** Arms swing upward briefly, then are medially rotated at the shoulder in a winging movement prior to takeoff. It appears that this movement is in reaction to loss of balance.

Step 3 **Bilateral assist.** The arms pump up and down together, usually in front of the line of the trunk. Any downward and backward motion of the arms occurs after takeoff. The arms may move parallel to each other or be held at different levels as they move up and down.

Step 4 **Semi-opposition.** The arm on the side opposite the swing leg swings forward with that leg and back as the leg moves down. The position of the other arm is variable, often staying in front of the body or to the side.

Step 5 **Opposing-assist.** The arm opposite the swing leg moves forward and upward in synchrony with the forward and upward movement of that leg. The other arm moves in the direction opposite to the action of the swing leg. The range of movement in the arm action may be minimal unless the task requires speed or distance.

Note. This sequence has been partially validated by Halverson & Williams (1985). From *Developing Children—Their Changing Movement* (pp. 56, 63) by M.A. Roberton & L.E. Halverson, 1984, Philadelphia, PA: Lea & Febiger. Copyright 1984 by Lea & Febiger. Reprinted by permission.

Remember that children might move through the levels of arm action and leg action at different rates. Two early hoppers are shown in Figures 4.10 and 4.11. The leg action of the hopper in Figure 4.10 is inefficient. The support leg is momentarily lifted from the floor by flexing rather than projecting the body up by leg extension and the swing leg is inactive. The arms are also inactive so that both leg and arm action fall into the first developmental step. The hopper in Figure 4.11 has achieved some leg extension and therefore is placed in the second step of leg action but still the first step of arm action.

Improvements Necessary for Mature Hopping Skill. The improvements these hoppers need to make include full extension of the support leg and assistance from the swing leg to lead the hop. The arms must also assist and act in opposition to the legs. The hopper in Figure 4.12 has made some of these improvements. The support leg extends at take-off, reflecting good force application. This leg flexes at landing to absorb the force of landing and to prepare for extension at the next take-off. The swing leg assists the hop but is still not used vigorously. The hopper in Figure 4.13 has made this improvement such

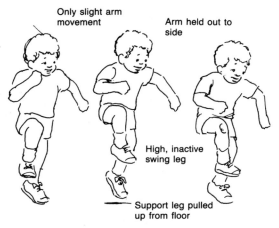

Only slight arm movement

Arm held out to side

High, inactive swing leg

Support leg pulled up from floor

Figure 4.10 An early hopping attempt exhibiting Step 1 leg action and Step 1 arm action. The support leg is pulled off the floor to produce only momentary flight. The swing leg is held high and remains inactive in the hop. The arms are high and one is held out to the side. They are not working in "opposition." Redrawn from the longitudinal film collection, Motor Development and Child Study Laboratory, Department of Physical Education and Dance, University of Wisconsin-Madison.

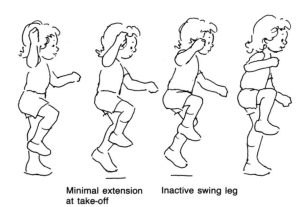

Minimal extension at take-off

Inactive swing leg

Figure 4.11 This girl uses some leg extension to leave the ground, but her swing leg is still inactive. She is in Step 2 of the developmental levels of leg action. Redrawn from the longitudinal film collection, Motor Development and Child Study Laboratory, Department of Physical Education and Dance, University of Wisconsin-Madison.

that the swing leg leads the take-off, allowing the momentum of several body parts to be chained together, then swings back behind the support leg in order to lead the next take-off. The hopper in Figure 4.12 moves the arm opposite the swing leg in opposition, but the other arm is variable. The advanced hopper

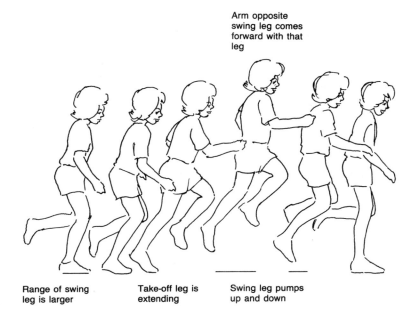

Arm opposite
swing leg comes
forward with that
leg

Range of swing
leg is larger

Take-off leg is
extending

Swing leg pumps
up and down

Figure 4.12 A more advanced hop, Step 3 in the developmental sequence of leg action, Step 4 in arm action. The swing leg leads the hop. While the range of the swing leg is larger and it is seen behind the support leg at landing, it could be still larger. The arm opposite the swing leg comes forward with that leg, but the other arm is not working in opposition. Redrawn from the longitudinal film collection, Motor Development and Child Study Laboratory, Department of Physical Education and Dance, University of Wisconsin-Madison.

in Figure 4.13 assists the hop with both arms moving in opposition to the legs, in accordance with the mechanical law of action and reaction.

Few children under age 3 can hop repeatedly (Bayley, 1969; McCaskill & Wellman, 1938). The preschool years are often cited as the time children become mature or proficient hoppers (Gutteridge, 1939; Sinclair, 1973; Williams, 1983). Yet, Halverson and Williams (1985) found that over half a group of sixty-three 3-, 4-, and 5-year-olds were in step 2 of both arm and leg action. Few attempts were observed that could be classified at the advanced levels, and hopping on the nonpreferred leg was developmentally behind hopping on the preferred leg. If the children in this study are representative of 3-, 4-, and 5-year-olds, the development of hopping extends well past the age of 5.

Assessing Hopping. As with the other locomotor skills, hopping assessment requires practice for a novice observer. Halverson (1983; see also Roberton & Halverson, 1984) suggests a systematic pattern of observation that focuses

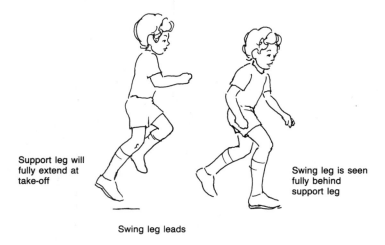

Support leg will
fully extend at
take-off

Swing leg is seen
fully behind
support leg

Swing leg leads

Figure 4.13 This boy demonstrates Step 4 leg action because the range of the swing leg is sufficient to carry it completely behind the support leg. Redrawn from the longitudinal film collection, Motor Development and Child Study Laboratory, Department of Physical Education and Dance, University of Wisconsin-Madison.

on the body parts one at a time. Leg action should be observed from the side. Attention should be given initially to the swing leg. Is it active? If so, does it move up and down or swing past the support leg? The support leg should be observed next. Does it extend at take-off? Does it flex upon landing and extend during the next hop? Arm action should be observed from both the side and the front. The observer should watch first to see whether the arm movement is bilateral or opposing. If it is bilateral, movements can then be categorized as inactive, reactive, or backward in direction. If it is opposing, note whether one or both arms move synchronously with the legs.

Galloping, Sliding, and Skipping

Galloping, sliding, and skipping are all locomotor movements that involve the fundamental movements of stepping, hopping, or leaping. Galloping and sliding consist of a step on one foot, then a leap-step of the other foot. The *same* leg always leads with the step. The difference between galloping and sliding is the direction of movement. Galloping is movement forward, and sliding is movement sideways. Skipping is a step then hop on the same foot, with the feet alternating: step-hop (on right foot), step-hop (on left foot), step-hop (on right foot), and so on. Movement is usually forward.

Early attempts at these skills are usually arhythmical and stiff. The arms are rarely involved in projecting the body off the floor. They might be held stiffly in the high guard position or out to the side to aid balance. The stride or step length is short, and landings are flat-footed. Little trunk rotation is used, and vertical lift is exaggerated. In early galloping attempts, the trailing leg may land ahead of the lead leg. In contrast, proficient galloping, sliding, and skipping are rhythmical and relaxed. The arms are no longer needed for balance. In skipping, arms swing rhythmically in opposition to the legs and provide momentum. The arms can be used for another purpose during galloping and sliding, such as clapping. Heel-forefoot or forefoot landings are prevalent. The knees "give" on landing, remaining flexed during support of the body weight, and then extend at take-off, especially for speedy traveling.

Galloping is the first of these three patterns to emerge. It develops sometime after the running pattern is established (around age 2) and usually before hopping is attempted at age 3 or 4. Sliding is mastered next, and skipping last, typically between 4 and 7 years of age. The ability to lead with the non-dominant leg in galloping and sliding is developed much later than the emergence of the pattern with the dominant leg. Girls typically perform these locomotor skills at an earlier age than boys, perhaps reflecting their slight edge in biological maturity for chronological age, imitation of other girls, or possibly encouragement from family and friends.

Ballistic Skills

The ballistic skills—throwing, kicking, and striking—have similar developmental pattern characteristics because the mechanical principles involved in projecting objects are basically the same. The ballistic skill that has received the most study is the forceful overhand throw for distance. Much of the discussion on throwing also applies to kicking and striking, which will be examined next.

Overarm Throwing

There are many forms of throwing. The two-handed underhand throw (wind-up between the legs) and one-handed underhand throw are common among young children. There is also a sidearm throw and a two-handed overarm throw. The type of throw used often depends upon the size of the ball, especially with children. Our focus, though, is on the one-handed *overarm* throw. It is the most common type of throw used in sport games and has been studied more widely than other types. Many of the mechanical principles involved in the overarm throw also apply to other types of throws.

Product assessments using accuracy, distance, and ball velocity as criteria are often used to gauge throwing skill development. However, there are several drawbacks to product measures. An accuracy assessment task often must be changed when working with children of different ages. Young children must be given a short distance over which to throw in order to reach the target. A short distance, though, makes the task too easy for older children who might all score perfectly. So the distance must be increased or the target size decreased for older groups. Also, scores on throws for distance often reflect factors such as body size and strength in addition to throwing skill. Two children may be equal in throwing skills but have quite different distance scores, because one child is bigger and stronger. Lastly, the measurement of ball velocity at release requires specialized equipment, which may not be readily available. Thus, one could argue that product scores are not as useful to instructors of throwing skill as knowing *how* a child throws. Let's now turn our attention to the *quality* of the throwing pattern.

Characteristics of Advanced Throwing Skill. It is helpful to contrast an advanced overarm throw with children's early attempts to throw. The throwing pattern of young children tends to be restricted to arm action alone. As depicted in Figure 4.14, the young boy does not step into the throw nor does he use much trunk action. The upper arm is merely positioned, often with the elbow up or forward, and the throw executed by elbow extension alone. Figure 4.15 shows more movement, but little gain in mechanical efficiency. Obviously, these boys demonstrate minimal throwing skill. By studying the characteristics of a proficient throw, the inefficiencies in early throwing attempts can be identified. Thus, an advanced, forceful throw for distance has the following movement patterns:

- The weight shifts to the back foot, the trunk rotates back, and the arm makes a circular, downward backswing in a "wind-up."
- The leg opposite the throwing arm steps forward to increase the distance over which force is applied to the ball and to allow full trunk rotation.
- The trunk rotates forward to add force to the throw. To achieve maximal force, trunk rotation is *differentiated*. That is, the lower trunk (pelvis) actually begins its rotation forward while the upper trunk (spine) is still "winding up" or moving backward. This type of action is also termed "opening up," and describes any action in which body parts move in opposite directions to exert force ultimately in one direction.
- The trunk bends laterally, away from the side of the throwing arm.
- The upper arm forms a right angle with the trunk and comes forward just as (or slightly after) the shoulders rotate to a front-facing position. This means that from a side view the upper arm is seen within the outline of the trunk.

- The elbow is held at a right angle during the forward swing, extending when the front-facing position is reached. Extending the arm just before release lengthens the radius of the throwing arc.
- The forearm lags behind the trunk and upper arm during the forward swing. While the upper trunk is rotating forward, the forearm and hand appear to be stationary or to move downward or backward. The forearm "lags" until the upper trunk and shoulders actually rotate to the direction of the throw (front-facing).
- The force of the throw is dissipated over distance by the follow-through. The greater portion of wrist flexion comes during follow-through, after the ball is released. Dissipating force after release allows maximal speed of movement while the ball is in the hand.
- The movements of the body segments are carried out sequentially, progressively adding the contributions of each part to the force of the throw. Generally, the sequence is: step forward and pelvic rotation; upper spine rotation and upper arm swing; upper arm inward rotation and elbow extension; release; and follow-through.

Developmental Sequences of Overarm Throwing. Now that the characteristics of an advanced, forceful throw have been discussed, the developmental steps of individual progression from initial throwing attempts toward advanced throwing skill can be examined. Several developmental sequences of overarm throwing development have been proposed, beginning with a sequence outlined by Wild in 1938 and including that of Seefeldt, Reuschlein, and Vogel in 1972. More recently, Roberton proposed a developmental sequence for the overarm throw using the body component approach. Two of the component sequences, arm action and trunk action, have been validated as developmental sequences (Roberton, 1977, 1978a; Roberton & DiRocco, 1981; Roberton & Langendorfer, 1980). Careful study of the developmental overarm throw sequence outlined in Table 4.6 will help to compare these steps with the different body components of throwers depicted in Figures 4.14 to 4.19.

Begin the comparison by focusing on the trunk action component. In the first step of the developmental sequence, no trunk action or forward-backward movements can be seen prior to releasing the ball (see Figures 4.14 and 4.15). In the second step, individuals proceed to a *block rotation* of the trunk; that is, the upper and lower trunk rotate together, or the upper trunk simply rotates alone. Block rotation occurs between the third and fourth positions in Figure 4.17. The most advanced trunk action, *differentiated rotation*, often can be identified in pictures of baseball pitchers. In Figure 4.19, the pitcher has started to rotate the lower trunk while the upper trunk is still twisting backward in preparation to throw.

To analyze the complexity of arm movements in throwing, the preparatory backswing is first studied, then the upper arm (humerus) motions, and

Table 4.6 Developmental Sequence for Throwing

Trunk action in throwing and striking for force

Step 1 **No trunk action or forward-backward movements.** Only the arm is active in force production. Sometimes, the forward thrust of the arm pulls the trunk into a passive left rotation (assuming a right-handed throw), but no twist-up precedes that action. If trunk action occurs, it accompanies the forward thrust of the arm by flexing forward at the hips. Preparatory extension sometimes precedes forward hip flexion.

Step 2 **Upper trunk rotation or total trunk "block" rotation.** The spine and pelvis both rotate away from the intended line of flight and then simultaneously begin forward rotation, acting as a unit or "block." Occasionally, only the upper spine twists away, then toward the direction of force. The pelvis, then, remains fixed, facing the line of flight, or joins the rotary movement after forward spinal rotation has begun.

Step 3 **Differentiated rotation.** The pelvis precedes the upper spine in initiating forward rotation. The child twists away from the intended line of ball flight and, then, begins forward rotation with the pelvis while the upper spine is still twisting away.

Backswing, humerus, and forearm action in the overarm throw for force

Preparatory arm backswing component

Step 1 **No backswing.** The ball-in-the-hand moves directly forward to release from the arm's original position when the hand first grasped the ball.

Step 2 **Elbow and humeral flexion.** The ball moves away from the intended line of flight to a position behind or alongside the head by upward flexion of the humerus and concomitant elbow flexion.

Step 3 **Circular, upward backswing.** The ball moves away from the intended line of flight to a position behind the head via a circular overhead movement with elbow extended, or an oblique swing back, or a vertical lift from the hip.

Step 4 **Circular, downward backswing.** The ball moves away from the intended line of flight to a position behind the head via a circular, down and back motion, which carries the hand below the waist.

Humerus (upper arm) action component during forward swing

Step 1 **Humerus oblique.** The humerus moves forward to ball release in a plane that intersects the trunk obliquely above or below the horizontal line of the shoulders. Occasionally, during the backswing, the humerus is placed at a right angle to the trunk, with the elbow pointing toward the target. It maintains this fixed position during the throw.

Step 2 **Humerus aligned but independent.** The humerus moves forward to ball release in a plane horizontally aligned with the shoulder, forming a right angle between humerus and trunk. By the time the shoulders (upper spine) reach front facing, the humerus (elbow) has moved independently ahead of the outline of the body (as seen from the side) via horizontal adduction at the shoulder.

Table 4.6 (cont.)

Step 3 **Humerus lags.** The humerus moves forward to ball release horizontally aligned, but at the moment the shoulders (upper spine) reach front facing, the humerus remains within the outline of the body (as seen from the side). No horizontal adduction of the humerus occurs before front facing.

Forearm action component during forward swing

Step 1 **No forearm lag.** The forearm and ball move steadily forward to ball release throughout the throwing action.

Step 2 **Forearm lag.** The forearm and ball appear to "lag," that is, to remain stationary behind the child or to move downward or backward in relation to him/her. The lagging forearm reaches its furthest point back, deepest point down, or last stationary point before the shoulders (upper spine) reach front facing.

Step 3 **Delayed forearm lag.** The lagging forearm delays reaching its final point of lag until the moment of front facing.

Action of the feet in forceful throwing and striking

Step 1 **No step.** The child throws from the initial foot position.

Step 2 **Homolateral step.** The child steps with the foot on the same side as the throwing hand.

Step 3 **Contralateral, short step.** The child steps with the foot on the opposite side from the throwing hand.

Step 4 **Contralateral, long step.** The child steps with the opposite foot a distance of over half the child's standing height.

Note. Validation studies support the trunk sequence (Roberton, 1977; Roberton, 1978a; Roberton & Langendorfer, 1980; Langendorfer, 1982; Roberton & DiRocco, 1981). Validation studies support the arm sequences for the overarm throw (Halverson, Roberton, & Langendorfer, 1982; Roberton, 1977; Roberton, 1978a; Roberton & Langendorfer, 1980; Roberton & DiRocco, 1981) with the exception of the preparatory arm backswing sequence, which was hypothesized by Roberton (1983) from the work of Langendorfer (1980). Langendorfer (1982) feels the humerus and forearm components are appropriate for overarm striking. The foot action sequence was hypothesized by Roberton (1983) from the work of Leme and Shambes (1978), Seefeldt, Reuschlein, and Vogel (1972), and Wild (1937). From *Developing Children—Their Changing Movement* (pp. 103, 106, 107, 118) by M.A. Roberton and L.E. Halverson, 1984, Philadelphia, PA: Lea & Febiger. Copyright 1984 by Lea & Febiger. Reprinted by permission.

finally the forearm motions. Unskilled throwers often use no backswing (Figure 4.14). At the next step of the developmental sequence they flex the shoulder and elbow in preparation for elbow extension, as in Figure 4.15. A more advanced preparation is to use an upward backswing, but the most desirable

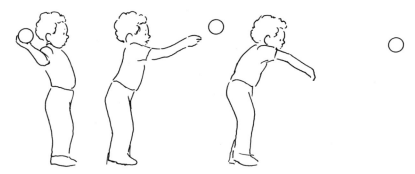

Figure 4.14 A beginning thrower who simply brings the hand back with the elbow up and throws by extending the elbow without taking a step. Redrawn from film tracings provided by the Motor Development and Child Study Laboratory, Department of Physical Education and Dance, University of Wisconsin-Madison.

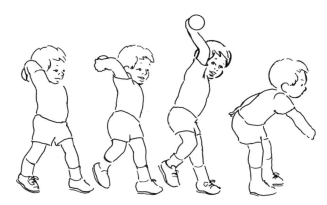

Figure 4.15 A beginning thrower. Note the trunk flexion, rather than rotation, with the throw. Redrawn from film tracings provided by the Motor Development and Child Study Laboratory, Department of Physical Education and Dance, University of Wisconsin-Madison.

backswing is circular and downward. This is used by the thrower pictured in Figure 4.17.

As unskilled throwers begin to swing their upper arm forward to throw, they often swing it at an angle oblique to the line of the shoulders, that is, with the elbow pointed up or down. A desirable advancement is to align the upper arm horizontally with the shoulders, forming a right angle with the trunk, as seen in Figure 4.16. Even so, the upper arm may move ahead of the trunk's outline, as seen in Figure 4.16. This movement results in a loss of some of the momentum gained from sequential movement of the body parts for a force-

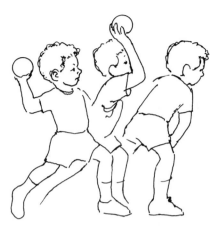

Figure 4.16 A thrower with Step 2 arm action. The forearm reaches its farthest point back before the shoulders rotate to front facing, but the humerus then swings forward before the shoulders and the elbow is consequently seen outside the body outline.
Note the right angle between the humerus and trunk. Redrawn from film tracings
provided by the Motor Development and Child Study Laboratory, Department of
Physical Education and Dance, University of Wisconsin-Madison.

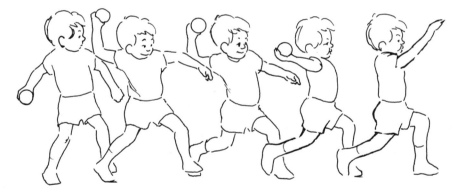

Figure 4.17 A relatively advanced thrower. Arm, leg, and preparatory action are characteristic
of the most advanced step, but the trunk action is characteristic of Step 2, or block
rotation, rather than differentiated rotation. Redrawn from film tracings provided
by the Motor Development and Child Study Laboratory, Department of Physical
Education and Dance, University of Wisconsin-Madison.

ful throw. In the most advanced pattern, the upper arm lags behind so that,
from a front-facing position, the elbow is seen from the side within the outline of the trunk, as in Figure 4.17.

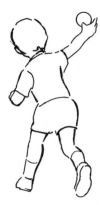

Figure 4.18 From the rear it can be seen that this advanced thrower flexes the trunk laterally away from ball at release. Redrawn from film tracings provided by the Motor Development and Child Study Laboratory, Department of Physical Education and Dance, University of Wisconsin-Madison.

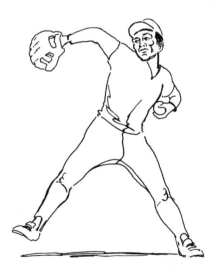

Figure 4.19 This still drawing of a baseball pitcher captures differentiated rotation. Redrawn from film tracings provided by the Motor Development and Child Study Laboratory, Department of Physical Education and Dance, University of Wisconsin-Madison.

It is also desirable for the forearm to lag behind. The thrower in Figure 4.16 has some forearm lag, but the deepest lag comes before rather than at front-facing. The thrower in Figure 4.17 demonstrates the advanced pattern of delayed forearm lag.

Most unskilled throwers throw without taking a step, as with the boy in Figure 4.14. When the step is learned, it is often taken with the homolateral leg, that is, the leg on the same side of the body as the throwing arm. This reduces the extent of trunk rotation and range of motion needed for a forceful throw. When the advanced pattern of a contralateral step is acquired, the step may initially be a short one, as in Figure 4.15. A long step (more than half the thrower's height) is desirable.

The body component analysis of overarm throwing demonstrates that individuals do not achieve the same developmental step for all body components at the same time. For example, the thrower in Figure 4.15 is in Step 1 of trunk, humerus, and forearm action, but Step 3 of foot action. The thrower in Figure 4.17 is in Step 3 of humerus, forearm, and foot action, but Step 2 of trunk action. Individuals of the same ages may be at various levels of the body component sequences, so that they look different from one another as they advance through the developmental sequence.

Differences in Rate of Progress. It is desirable for all individuals to move through the various developmental steps during childhood to achieve an advanced throwing pattern. In fact, several authors have noted that children are skillful in throwing pattern by age 6 (DeOreo & Keogh, 1980, p. 76; McClenaghan & Gallahue, 1978, p. 45; Zaichkowsky, Zaichkowsky, & Martinek, 1980, p. 40). At least two studies demonstrate that such is not the case. Halverson, Roberton, and Langendorfer (1982) filmed a group of 39 children in kindergarten, 1st, 2nd, and 7th grade and classified them according to Roberton's developmental sequence. Their analysis of upper arm action demonstrated that at a young age most boys were already at Step 2 of humerus action, and by grade 7, over 80% had achieved the most advanced level (Step 3). In contrast, approximately 70% of the girls were still in Step 1 of humerus action when initially filmed. By grade 7, only 29% of the girls had reached Step 3. This trend was also apparent for forearm action. Almost 70% of the boys demonstrated Step 2 forearm action when initially filmed. Some were still in this level by Grade 7, but considerably more, 41%, had reached Step 3. Over 70% of the girls began in Step 1 and the majority, 71%, were only at the second level in Grade 7. Gender differences in developmental throwing progress were even more apparent for trunk action. Almost all the boys started in Step 2 and 46% advanced to Step 3 by Grade 7. Similarly, almost 90% of the girls were in Step 2 in kindergarten, but by Grade 7, *all* the girls remained in Step 2, none having advanced to Step 3.

Another study (Leme & Shambes, 1978) focused on throwing patterns in adult women. The 18 persons were selected because they had very low throwing velocities. All of the women demonstrated immature throwing patterns, including block rotation, the lack of a step forward with the throw, and lack of upper arm lag. While these women were unique because of their low throwing velocity, the study certainly demonstrates that not all adults achieve an advanced throwing pattern. Perhaps these women lacked practice opportunities or good instruction in childhood. Together, these two studies suggest that progress through the developmental levels is not automatic and may not be complete during childhood or even adolescence.

Overhand throwing is complex and difficult to observe in detail. The best procedure is to focus on a small number of components, or even a single component, at any one time. Some characteristics are best observed from the front or back: the trunk/upper arm angle, the elbow angle, and lateral trunk bend. Others can be seen from the (throwing) side: the step, trunk rotation, and lagging of the upper arm and forearm. Videotaping is particularly helpful in learning to observe the overarm throw.

Kicking

As with throwing, unskilled kicking tends to be a single action, rather than a sequence of actions, and tends to be mechanically inefficient. As seen in Figure 4.20, there is no step forward with the nonkicking leg and merely a push of the kicking leg forward at the ball. The knee of the kicking leg is bent at contact, and some unskilled kickers even retract their leg immediately after contacting the ball. The trunk does not rotate, and the arms are held stationary at the side. The boy in Figure 4.21 demonstrates better kicking skill by stepping forward with the nonkicking foot, thus putting the kicking leg in a cocked position. Compare these two figures with the advanced kicker pictured in Figure 4.22. The advanced kicker

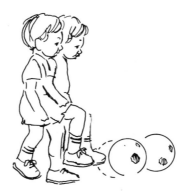

Figure 4.20 A beginning kicker performs the kick as a simple push of the leg forward. Redrawn from film tracings provided by the Motor Development and Child Study Laboratory, Department of Physical Education and Dance, University of Wisconsin-Madison.

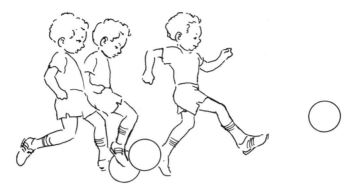

Figure 4.21 This kicker has made some improvements in his kick compared to the beginning kicker. He steps forward, putting the leg in a cocked position, but the leg swing is still minimal. The knee is bent at contact and some of the momentum of the kick is lost. Redrawn from film tracings provided by the Motor Development and Child Study Laboratory, Department of Physical Education and Dance, University of Wisconsin-Madison.

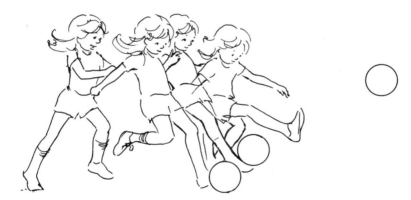

Figure 4.22 An advanced kicker. Note the full range of leg motion, trunk rotation, and arm opposition. Redrawn from film tracings provided by the Motor Development and Child Study Laboratory, Department of Physical Education and Dance, University of Wisconsin-Madison.

- starts with a preparatory "wind up." This position, trunk rotated back and the kicking leg cocked, is achieved by leaping or running up to the ball. As a natural consequence of the running stride, the trunk is rotated back, and the knee of the kicking leg is flexed just after the push-off of the rear leg. Hence, maximal force application over the greatest distance is obtained. The run also contributes momentum to the kick.

- uses sequential movements of the kicking leg. The thigh rotates forward, then the lower leg extends (knee straightens) just before contact with the ball to increase the radius of the arc through which the kicking leg travels. The straightened leg continues forward after contact to dissipate the force of the kick in the follow-through.
- swings the kicking leg through a full range of motion at the hip.
- uses trunk rotation to maximize range of motion. As a result of complete leg swing, the kicker compensates by leaning backward at contact.
- uses the arms in opposition to the legs, as a reaction to trunk and leg motion.

The study of kicking development in children has not been as extensive as educators would like. Although the overall changes children must undergo to perform an advanced kick are known, the qualitative changes made by each body part are not well documented. Recently, Haubenstricker, Seefeldt, and Branta (1983) found that only 10% of the 8.5- to 9.0-year-old children they studied exhibited advanced kicking form. So, there is reason to speculate that proficient kicking, like throwing, is not automatically achieved in childhood.

Observation of individual children is especially important to provide adequate instruction in kicking skills. From the side, a teacher can look for placement of the support foot, range of motion and precontact extension in the kick leg, range of trunk motion, and arm opposition. A special form of kicking is called punting; contact is made with the ball after it is dropped from the hand(s) but before it reaches the ground. Punting is more difficult than place kicking, because the kick must be timed to the falling ball, hence it naturally develops later than place kicking. The mechanical principles involved in punting are quite similar to those of place kicking, hence, further discussion is not undertaken here.

Sidearm Striking

Although many sports and physical activities require the use of a striking implement, there is a decided lack of research data on the development of striking. Striking is a term that encompasses numerous skills carried out with various body parts or implements in a variety of relationships to the body's orientation. Here in our discussion the focus is on one-handed sidearm striking with an implement. Additionally, striking of a stationary ball is illustrated. Striking involves the most difficult perceptual judgment of the basic skills discussed so far. Success in meeting a moving object is limited in early childhood; therefore, it is difficult to assess striking of a moving object at these ages. The mechanical principles and developmental aspects of one-handed striking of a stationary object can be applied to other types of striking tasks. Keep this in mind as we examine development of the striking pattern.

Unskilled attempts to execute sidearm striking often look like unskilled attempts to throw overhand! Strikers chop at the oncoming ball by extending at the elbow, using little leg and trunk action. Like the girl in Figure 4.23, they often face the ball. A complete developmental sequence for sidearm striking has not been validated, but the sequences for foot and trunk action in the overarm throw are applicable to striking (see Table 4.6). Additionally, some of the qualitative changes individuals make in the arm action of sidearm striking are known. Langendorfer (1982) feels that overarm striking development is quite similar in arm action to overarm throwing development. The arm action in sidearm striking is distinct from overarm striking, but many of the same mechanical principles apply to both forms of striking as well as to underarm striking such as the golf swing. From the known qualitative changes in arm action of sidearm striking and the mechanical principles involved, common developmental changes can be outlined.

Developmental Changes in Sidearm Striking. The first obvious change in sidearm striking from that shown in Figure 4.23 occurs when strikers stand sideways to the ball. By transferring their weight to the rear foot, taking a step

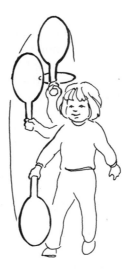

Figure 4.23 This young girl executes a striking task with arm action only. She faces the ball and swings down rather than sideways. Redrawn from film tracings provided by the Motor Development and Child Study Laboratory, Department of Physical Education and Dance, University of Wisconsin-Madison.

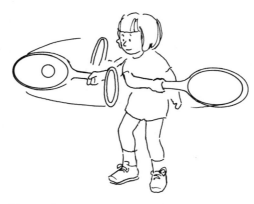

Figure 4.24 This girl has made improvements compared to the beginning striker. She stands sideways and executes a sidearm strike, but does not involve the lower body. Redrawn from film tracings provided by the Motor Development and Child Study Laboratory, Department of Physical Education and Dance, University of Wisconsin-Madison.

forward and transferring their weight forward at contact, strikers are able to improve their striking skills. The girl in Figure 4.24 turns sideways but has not yet learned to step into the strike. A second beneficial change is the use of trunk rotation. Individuals first use block rotation before advancing to differentiated (pelvic then spinal) rotation, a developmental sequence similar to throwing.

Strikers also progressively change the plane of their swing from the vertical "chop" seen in Figure 4.23 to an oblique plane, and finally to a horizontal plane, as seen in Figure 4.24. They eventually obtain a longer swing by holding their elbows away from their sides and extending their arms just before contact. Beginning strikers frequently hold a racket or paddle with a "power grip," where the handle is placed in the palm like a club (Napier, 1956). With this grip the striker tends to keep the elbow flexed during the swing and to supinate the forearm, thus undercutting the ball. While children often use this grip with any striking implement, it is common for them to adopt the power grip when given an implement that is too big and heavy. Educators can promote use of the proper "shake hands" grip by providing striking implements of appropriate weight (Roberton & Halverson, 1984).

Characteristics of Advanced Sidearm Striking. An advanced sidearm strike incorporates many of the characteristics of an advanced overarm throw. These characteristics as well as arm actions consistent with the mechanical principles can be identified in Figure 4.25. They include the following movements:

- Stepping into the hit, thus applying straight-line force to the strike. The step should be a distance more than half the individual's standing height

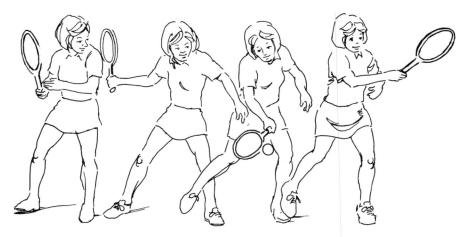

Figure 4.25 An advanced striker. The swing arm moves through a full range of motion. The striker steps into the swing and uses differentiated trunk rotation. Redrawn from film tracings provided by the Motor Development and Child Study Laboratory, Department of Physical Education and Dance, University of Wisconsin-Madison.

(Roberton, 1984). The preparatory stance should be sideways to allow for this step and the sidearm swing.

- Using differentiated trunk rotation to permit a larger swing and more force contribution through rotary movement.
- Swinging through a full range of motion to apply the greatest force practical.
- Swinging in a roughly horizontal plane and extending the arms just prior to contact.
- Chaining the movements together to achieve the greatest force possible. The sequence is: backswing and step forward, pelvic rotation, spinal rotation and swing, arm extension, contact, and follow-through.

As with many of the previous skills, studying a child's swing from two locations yields the most information. From the "pitching" position the direction of the step, plane of the swing, and arm extension can be observed. From a side position the step, trunk rotation, and extent of swing can be checked.

Catching Skills

Several "reception" skills are basic to sport performance. The most common is catching. "Trapping" a soccer ball is another skill where the ball's momentum is absorbed by the body or foot such that it remains in a player's control and doesn't bounce away. "Fielding" in hockey also keeps the ball (or puck in ice hockey) under control. Little research data are available for reception skills other than catching. However, many of the mechanical principles involved in catching are applicable to these other reception skills, and a discussion of the development of catching provides an overview of reception skills.

Development of Catching

A child's initial catching attempts involve little force absorption. The young boy pictured in Figure 4.26 has his hands and arms positioned rigidly. The ball is trapped against his chest rather than caught in his hands. It is common to see children turn away and close their eyes in anticipation of the ball's arrival. To become more proficient, novice catchers must learn to "give" with the ball, thus gradually absorbing the force of the ball. Also to be mastered is the ability to move to the left or right, to move forward, or to back up to catch a ball. Catchers must also learn to point the fingers up when catching a high ball but down when catching a low ball.

Haubenstricker, Branta, and Seefeldt (1983) have conducted a preliminary validation of a five-step sequence for the arm action in two-handed catching development. The sequence, originally outlined by Seefeldt, Reuschlein, and Vogel (1972), is summarized in Table 4.7. At 8 years of age most of the boys and almost half of the girls tested by these investigators were at the highest level of catching. Virtually all of the children had passed through Steps 1 and

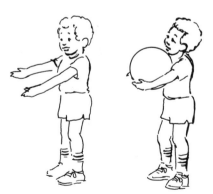

Figure 4.26 This young boy holds his arms and hands rigidly rather than "giving" with the ball to gradually absorb its force. Instead of catching the ball in his hands, he traps it against his chest. Redrawn from film tracings provided by the Motor Development and Child Study Laboratory, Department of Physical Education and Dance, University of Wisconsin-Madison.

Table 4.7 Two-Handed Catching Development

Step	Brief Description
1. Little response	Arms are extended forward, but there is little movement to adapt to ball flight; ball usually trapped against chest
2. Hugging	Arms are extended sideways to encircle the ball (hugging); ball is trapped against chest
3. Scooping	Arms are extended forward again but move under object (scoop); ball is trapped against chest
4. Arms "give"	Arms extend to meet object with the hands; arms and body "give"; ball is caught in hands
5. Movement to catch	Child moves to catch a ball not thrown directly to him or her; catcher may regress briefly to "scooping"

Note. Adapted from "Standards of Performance for Throwing and Catching" by J.L. Haubenstricker, C.F. Branta, & V.D. Seefeldt, 1983. Paper presented at the annual conference of the North American Society for Psychology of Sport and Physical Activity, Assilimar, CA. Based on "Sequencing Motor Skills Within the Physical Education Curriculum" by V. Seefeldt, S. Reuschlein, & P. Vogel, 1972. Paper presented at the annual conference of the American Association for Health, Physical Education, and Recreation, Houston, Texas.

2 by this time. Slightly higher percentages of boys than girls performed at higher levels at any given age, but overall catching tended to be well developed in this group by age 8.

Visual Perception in Catching

Catching, like striking, involves complicated perceptual judgments. Many aspects of visual perception are needed at a refined level to judge an oncoming object. These perceptual abilities will be discussed in chapter 5, but as an example, figure-ground perception is needed to pick out a moving object (figure) from a moving or stationary background. Certain combinations of ball and background color have been shown by Morris (1976) to affect the catching accuracy of young children, age 7 years. Blue balls against a white background were more accurately caught, for example, than white balls against a white background. The effect of these color combinations, however, diminished with older groups up to age 11 years. Certainly skills such as catching can improve as visual perception is refined. Perfect perceptual judgment, however, does not guarantee task success because the necessary movements must be properly executed in addition to accurately perceiving the object to be caught.

Factors Influencing Catching Task Difficulty

Characteristics of a catching task, such as the trajectory of the approaching ball, can affect catching accuracy because the difficulty of the perceptual judgment is affected. Young children whose visual perception is not yet refined to adult levels and who have relatively little experience and practice with catching tasks can be particularly affected. Ball velocity, ball size, and ball trajectory and direction affect catching and interception (as in striking a moving object) accuracy. The relationship between such factors and accuracy, however, is not as simple as might be assumed. For example, larger balls are easier for children to catch than smaller ones, to a point (McCaskill & Wellman, 1938), whereafter, large balls promote poorer catching form because individuals scoop very large balls rather than catching them in the hands (Victors, 1961). Additionally, faster velocities make interception more difficult than slower velocities, but young children in particular often have difficulty delaying their response to a very slow velocity, and respond early (Haywood, 1977; Haywood, Greenwald, & Lewis, 1981). One investigation (Bruce, 1966) found that the different ball trajectories produced by 30° and 60° angle projections did not affect the catching accuracy of 7-, 9-, and 11-year-old children; yet it is common for individuals to have difficulty catching balls with a very high trajectory compared with a slightly arched trajectory. Ball velocity, size, and trajectory have specific effects on tasks such as catching. Educators must carefully manipulate these factors to make catching tasks easier or more difficult as the skill level of individual children demands.

When observing catching skills it is important to remember that performance varies with such factors as ball size, velocity, and trajectory. If children are periodically classified into developmental stages and their previous performance is compared with their current performance, it is important to have these factors, especially ball size, as consistent as possible from session to session.

Observing Motor Skill Patterns

The ability to critically observe children's skill patterns is essential for an instructor of motor skills. It is necessary to provide students with feedback and further practice experiences, or to formally assess their skills. The observation process requires disciplined, systematic focus on the critical features of a skill pattern rather than the tendency to focus on the outcome or product of a skill. Observation techniques must be learned and practiced like any other skill before they become automatic.

Barrett (1979) has provided a guide for improving the observation skills of instructors and coaches based on three principles: analysis, planning, and positioning. To analyze developmental movement, the observer first must know the developmental sequences of the skill, including the critical features that characterize a given developmental step, and the mechanical principles involved in proficient performance. Observers must organize and plan their observation to prevent their attention from wandering once the activity begins. It may be helpful to have written observation guidelines, many of which are provided by the formal qualitative assessment tools discussed in chapter 5. However, suitable observation guidelines could be designed by simply listing the critical features of the skill to be watched. It might also be helpful to watch a given feature of a skill many times (two tries, three, etc.). The third principle is *positioning*. Many new observers rivet themselves to one location and attempt to watch everything from there. As was indicated earlier in this chapter, some critical features of motor skills can be seen only from the side and others seen best from the front or back position. It is important, then, for the observer to move about to be able to watch a skill from several angles. The process of motor skill observation demands focused attention: New observers must plan ahead, know the critical features of the skill to be watched, position themselves properly, and practice.

Summary 4.2—Developmental Sequences for Motor Skills

During childhood, basic skill performance improves. Much of this improvement is accomplished by increased mechanical efficiency. That is, children's movements are gradually refined to conform with the laws of motion and stability. This transition is marked by qualitative changes in the movement pattern. These qualitative changes can then be used to outline a developmental sequence. Several such sequences have been proposed and a few have been validated. A useful feature of many developmental sequences is the categorization of qualitative change by body component. Individuals do not necessarily move to the next developmental step through simultaneous change in all body components. Hence, sequencing by body component allows an assessment of developmental level that recognizes these variations. Children do not look the same as they advance through the developmental sequences because some may have more refined leg action than arm action, some more refined arm action than leg action, and so on.

Ideally, refinements in the basic skills are made in childhood. During adolescence individuals can continue to improve the product of their performance, learn to combine basic skills, and perform skills in a wide variety of situations. Chapter 5 turns to motor development during adolescence.

Suggested Readings

Espenschade, A.S., & Eckert, H.D. (1980). *Motor development* (2nd ed.). Columbus, OH: Charles E. Merrill.

Roberton, M.A. (1984). Changing motor patterns during childhood. In J.R. Thomas (Ed.), *Motor development during childhood and adolescence* (pp. 48-90). Minneapolis, MN: Burgess.

Roberton, M.A., & Halverson, L.E. (1984). *Developing children—Their changing movement*. Philadelphia, PA: Lea & Febiger.

Wickstrom, R.L. (1983). *Fundamental motor patterns* (3rd ed.). Philadelphia, PA: Lea & Febiger.

Motor Behavior in Preadolescence Through Adulthood

The preadolescent and adolescent years typically bring improvement in the product of skilled performance: running speed, throwing distance, jumping height, and so on. Part of this quantitative improvement is the result of continued growth, especially during the adolescent growth spurt, and accompanying increases in strength and endurance. Improved coordination undoubtedly contributes to skill improvement, too. This is not to say that all children automatically emerge from the 2- to 8-year age period having achieved the highest developmental step of qualitative change in skill pattern. Although childhood is a period of great progress in basic skill performance and movement pattern many adolescents and adults do not perform basic skills efficiently (Halverson et al., 1982; Haubenstricker et al., 1983; Zimmerman, 1956). Thus the preadolescent and adolescent years ideally are years when remaining deficits in motor pattern efficiency are overcome. Preadolescents and adolescents who have acquired relatively advanced basic skills begin learning to combine and sequence the basic skills into more complex sport-related skills. For example, an infielder runs to catch a bouncing ball, pivots and throws it to first base, not as three individual skills, but as one continuous movement. Performance of sport-related skills also demands the ability to adapt the basic movements to a wide variety of situations. Thus the adolescent years can be a period of great progress in skill performance that brings individuals to a level of proficient performance in a variety of enjoyable activities.

Concept 5.1 During the preadolescent and adolescent years the product (quantity) of skill performance improves.

A variety of motor skills have been studied which describe motor development during the 7- to 18-year age span. Usually these skills are assessed by quantitative measures of skill performance. Changes in basic skills, such as running, jumping, and throwing, when measured for performance, speed, distance, or accuracy reflect quantitative improvement in motor performance. Similarly, measures of functional strength (e.g., the flexed arm hang) and flexibility (e.g., the sit-and-reach test) indicate changes in motor performance in adolescence (Branta, Haubenstricker, & Seefeldt, 1984). Although specific performance scores are reviewed in this section, the emphasis is on the *trends* in improved performance such scores outline rather than actual scores in feet or seconds; specific scores are easily influenced by test administration procedures, type of equipment (size and weight), and even the clothing and shoes worn by participants. Thus, from a developmental perspective, the discussion focuses on relative changes in motor performance during this period.

Quantitative Improvement in Motor Performance

Running

The common quantitative measures of running ability are speed over a short distance (such as 30 yd) and speed in an agility run. The agility run requires, in addition, frequent change of direction. After reviewing studies of dash performance in 1960, Espenschade concluded that running speed increased in boys and girls from an average rate of just under 4 yd/sec at age 4 to just over 6 yd/sec at age 12 (see Figures 5.1 and 5.2). Boys continued to improve to just over 7 yd/sec by age 17, but girls leveled off and actually regressed slightly during this age period. A later review by Branta et al. (1984)

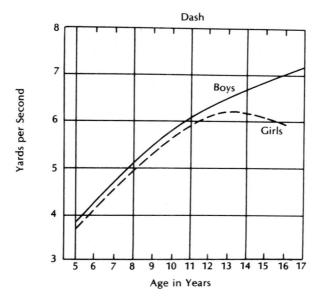

Figure 5.1 Running (dash) performance by boys and girls. From "Motor Development" by A. Espenschade & H. Eckert, 1974, in *Science and Medicine of Exercise and Sport* (p. 329) by W.R. Johnson & E.R. Buskirk (Eds.), New York, NY: Harper & Row. Copyright 1974 by Warren R. Johnson and Elsworth R. Buskirk. Reprinted by permission of Harper & Row, Publishers, Inc.

has confirmed this trend for boys. Recently collected scores for girls, however, have been higher. For example, Branta et al. report a speed of 6.7 yd/sec for 14-year-old girls. Additionally, recent data have not shown the regression in girls' performance that was reported in earlier studies. This trend may reflect increased opportunities for girls to practice, improved instruction, and broadened social acceptance of an all-out effort in activity by girls.

Running agility tests are quite variable in design. The length of such tests can range from 120 to 400 ft with variations in the number and type of directional changes. Such variations hinder comparison among the studies reporting adolescents' performance. Among those using the 120-ft shuttle run, a consistent improvement for boys between 5 and 18 years has been reported, with times of approximately 13 to 16 sec at 5 years improving to approximately 10 sec in the midadolescent years. The trend and scores for girls were similar, although the best average score in midadolescence was approximately 11 sec (Branta et al., 1984). Two cross-sectional studies reported a regression in girls' scores in early adolescence (AAHPERD, 1976; Campbell & Pohndorf, 1961), but longitudinal studies have found improvement at all ages (Branta

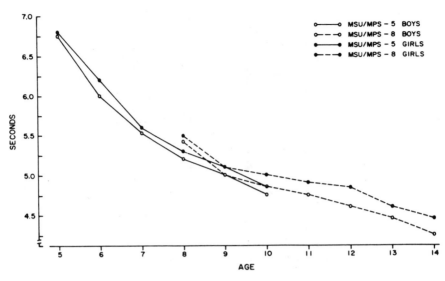

Figure 5.2 Running (dash) performance in boys and girls from two groups measured longitudinally from 5 to 10 or 8 to 14 years of age. From "Age Changes in Motor Skill During Childhood and Adolescence" by C. Branta, J. Haubenstricker, & V. Seefeldt, 1984, in *Exercise and Sport Science Reviews* (p. 485) by R.L. Terjung (Ed.), Lexington, MA: Collamore Press. Copyright 1984 by Collamore Press, Macmillan Publishing. Reprinted by permission.

et al., 1984). Average running performance on both dashes and agility runs, then, improves during preadolescence and adolescence for both boys and girls.

Jumping

The most commonly used jumping tests are the horizontal and vertical jumps. Espenschade (1960) determined that boys and girls improved the distance they could jump horizontally from approximately 33 in. at 5 years of age to 60 in. at 10 to 11 years of age. Thereafter, boys continued to improve to approximately 90 in. at age 17 years, while girls plateaued at 64 in. (see Figures 5.3 and 5.4). This trend has been confirmed by more recent studies (see Branta et al., 1984, for a review), although the scores reported for girls have often been higher and not as far below the average performance of boys as those scores reported in earlier studies. Vertical jumping performance follows a similar trend, improving from approximately 2 in. at age 5 to almost 17 in. in 17-year-old boys and approximately 12 in. in 16-year-old girls (Espenschade, 1960).

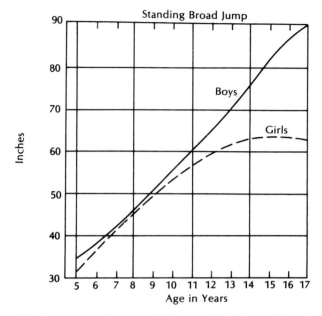

Figure 5.3 Standing long jump performance by boys and girls. From "Motor Development" by A. Espenschade & H. Eckert, 1974, in *Science and Medicine of Exercise and Sport* (p. 330) by W.R. Johnson & E.R. Buskirk (Eds.), New York, NY: Harper & Row. Copyright 1974 by Warren R. Johnson and Elsworth R. Buskirk. Reprinted by permission of Harper & Row, Publishers, Inc.

Throwing

Throwing distance is most often used to measure throwing performance, although speed and accuracy have also been assessed. Distance throw performance differs from running and jumping performance in that differences between boys' and girls' performance exist from even young ages. For example, Espenschade (1960) found that boys improved from approximately 24 ft at 5 years of age to 153 ft at 17 years of age. In contrast, girls threw only 14.5 ft at age 5 years, then improved to 75.7 ft at 15 years, but declined to 74.0 ft at 16 years (see Figure 5.5). While both sexes improve dramatically from childhood to adolescence, differences in performance level are large and have been reported in many studies. Additionally, there has been no trend of improved scores for girls in later studies (see Branta et al., 1984, for a review). Recall from concept 4.1 that the study by Halverson et al. (1982) noted significant gender differences in efficiency of the throwing process in 7th grade (approximately 13 years of age).

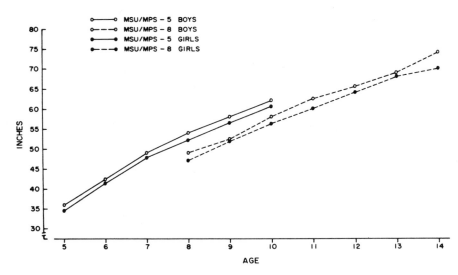

Figure 5.4 Standing long jump performance by boys and girls from two groups measured longitudinally from 5 to 10 or 8 to 14 years of age. From "Age Changes in Motor Skill During Childhood and Adolescence" by C. Branta, J. Haubenstricker, & V. Seefeldt, 1984, in *Exercise and Sport Science Reviews* (p. 485) by R.L. Terjung (Ed.), Lexington, MA: Collamore Press. Copyright 1984 by Collamore Press, Macmillan Publishing. Reprinted by permission.

Few studies have measured changes in throwing speed over age, but Roberton, Halverson, Langendorfer, and Williams (1979) have reported that boys improve their throwing speed 5.45 ft/sec per year from kindergarten to 7th grade. Girls improve at a rate of 3.88 ft/sec per year over the same span. Hence, the trend of dramatic improvement but large gender differences in throwing speed parallels the results of distance throw studies.

Quantitative Versus Qualitative Assessment

In studying the basic skills, you saw repeatedly that skill development could be assessed by the *quality* or process of the skill or by the *quantity* or product of the skill. That is, the performer can be classified into developmental steps relative to each body component, or the distance of a jump or the speed of a throw can be measured. When faced with assessing children, which method should be used, qualitative or quantitative? It depends upon both the children and the purpose of assessing them. If the purpose is to plan instructional experiences for children, qualitative assessment is the better method.

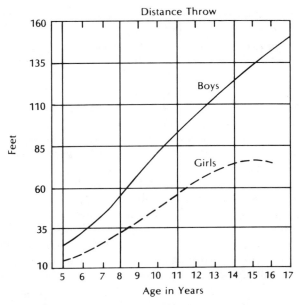

Figure 5.5 Distance throw performance by boys and girls. From "Motor Development" by A. Espenschade and H. Eckert, 1974, in Science and Medicine of Exercise and Sport (p. 330) by W.R. Johnson & E.R. Buskirk (Eds.), New York, NY: Harper & Row. Copyright 1974 by Warren R. Johnson and Elsworth R. Buskirk. Reprinted by permission of Harper & Row, Publishers, Inc.

Qualitative assessment is particularly useful as a *formative* evaluation, because it can be used to provide appropriate educational experiences for children or to instruct them in an appropriate movement pattern. For example, qualitative assessment will indicate whether the child is taking a step with the throw, extending at the take-off of a jump, and so on. Scores provided by quantitative assessment, such as the distance a child can throw a ball, give status quo information about a child that is useful for comparisons with other children. However, the quantitative score alone does not indicate *how* a child threw the ball. Particularly in the case of poor throwing ability, a qualitative assessment is needed to provide instructional experiences and feedback to children on the skill pattern used. In contrast, once children have relatively mature form, a quantitative assessment, especially one repeated at regular intervals, may chart a child's progress and allow comparisons to norms for children of the same age and gender.

Most of the assessment instruments available to educators yield quantitative scores (Herkowitz, 1978a), because quantitative measurement is straightforward. The qualitative changes in skills during development have only recently been researched as a result of technical advances in high-speed filming and widespread availability of equipment.

The Lincoln-Oseretsky Motor Development Scale is a well-known example of a quantitative assessment. The Scale was first published in 1923 in Russian and has been revised several times (Bailer, Doll, & Winsberg, 1973; DaCosta, 1946; Sloan, 1955). It is intended to assess children during the 5- to 15-year age span and contains both hand and arm movement tests as well as gross motor tests (seven for balance, four for jumping). Hence it is an assessment of overall motor development. The original Oseretsky scale has been revised as the Bruininks-Oseretsky Test of Motor Proficiency (Bruininks, 1978), and this revision is widely available. In the Bruininks-Oseretsky test are eight subtests for both gross and fine motor skill, but a short form is also available. Other well-known examples of multiskill quantitative instruments are the Denver Developmental Screening Test (birth to 6 years), the Gesell Developmental Schedules (4 weeks to 6 years), and the Bayley Scales of Infant Development (2 months to 2.5 years) discussed in chapter 3 (Frankenburg & Dodds, 1967; Bayley, 1969; Gesell & Amatruda, 1949). All of these quantitative assessment instruments establish levels of normative skill performance deemed appropriate for a specified chronological age. They are generally well standardized, but their motor items have lower reliability and validity measures than desirable. In this sense they are useful but limited in the information they provide about motor development (Herkowitz, 1978a).

In contrast to these well-known quantitative assessments, qualitative assessment instruments are relatively new. Most provide descriptions of the developmental steps of a particular skill to which a child's pattern of performance is then compared. Of concern to motor development instructors is the variance among qualitative assessment tools in the number of developmental steps or levels proposed for the same skill. For example, the Fundamental Movement Pattern Assessment Instrument (McClenaghan & Gallahue, 1978) describes three steps for each of five motor patterns (running, long jumping, kicking, throwing, and catching). The motor pattern descriptions are made relative to body components. In a second measure, descriptions of four levels for each of 11 motor skills are provided in the OSU Sigma Test (Loovis, 1976). The Developmental Sequences of Fundamental Motor Skills (Seefeldt, 1973, cited in Herkowitz, 1978c) categorizes each of 10 motor skills into four or five steps. In yet another measure, DeOreo's Fundamental Motor Skills Inventory (DeOreo, 1974) evaluates both the product and process of 11 basic skills.

These assessment tools are initial attempts to provide a means for process evaluation of children's performance. They must be used with caution, however, because little information is available on their standardization procedures. Further, little is known about their validity, and only a few have been examined for reliability (Herkowitz, 1978c). Although further work on these assessments is needed, they represent a positive step toward providing instructors with qualitative assessment tools.

Teachers can devise their own written records to chart children's progress from the sequences outlined in chapter 4. For example, the steps for each component of the overhand throw can be listed on a page. As each child is observed, a checkmark can be placed next to the appropriate step. By repeating this evaluation throughout the school year, each child's progress can be charted. An example of a checklist for hopping performance of an individual child is given in Figure 5.6.

Factors Influencing Quantitative Performance

Motor performance on the skills discussed clearly improves during preadolescence and adolescence, but it must be remembered that performance reflects many factors such as the developmental pattern used, body size and physique, body composition, strength, and coordination. These factors are apparent particularly at the extremes of the performance continuum (Malina, 1980). For example, an overweight or very weak child will score poorly on quantitative tests. An early maturing, muscular child will score well. In addition, a quantitative score often confounds several factors. For example, a throw for distance confounds force and angle of projection. Some children score poorly because they have poor force production, while others score poorly because they throw at a disadvantageous projection angle.

The one exception to steady improvement in motor performance at all ages has been the plateau or regression of girls' scores in midadolescence (Espenschade & Eckert, 1974). Recall that teenage girls between 14 and 17 are typically past menarche and have achieved their adult stature. An aspect of this maturation process is the accumulation of at least some additional fat weight. The earlier attainment of adult size may explain the early plateau in girls' scores when compared to boys'. The smaller average size and greater average percent body fat may explain lower performance levels, but what about the regression in some scores? It might be that psychosocial rather than physical factors account for this decline. That is, some girls may lose interest in physical activities or come to feel, through contact with significant friends and relatives, that a maximal effort on such activities is no longer appropriate to their gender role. The latter factor might have been particularly significant in groups tested before the 1970s. The social factors that affect performance are discussed more fully in chapter 9, but for now, keep in mind that such factors could account in part for the gender differences observed in performance. Remember, too, that these differences are stated in the average scores of groups of adolescent girls. Scores vary considerably within a group, and

Child: <u>Jones, Randy</u>   Classroom: <u>S. Johnson</u>
Motor Task: <u>Hopping</u>

Level Observed

Movement Component: Leg Action	Jan. 4		
Step 1. Momentary flight			
Step 2. Fall and catch; Swing leg inactive			
Step 3. Projected takeoff; Swing leg assists	✔		
Step 4. Projection delay; Swing leg leads			
Movement Component: Arm Action			
Step 1. Bilateral inactive			
Step 2. Bilateral reactive			
Step 3. Bilateral assist			
Step 4. Semi-opposition	✔		
Step 5. Opposing assist			
Overall Movement Profile Legs	3		
Arms	4		
Movement Situation Teacher selected			
Child selected	✔		
Observation Type Direct	✔		
Video-tape			
Film			
Comments:			

Figure 5.6   A checklist for hopping based on the component sequences in Table 4.5 (p. 116). Such checklists can be designed from any of the component sequences available. From *Developing Children—Their Changing Movement* (p. 54) by M.A. Roberton and L.E. Halverson, 1984, Philadelphia, PA: Lea & Febiger. Copyright 1984 by Lea & Febiger. Reprinted by permission.

some girls probably continue to improve their performance. The more recent findings of higher and improved running and jumping by adolescent girls might indicate a change in social attitudes toward girls' motor performance. Additionally, such improvements may reflect a secular trend toward early maturation or larger body size. Most of the recent studies have tested adolescent girls only to the midadolescent years. Continued measurement of girls into late adolescence in future studies will help place many of these contributing factors in perspective.

Another aspect to consider when examining gender differences in performance is the *type* of skill involved. Gender differences in the absolute level of performance are typically small before boys enter their adolescent growth spurt. When boys do surpass girls in body size, they have an advantage in *some* motor activities because of their greater height, longer limb length, leaner body composition, and greater amount of muscle tissue and strength. When these physical size advantages exist, an average boy has a performance edge over an average girl in many gross motor skills such as sprinting, jumping, and throwing (Espenschade & Eckert, 1974). But what about other motor skills that require fine coordination and precision? Girls have outperformed boys on skills demanding speed and exactness of grasping (Yarmolenko, 1933) as well as hopping (Halverson & Williams, 1985; Jenkins, 1930). So, performance differences between the sexes depend in part upon the type of motor task involved. Individual variability is still the overriding rule, and considerable overlapping exists in the performance abilities of boys and girls.

Stability in Motor Behavior

Some educators and coaches would like to identify the young boys and girls who have the potential to become elite athletes. These children could then be given special training and coaching to prepare them for Olympic or professional competition. Is this possible? Several investigators have examined this issue objectively by testing groups of children periodically and calculating correlation coefficients of the scores obtained at different ages. The closer any coefficient is to 1.0, of course, the more children tend to maintain their relative position in the group over the growth period. That is, the better children at a young age will tend to be the better performers when the group is again tested years later. The closer a coefficient is to 0.0, the more children tend to trade relative positions within the group during the intervening time span. Rarick and Smoll (1967) repeated several motor tests—the long (broad) jump, 30-yd dash, and throw-for-velocity—with a group at every age between 7 and 12 and then again at 17 years. In general, the correlations were moderate (see Table 5.1). They were a bit higher over the late childhood years from 7 to 12, from .115 to .924, than over the entire age span of 7 to 17, from .127 to .596. Also, the coefficients were higher between two close ages, such as 11 and 12, than between two widespread ages, such as 7 and 17. Glassow and Kruse (1960) found that long jump and 30-yd dash performance were moderately correlated, .74 and .70, respectively, between 6 to 7 years and 12 to 13 years. Espenschade (1940) obtained correlations ranging from .29 to .66 for boys and .36 to .84 for girls on performance of a variety of tasks between 13 and 16 years. In summary, age-to-age correlations of motor performance during the preteen and teen years tend to be positive. Yet, most

Table 5.1 Age-to-Age Correlations of Motor Performance Measures

Measures	Age-to-Age Correlations (Childhood)					Age-to-Age Correlations (Childhood to Adolescence)					
	7 to 12	8 to 12	9 to 12	10 to 12	11 to 12	7 to 17	8 to 17	9 to 17	10 to 17	11 to 17	12 to 17
Boys											
Broad jump	.484	.534	.663	.849	.780	.596	.563	.694	.788	.665	.728
30-yd dash	.386	.424	.460	.694	.780	.181	.138	−.073	.381	.354	.517
Velocity throw	.501	.308	.479	.580	.501	.278	.136	.378	.455	.330	.404
Girls											
Broad jump	.709	.705	.755	.807	.896	.502	.804	.704	.745	.714	.661
30-yd dash	.924	.830	.784	.915	.933	.562	.699	.765	.718	.710	.696
Velocity throw	.115	.534	.462	.361	.552	.127	.252	.204	.225	.290	.295

Note. From "Stability of Growth in Strength in Motor Performance From Childhood to Adolescence," 1967, by G.L. Rarick & F.L. Smoll, *Human Biology*, **39**, pp. 299, 301, 302. Copyright 1966 by Wayne State University Press. Reprinted by permission.

of the correlations obtained are not high enough to be used for *prediction*, because too many incorrect judgments would be made. Instructors are wise to avoid definitive judgments about the long-term skill potential of children based on their status in late childhood.

Skill Refinement

Improvement in the quantity of performance is only one aspect of skill progress that must be made during the teen years to achieve proficient skill. Children must learn to combine the basic skills into integrated sequences and to respond to increasingly more dynamic environments. For example, it is desirable to improve in throwing velocity during the preteen and teen years, but what is more, a young ball player must learn to catch a bouncing ball, step on second base, turn, and throw quickly to first base over an oncoming runner. Unfortunately, educators do not presently have effective tools for systematically measuring these complex aspects of performance. Hence, not much is known about how these aspects of skill are acquired; it is just known that young athletes improve in their ability to combine skills as needed to meet the challenge of a dynamic environment.

Another necessary improvement in skill performance is the ability to adapt a movement to any one of a wide range of task demands and conditions. Basketball players making lay-up shots must adapt their movement to their starting position in relation to the basket and the positions of other players on the court, which might even be changing during the lay-up. As with movement combinations, no system for comprehensively evaluating the development of this ability exists.

Educators can, however, specify the range of conditions that affect skill performance. For example, Herkowitz (1978b) has suggested a developmental task analysis in which a chart is created to list the factors involved in a specific task and the continuums along which the factors vary. Examples for striking and throwing are given in Figures 5.7 and 5.8. The dotted lines in Figure 5.7 outline a relatively simple striking task, and the solid lines outline a complex task; note how the characteristics of the object struck and the implement used varies between the levels of task difficulty.

Using such an analysis, many levels of difficulty can be generated. Research has not yet been conducted to show which factors are mastered first by developing children or what levels along the continuums are easily achieved in any but a few specific cases. It is clear that such variations are mastered with sufficient guidance, experience, and practice and that such mastery is needed for sport and dance performance.

Educators can use a developmental task analysis to provide students with a variety of environmental situations. It is likely that children and adolescents achieve an advanced movement pattern in a simple task before they achieve

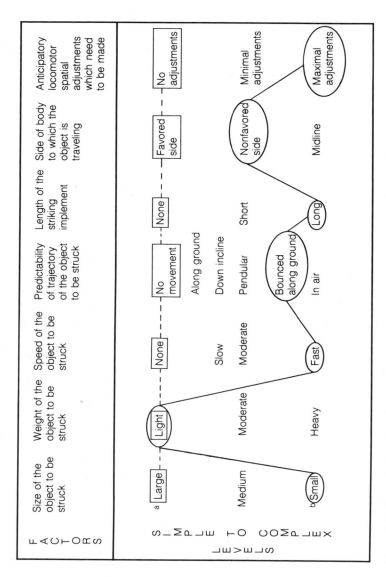

Figure 5.7 General task analysis for striking behavior: (a) profile of a general task analysis for a relatively simple striking task (dotted line); (b) profile of a general task analysis for a relatively complex striking task (solid line). From "Developmental Task Analysis: The Design of Movement Experiences and Evaluation of Motor Development Status" (p. 141) by J. Herkowitz, 1978, in *Motor Development* by M.V. Ridenour (Ed.), Princeton, NJ: Princeton Book Company. Copyright 1978 by Princeton Book Company. Reprinted by permission.

FACTORS	Size of the object being thrown	Distance object must be thrown	Weight of the object being thrown	Accuracy required of the throw	Speed at which target being thrown at is moving	Acceleration and deceleration characteristics of the target being thrown	Direction in which target being thrown at is moving
SIMPLE	Small	Short	Moderately light	None	Stationary	No movement	No movement
		Moderately	Little heavy	Slow	Steady	Left to right speed	of thrower
LEVELS OF	Medium	Medium					Right to left of thrower
COMPLEXITY			Light	Moderate	Moderate	Decelerating	Toward thrower
	Large	Long	Heavy	Much	Fast	Accelerating	Away from thrower

Figure 5.8 General task analysis for throwing behavior. From "Developmental Task Analysis: The Design of Movement Experiences and Evaluation of Motor Development Status" (p. 149) by J. Herkowitz, 1978, in *Motor Development* by M.V. Ridenour (Ed.), Princeton, NJ: Princeton Book Company. Copyright 1978 by Princeton Book Company. Reprinted by permission.

it in a complex task; also, skilled performers given a simple task may use a developmental pattern less efficient than the one they are capable of in a challenging situation. That is, task complexity can drive the developmental level demonstrated in a given performance. The quantity of skill performance is also affected by the environmental situation. One task can elicit a fast sprint, while another elicits an easy run. Educators can design educational experiences at the appropriate and desired level by manipulating task characteristics.

Summary 5.1—Quantitative Improvements in Skill Performance

Steady, continued improvement is made during the preadolescent and adolescent years in quantitative skill performance. Before adolescence gender differences in performance are minimal in running and jumping but are large in throwing. During adolescence the gap widens, in part because girls may plateau or even regress. Some recent studies have noted improved performance by adolescent girls, possibly reflecting environmental factors that affect girls' performance, such as increased acceptance of maximal efforts in physical endeavors or increased opportunities for practice. Additionally, the type of skill determines performance differences between the sexes. In skills involving strength, boys as a group have an advantage over girls as a group, and in other skills, girls outperform boys. In all such cases, there is considerable overlapping of the boys and girls in performing these skills. The overlapping of skilled performance stresses how important it is to consider each adolescent as an individual. Little is known about the specific way adolescents improve their ability to combine skills and respond to dynamic environments. Yet, adolescence is a period of dramatic improvement in motor performance when adequate instruction and experience are provided. When adolescents maximize their opportunities to learn skills well, they enter adulthood at a skill level that can provide many enjoyable and beneficial experiences with physical activities.

Quantitative improvement in skill performance accompanies qualitative improvement and growth in size and strength. Both the quantity and the quality of skill can be assessed. Qualitative assessment is helpful in planning practice experiences and in providing formative feedback. Once a movement pattern is relatively mature, quantitative assessment can be used for comparison to other performers or to one's own previous performance.

Concept 5.2   Skill performance can be refined and perfected in adulthood, but it is affected by the aging process.

Once young adults attain a given level of performance on a well-practiced skill, will they be able to maintain or improve that level in middle and older adulthood? This is a complex question because the performance of skills is multifaceted. Some skills require accuracy, others speed, others both accuracy and speed. Strength is a major factor in some skills, while endurance or flexibility is emphasized in the performance of others. Then, too, it is possible to use either the movement process, the movement product, or both as the gauge for maintenance and improvement. It is likely that the question about middle and older adult performance can be answered differently for various skills and methods of assessment because these factors are affected differently by the aging process. That is, skills whose major component is speed may not be retained at a young adult level, but skills emphasizing accuracy may be improved. Or the quality of performance may be maintained, but the quantity may decline.

Some types of skill performance by middle and older adults have received little attention. For example, few studies have examined the movement patterns of older adults. In contrast, the cardiovascular and memory functions of older adults have been more widely studied. As a result, generalizations can be formed about some aspects of adult skill performance, while questions remain unresolved on other aspects. Since perception, fitness, and learning and memory will be discussed later, the following discussion focuses upon the qualitative and quantitative skill performance of adults. In many cases, only tentative conclusions regarding adult skill performance can be made.

Motor Performance in Adulthood

A prevailing stereotype of the motor performance of middle and older adults has been one of declining performance. To an extent this stereotype is understandable. Recall from chapter 2 that physical changes are known to occur with aging, such as a loss of bone and muscle mass. One could speculate that such changes affect the mass of the various body parts, altering in turn the mechanical nature of the skill to be performed. The central nervous system seems to be less adaptable in old age, and reaction and movement times tend to slow with increasing age. All of these factors might affect a change in movement patterns established in younger years.

On the other hand, it is difficult to know if these changes are inevitable or the result of declining activity levels or declining expectations of performance levels. That is, middle-aged adults who believe they are destined to declining performance fulfill their own beliefs. In fact, the physical changes associated with aging are often shown to be minimal in older adults who remain fit and active and continue their participation in physical activities. Whether or not small physical changes are significant enough to cause noticeable changes in movement pattern during execution of a skill is unclear at this time. Care must be taken in examining research on adult motor performance to recognize that results often reflect the sample of subjects studied. The range of abilities among an older adult sample is more variable than among other age-groups. For example, one might study older adults confined to a nursing home or older adults of the same age living independently and participating in a regular exercise program for seniors in the community. As such, those studies showing significant declines in performance may reflect the effects of a sedentary lifestyle or of various disabilities and not the potential for older adult performance.

Age at Peak Performance

One method to examine the course of skill performance in adulthood is to document the ages of athletes in elite competitive events or at the time of their peak performance. This was done by de Garay, Levine, and Carter (1974) for performance at the 1968 Olympics and Malina, Bouchard, Shoup, and Lariviere (1982) at the 1976 Olympics. Partial results of these surveys are presented in Table 5.2. It can be seen that the ages of these elite performers vary considerably depending upon the type of skill and gender of the participant. For example, the men ranged in age between 14 and 49; swimmers and divers were typically the youngest, and weight lifters, fencers, and wrestlers were the oldest. Ages for women ranged between 12 and 38 years; gymnasts and swimmers were among the youngest, and divers and canoeists/rowers among the oldest.

A consideration of the factors associated with this variability in ages clarifies the pattern of adult physical performance. First, the fitness component factors influence the pattern of age variability in elite performance. Some sports such as weight lifting require peak strength for peak performance. Because peak strength is achieved in the 20s (Burke, Tuttle, Thompson, Janney, & Weber, 1953), peak performance in weight lifting can be expected in the 20s or early 30s. In contrast, performance in activities such as rifle and pistol shooting requires less strength but benefits from years of practice and experience. This trend was confirmed in an early survey of ages at which championships were won (see Table 5.3; Lehman, 1953). While specific changes may have occurred over the years since this survey, it is still likely today that the more physically demanding sports have younger champions than activities that are less physically demanding.

Social and cultural factors are likely to play a role in the age patterns of adult performance. Adults are expected to conform to societal norms, and these norms have often included "retirement" from sports and games by middle adulthood, especially for women. Recent emphasis on exercise and fitness over the life span may have begun to change such norms. It will be

Table 5.2 Ages of Performers in Various Olympic Events

Event	Year	Men			Women		
		N	M	Range	N	M	Range
Swimming	1968	67	19.2	14-25	32	16.3	12-23
	1976	44	19.8	14-26	33	16.7	12-26
Diving	1968	16	21.3	16-30	7	21.1	16-38
Water polo	1968	71	22.9	16-37			
Boxing	1968	142	22.9	17-35			
	1976	20	23.6	19-31			
Cycling	1968	104	23.6	17-32			
	1976	22	22.8	17.32			
Gymnastics	1968	28	23.6	18-31	28	23.6	18-31
	1976	11	24.8	20-33	15	17.0	13-20
Basketball	1968	63	24.0	18-38			
Track	1968	246	24.3	16-42	82	20.8	15-29
Track and field	1976	43	24.1	17-32	34	21.7	14-27
Canoeing	1968	49	24.2	18-38	4	22.0	18-25
Rowing	1968	86	24.3	18-40			
	1976	88	24.3	18-36	59	23.4	16-30
Wrestling	1968	90	25.8	17-37			
	1976	16	21.9	17.27			
Weight lifting	1968	59	26.7	17-49			
	1976	11	27.8	22-34			

Note. Adapted from data in *Genetic and Anthropological Studies of Olympic Athletes* (pp. 82-145) by A.L. deGaray, L. Levine, & J.E.L. Carter, 1974, New York, NY: Academic Press and from "Age, Family Size and Birth Order in Montreal Olympic Athletes" (p. 20) by R.M. Malina, C. Bouchard, R.F. Shoup, & G. Lariviere, 1982, in *Physical Structure of Olympic Athletes, Part I* by J.E.L. Carter (Ed.), Basel, Switzerland: S. Karger.

interesting to study changes in the participants' ages in elite competitions as attitudes change toward lifelong activity for men and women.

Data on the age of champions or elite performers reflect the performance of the "best of the best." Certainly many middle-aged athletes excel in competitive events below national and international levels, and many outperform the majority of younger adults. The decline in average performance levels of middle and older adults is often very slight, and individuals sometimes achieve their personal best in middle or later adulthood. An examination of the quantitative performance levels in middle and older adulthood illustrates how small the decline in performance really is.

Table 5.3 Ages (yrs) at Which 1,175 Championships Were Won

Type of Skill	N of Cases	Median Age	Mean Age	Years of Maximum Proficiency
U.S.A. outdoor tennis champions	89	26.35	27.12	22-26
Runs batted in: annual champions of the two major baseball leagues	49	27.10	27.97	25-29
U.S.A. indoor tennis champions	64	28.00	27.45	25-29
World champion heavy-weight pugilists	77	29.19	29.51	26-30
Base stealers: annual champions of the two major baseball leagues	31	29.21	28.85	26-30
Indianapolis-Speedway racers and national auto-racing champions	82	29.56	30.18	27-30
Best hitters: annual champions of the two major baseball leagues	53	29.70	29.56	27-31
Best pitchers: annual champions of the two major baseball leagues	51	30.10	30.03	28-32
Open golf champions of England and of the U.S.A.	127	30.72	31.29	28-32
National individual rifle-shooting champions	84	31.33	31.45	32-34
State corn-husking champions of the U.S.A.	103	31.50	30.66	28-31
World, national, and state pistol-shooting champions	47	31.90	30.63	31-34
National amateur bowling champions	58	32.33	32.78	30-34
National amateur duck-pin bowling champions	91	32.35	32.19	30-34
Professional golf champions of England and of the U.S.A.	53	32.44	32.14	29-33
World record-breakers at billiards	42	35.00	35.67	30-34
World champion billiardists	74	35.75	34.38	31-35

Note. From *Age and Achievement* (p. 256) by H.C. Lehman, 1953, Princeton, NJ: Princeton University Press. Copyright 1953 by the American Philosophical Society. Reprinted by permission.

Quantitative Performance in Middle and Older Adulthood

The recent emphasis on lifetime exercise and fitness has made participation in Master's competition and Senior Olympics popular. This in turn has provided information on the quantitative levels of achievement attainable in middle and older adulthood. A set of regional Senior Olympic records for selected events is summarized in Table 5.4. While the records decline with increasing age in almost every case, the decline over approximately 20 years is relatively small in most of the events.

The time of 16.8 sec in the 100-m dash, 65- to 69-year-old women, was set by Helen Stephens, who won the 1936 Olympic gold medal in the same event with a time of 11.5 seconds. That performance set an Olympic record, which stood until 1960. The difference between Helen Stephens' superior performance as an 18-year-old and her time in the same event over 45 years later was 5.3 sec. This is a relatively small decline over the middle and older adulthood years.

In our discussion of motor development in childhood and adolescence, the relationship between quantitative performance levels and qualitative change in the movement pattern was emphasized. It is possible that the slight declines in quantitative performance level during older adulthood are related to qualitative changes in movement. Or the movement patterns might be stable, and the declines may be related to fitness factors such as a loss of strength, or to societal norms that predict a decline and become a self-fulfilling prophecy. The following discussion examines the movement patterns of older adults. Fitness and social factors will be discussed in later chapters.

Qualitative Performance in Middle and Older Adulthood

It is unfortunately the case that research studies of the movement patterns of middle and older adults are few. In part this lack of research reflects the recency of technical advances allowing faster data analysis, but it also reflects the tendency of motor developmentalists to study children first. Too, older adults have been stereotyped as having a sedentary lifestyle and little interest in activity.

A large number of the existing studies on the movement patterns of older adults have focused on walking. Murray and her coworkers (Murray, Drought, & Kory, 1964; Murray, Kory, Clarkson, & Sepic, 1966; Murray, Kory, & Sepic, 1970) conducted a series of studies on gait patterns in older men and women by measuring the linear and rotary displacements and the velocities of the limbs during walking. They found that the older men walked in a pattern similar to younger men but with these differences: The step length of the older men was approximately 3 cm shorter, the older men toed out approximately 3° more than younger men, the degree of ankle extension was reduced, and pelvic rotation was diminished. Older women also showed greater outtoeing, shorter stride length, and less pelvic rotation than younger women. Schwanda (1978) confirmed the finding of a shorter stride length among older men and

Table 5.4 Regional Senior Olympic Records Set Between 1980 and 1984

Event	Men					Women			
	55 to 59	60 to 64	65 to 69	70 to 74	75+	55 to 59	60 to 64	65 to 69	70 to 74
Standing broad jump (ft-in.)	8 3-1/2	7 11	7 8-5/8	7 1/4	6 7-3/4	5 11-1/2	5 11-7/8	7 4-1/2	8 6
Softball distance throw (ft-in.)	220 7	177 1	165 0	135 0	118 6	122 0	86 7	84 0	83 0
Running, 50-m dash (s)	6.90	6.59	7.28	8.01	8.65	8.16	8.58	8.70	9.60
Running, 10,000-m run (min:s)	38:10	42:38	48:31	55:62	—	50:11	56:38	—	75:33
Swimming, 50-yd freestyle (s)	29.30	28.88	29.49	35.81	35.35	33.34	39.50	45.67	44.71

Note. Adapted from *Senior Olympics Newsletter* (St. Louis, Missouri), **4**, September, 1984. Records were established at the Senior Olympics competition in St. Louis County, Missouri. The 1984 participation count for the entire event was 1,205.

further demonstrated that most other aspects of the walking pattern (stride rate, time for recovery leg swing, time on support leg, and vertical displacement of the center of gravity) remained similar to those of middle-aged men. It is likely that shortened stride length and greater outtoeing reflect uncertainty in balance. These and other studies (Adrian, 1982) indicate that older adults generally maintain a near-normal walking pattern.

A few other movement patterns in older adults have been studied. Nelson (1981) studied both the walking and running patterns of older women (ages 58 to 80). She asked the participants in her study to walk normally, walk as fast as possible, jog, and run as fast as possible. Average speed, stride length, and stride frequency all tended to increase over this sequence, but individuals were extremely variable in how they changed from walking to jogging. The older women generally achieved increased walking speed by lengthening their stride, but achieved increased running speed by increasing stride frequency as do young women. A major difference between younger and older women came in the *pattern* used for fast running: The older women did not tuck their "recovering" leg as completely, had a shorter stride length, and took fewer strides than younger women. The absolute *speed* of both jogging and running also differed among the age groups. Older women jogged more slowly (1.85 vs. 3.93 m/sec) and ran more slowly (2.60 vs. 6.69 m/sec) than a group of 20-year-old women (Nelson, 1981).

Klinger, Masataka, Adrian, and Smith (1980; cited in Adrian, 1982) included a vertical jump among several activities studied in women over 60. As with the Nelson study of running, the jumping pattern of the older women appeared normal in the sequence of movements. Their maximal range of knee flexion, though, was smaller than that typical of young adults, and the older women could not extend their legs as quickly. The speed of elbow extension in older women was recorded during throwing and striking tasks. The extension velocities achieved were again much slower than those recorded from performances of young women.

Although the number of studies providing information on the movement patterns of older adults is limited, several generalizations can be made. The movement patterns of older adults are generally well maintained from younger adulthood. Although one might suspect that older adults revert to the patterns used by children, the extent of any such regression appears limited. Also, the movements of older adults are not as fast as those of their younger counterparts. To what can slower speed be attributed? While physical factors such as strength could certainly be involved, Klinger et al. interestingly noted that half of the older women in the aforementioned study reported they had no sports background, and many indicated they had not attempted some of the activities performed since they were in high school. It is possible that lower limb velocities among these women reflect a lack of practice and experience during the adult years or, perhaps, that faster speeds were never attained in young adulthood. Adrian (1980) suggests that such lack of participation in sport activities might *precede* rather than *follow* bone, joint, and muscle changes with aging. If rapid movements through a large range of motion are rarely made, the bones, joints, and muscles are never subjected to the beneficial levels of "stress" that contribute to improved strength and integrity of the tissues.

Summary 5.2—Adult Motor Behavior and Aging

Ideally, individuals should perfect the basic skills during childhood and adolescence so that by adulthood they can demonstrate mastery of the skills. Adulthood, then, should be a period of skill refinement and recombination wherein additional practice and experience contribute to improved performance levels. In fact, this is true only for some adults. Others may never master the basic skills. Nevertheless, the level of skill pattern achieved appears to be relatively stable during middle and older adulthood. Some declines are evident, though, in the quantity of performance, depending in part on the physical or experiential demands of the specific skill. It is difficult to determine now how much of the decline in performance is related to an expectation that performance will decline or to a lack of practice and conditioning. Too, many of the adults studied may never have reached advanced movement patterns in young adulthood. As more research is done on the movement patterns of older adults, including more research on a variety of individual lifestyles, a better understanding of the potential for performance in older adulthood will be achieved.

Throughout our discussion of motor performance, we have mentioned factors related to the performance of skills, such as fitness and social norms. Our descriptions of growth, maturation, and motor development have often focused on the average or normal course of development, but factors related to skill performance introduce even more variation to the norm. Educators work with individual persons. To achieve a more complete perspective on the range of factors that determine the performance levels of individuals as well as their skill potential, an understanding of the correlates of motor development is desirable. It is to these factors that we direct our attention in the next chapters.

Suggested Readings

Adrian, M.J. (1980). Biomechanics and aging. In J.M. Cooper and B. Haven (Eds.), *Proceedings of the Biomechanics Symposium*. Indiana: Indiana State Board of Health.

Branta, C., Haubenstricker, J., & Seefeldt, V. (1984). Age changes in motor skill during childhood and adolescence. In R.L. Terjung (Ed.), *Exercise and sport science reviews* (Vol. 12) (pp. 467-520). Lexington, MA: Collamore Press.

Espenschade, A.S., & Eckert, H.D. (1980). *Motor development* (2nd ed.). Columbus, OH: Charles E. Merrill.

P A R T
2

Correlates of Motor Development

Part II is a survey of factors that affect motor development. The discussions focus on changes in other modes of behavior that are integrally related to motor development including perceptual change, physiological change in response to exercise, cognitive change, and sociocultural practices.

In chapter 6 the courses of visual, auditory, and kinesthetic development are described, and the integration of these systems is explained. Scientifically validated concepts and claims that remedial programs benefit academic achievement are presented. The methods of assessing perceptual-motor development are reviewed, and the chapter concludes with a discussion of the role of perceptual-motor activities in development.

Another correlate of motor development, the age-related changes in physiological response to exercise, is explored in chapter 7. Basic concepts of exercise physiology are reviewed including the physical fitness components of endurance, strength, flexibility, and body composition.

In chapter 8 the cognitive changes involved in processing information are investigated. Age-related changes in the various aspects of information processing, such as attention and response selection, are discussed as is the memory system. Part of the chapter is also devoted to changes in mental capacity, especially as it is viewed by neo-Piagetian theorists.

Sociocultural influences on motor development are discussed in the final chapter. Initially, the focus is on the socialization process as it affects participation in physical activities over the life span. The remainder of the discussion concentrates on the manner in which ethnic and cultural factors alter the environment for physical growth and motor development among children from black, white, and other ethnic backgrounds.

Perceptual-Motor Development

Almost every motor act in one sense is a *perceptual-motor* skill. That is, movements are based on information about the environment and a person's position or location in it. For example, a softball infielder sees the location of the pitch, the bat striking the ball, and the ball bouncing on the ground; he or she hears the hit and perhaps a runner on the basepath, and then feels the position of his or her body and arms. The player combines this *sensory* information with memories of previous experiences and *perceives* the surrounding world. Then, based on these perceptions, the infielder decides where and when the ball could be intercepted, where to move, how to position his or her body; and so the ball is caught, taken from the glove, and thrown to first base. These perceptions of environment and movements are added to the store of perceptions to help the infielder in future performance.

On the other hand, you might think platform divers could execute well-learned dives without hearing and without seeing the water below, because it is an established distance away. Yet, they must still feel the orientation of their bodies to the pull of gravity and the location of their trunk and limbs relative to one another both before and during the dive. Whether performance of a given skill relies predominantly on visual information as fielding does, or on kinesthetic information as diving does, it is evident that perception is important to skilled performance.

Some improvements children make in their motor skills as they grow and mature can be attributed to improvements in their sensory and perceptual functioning. As children learn to better select, process, organize, and integrate perceptual information and coordinate it with information from past experiences, their motor skills improve.The result is more refined motor skills and better performance. The term "perceptual-motor" is used to describe the age-related improvement in perception and the subsequent improvement in movements based on those perceptions. Perceptual-motor functioning, once refined, is believed to be maintained throughout adulthood. Very little is known about perceptual-motor changes in older adults, but many age-related changes in the sensory systems have been identified. Older adults probably adapt to many of the physical changes taking place in their sensory receptors and continue to perform well. Other changes may be detrimental to their performance so that attention to these changes is warranted. In the next section, age-related changes in vision, kinesthesis, and audition over the life span are reviewed. Later the integration of these systems is discussed as well as the importance of identifying perceptual-motor deficiencies in young performers.

Concept 6.1   Visual, kinesthetic, and auditory development contribute to skill development.

Visual Development

Vision plays a major role in most skill performance. To understand this role better, we need to examine age-related changes in both visual *sensation* and *perception*. These changes occur in the sensory system that transmits nerve signals to the brain as well as in the multistage perceptual process wherein the performer selects, processes, organizes, and integrates the neural information. During the 1st month of life, the visual system provides the infant with functionally useful, but unrefined vision at a level approximately 5% of eventual adult *acuity* level (sharpness of sight), or 20/800 on the Snellen scale of visual acuity (20/20 is desirable). The infant's resolution of detail is such that he or she can differentiate facial features from a distance of 20 in.; distant objects beyond this are probably not seen clearly.

During the first 6 months, the infant makes rapid improvements in accommodation, contrast sensitivity, and acuity (Atkinson & Braddick, 1981). *Accommodation* is the process that adjusts the shape of the eye's lens (see Figure 6.1) for viewing objects at varying distances, which is important for performing motor skills. Newborns do not control accommodation very well, but by 5 to 6 months of age they show an accurate accommodation response. *Contrast sensitivity* describes our sensitivity to distributions of light and dark as they are spatially arranged in our field of view. Improvements in acuity are related more to the increased number of neural connections in the visual cortex of the brain and to differentiation of the neurons in the part of the retina responsible for detailed vision (the fovea) than to changes in the size of the

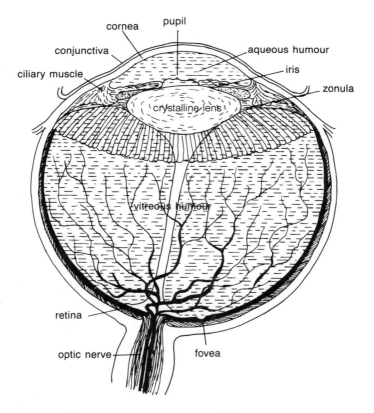

Figure 6.1 The human eye. From *Eye and Brain* (2nd ed.) (p. 34) by R.L. Gregory, 1972, New York, NY: World University Library, McGraw-Hill. Copyright 1972 by McGraw-Hill. Reprinted by permission.

eye or its lens. Taken together, contrast sensitivity and acuity indicate how detailed visual information appears to the infant.

At about 6 months of age, then, as infants are motorically ready to begin self-propelled locomotion, their visual system perceives adequate detail to assist in the task. Many infants exhibit astigmatism, that is, blurred vision due to an imperfect curvature of the cornea. This phenomenon appears to be transient, however, and its incidence declines between 6 and 18 months of age (Braddick & Atkinson, 1979). Visual sensation continues to improve during the childhood period, with slightly more rapid gains in acuity noted between 5 and 7 years of age and again between 9 and 10 years of age. On the average, infants 1 year old have visual acuity of about 20/100 to 20/50, children at 5 years of age about 20/30, and by age 10, children without a visual anomaly score at the desired level of 20/20. Refraction of light by the growing eye depends on the curvature of the cornea, the shape of the lens, and the axial length of the eye. It is likely these structures have a genetically determined growth target size, but they do not grow in synchrony. It has been suggested that growth is controlled so that variations in one structure are balanced by another, minimizing refractive errors during growth. The role of visual experience in this process is unclear, but deprivation of vision during development is known to induce refractive errors (Atkinson & Braddick, 1981).

Visual Perception

Turning now to the development of visual perception, we will discuss the aspects of visual perception important to motor skills, including perception of size constancy, figure-and-ground, whole objects versus parts, depth, spatial orientation, and movement. Although more detailed explanations of visual perception are available (c.f. Rosinski, 1977), our discussion is confined to these topics and their development in children.

Perception of Size Constancy. Consistent interpretation of the visual environment requires perceptual size constancy, that is, the ability to recognize that objects maintain a constant size even if their distance from the observer varies and their image takes up more or less space on the retina (Figure 6.2). Hence, two identical chairs are recognized as being the same size, even if one is nearby and the other is across the room. Similarly, the space or gap between two objects is perceived as constant whether they are near or far. Another aspect of perceptual size constancy is the ability to judge accurately the sizes of different objects that are varying distances away. Young children tend to overestimate the space between two objects as they are placed farther and farther away from them. Gradually, such perceptual judgments improve with age and are relatively mature in the average 11-year-old (Collins, 1976).

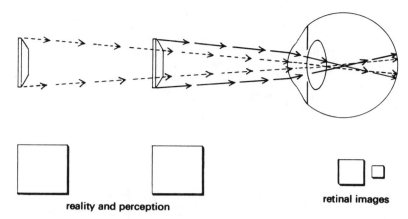

reality and perception   **retinal images**

Figure 6.2 Size constancy. The image of an object halves in size with each doubling of the distance of the object from the eye, but it does not *appear* to shrink so much—the brain compensates for the shrinkage of the image with distance by a process called constancy scaling. From *Eye and Brain* (2nd ed.) (p. 151) by R.L. Gregory, 1972, New York, NY: World University Library, McGraw-Hill. Copyright 1972 by McGraw-Hill. Reprinted by permission.

Perception of Figure-and-Ground. A second aspect of visual perception, called *figure-and-ground*, allows an observer to locate and focus on an object (figure) embedded in a distracting background (ground) (Figure 6.3). This ability to extract figures seems to improve in spurts in growing children, particularly between 4 and 6 years of age (Williams, 1983), and again between 6 and 8 years of age (Temple, Williams, & Bateman, 1979). Children can extract items from a background more successfully if the objects are familiar; they find considerable difficulty with abstract geometric forms. Refinement to a near-adult level of figure-ground perception is achieved after 8 years of age (Williams, 1983).

Perception of Whole-and-Parts. The ability to discriminate the parts of an object, or a picture, from the whole is another important aspect of visual perception. This process allows adults to look at a stick man of nuts and bolts and report seeing "a man made from nuts and bolts." A young child with immature whole-part perception may report seeing just the man, only the nuts and bolts, or report both but at different times. Later, by the age of 9, most children can integrate parts and the whole into the total picture (Elkind, 1975; Elkind, Koegler, & Go, 1964) (see Figure 6.4).

Perception of Depth. The perception of depth is particularly important for performing motor skills. It enables a person to judge the distance from the

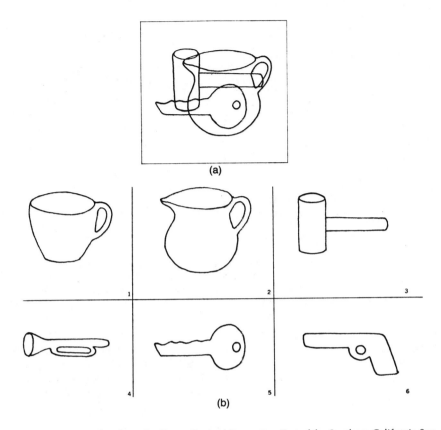

Figure 6.3 A test plate from the Figure-Ground Perception Test of the Southern California Sensory Integration Test. A child must identify which of the six objects in (b) are present, or "embedded," in picture (a). Copyright 1972 by Western Psychological Services. Not to be reproduced in whole or part without written permission of copyright owner. All rights reserved. Reprinted by permission of Western Psychological Services, 12031 Wilshire Blvd., Los Angeles, CA 90025.

body to an object and to recognize the three-dimensional nature of objects. The information one needs to judge depth results from a comparison of the two slightly different "pictures" viewed by each eye, because the eyes are in different locations and each eye sees the visual field from a slightly different angle. This is termed *retinal disparity* (see Figure 6.5). Depth perception requires good visual acuity, too, since the sharper the "picture" from each eye, the more information available for the comparison. Infants have at least some functional vision, and therefore the mechanics for some degree of depth perception. Indeed, the "visual cliff" studies reported by Walk in 1969 demon-

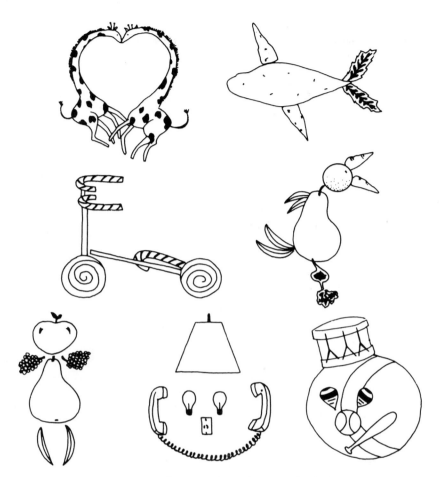

Figure 6.4 The drawings used by Elkind, Koegler, and Go to study whole-part perception. From "Studies in perceptual development: II. Part-whole perception," *Child Development*, **35**, 81-90. By D. Elkind, R.R. Koegler, and E. Go, 1964. Copyright 1964 by Society for Research in Child Development, Inc. Reprinted by permission.

strated depth perception ability in infants at 6 months. On the other hand, even 4-year-olds may err frequently in judging depth. Undoubtedly, as vision becomes more refined, so does depth perception. Recall that adult levels of visual acuity are reached around age 10. Hence, Williams (1968) found that 12-year-old boys judged depth as accurately as 16- and 20-year-olds.

Spatial Orientation. Spatial orientation is defined as the recognition of an object's orientation or arrangement in space. The importance of attending to

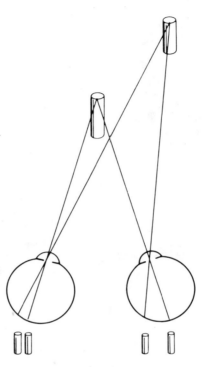

Figure 6.5 Retinal disparity. Images on the left retina are closer together than the images on the right retina. The observer sees the two rods in depth. From *Perception: The World Transformed* by Lloyd Kaufman. Copyright 1979 by Oxford University Press, Inc. Reprinted by permission.

or ignoring the orientation varies with the situation. In some cases, it is important to recognize that an object is identical even if it is tipped to one side, upside-down, or rotated. In other situations, an object's or symbol's orientation is critical to its meaning. Such is the case with letters such as *d* and *b*.

Many motor skills also must be performed in defined spatial dimensions or with objects oriented in a particular way. As such, perception of spatial orientation is important for both everyday and sport tasks. Children are able to attend to spatial orientation before they are able to ignore it in situations where spatial orientation is irrelevant (Gibson, 1966; Pick, 1979). Three- and 4-year-olds can learn directional extremes such as high/low, over/under, front/back, but they still consider intermediate orientations the same as the nearest extreme. Although children at this age can distinguish vertical from horizontal positions, they have difficulty with oblique lines and diagonals. By 8 years of age, most children have learned to differentiate obliques and diagonals, but may still confuse left and right (Naus & Shillman, 1976; Williams, 1973).

Perception of Movement.   The perception of movement in the environment is critical to motor skill performance. It involves the ability to detect and track a moving object with the eyes. Newborns can briefly track horizontally moving objects; they continue to acquire tracking ability in other spatial paths at a variety of ages but in a fixed sequence, beginning with vertical, diagonal, and then circular paths (Gallahue, 1983; Haith, 1966). Between 2 and 5 years of age, children improve in their eye-tracking abilities and in their control of eye movements (Williams, 1983). Their tracking abilities improve even further, so that they can accurately follow moving objects between the ages of 5 and 10 (Haywood, 1977).

The precise role of accurate eye tracking in performance of perceptual-motor skills is presently complicated by the additional ability to detect movement by peripheral vision. For example, a basketball player can judge a teammate's movement in order to throw a pass either (a) by following the player with movement of the eyes, or (b) by fixing the eyes on another point and perceiving the player's movement with peripheral vision. The ability to perceive a moving object and move in response to it is well established by age 12, as demonstrated by children who made quick and accurate movement decisions similar to those of 20-year-olds (Williams, 1968, 1983).

Changes With Aging

It is apparent that many perceptual processes involve judgments about visual stimuli from the environment. Once a performer can make relatively accurate judgments, the ability to do so is maintained throughout adulthood and depends upon the integrity of the visual system to deliver accurate information to the central nervous system. With increasing age, changes in the visual system occur naturally, and some conditions and diseases become more prevalent, especially in older adulthood. These changes may affect the quality of the visual information reaching the central nervous system. For example, the ability to see *nearby* images clearly decreases with aging, becoming clinically significant at around 40 years of age. Resting diameter of the pupil also decreases during the aging process, reducing retinal illuminance of a 60-year-old to one third that of the young adult, making glare a problem for older adults. Contrast sensitivity also declines with aging, and dark adaptation suffers. Cataracts, glaucoma, and age-related maculopathy (a disease affecting the retinal area that enables fine, detailed vision) are visual disturbances more prevalent in older adults. On the other hand, problems in depth perception appear to be related to visual acuity and may be abated when acuity losses are corrected by eyeglasses or contact lenses. Although the visual system can function well for most of adult life, especially with corrective lenses, changes in the eye itself may influence visual perception and, in turn, skill performance. For example, playing tennis at dusk can be difficult for the older adult because retinal illuminance is reduced, which makes visual judgments in dimly lit settings difficult (Haywood & Trick, 1983).

Persons working with children or with older adults can look for certain signs that may indicate a performer has a visual problem. These include a lack of coordination in hand-eye tasks, squinting the eyes, under- or over-reaching for objects, and unusual head movements to line up one's gaze with a particular object. Activity leaders should try to minimize the effect of visual problems on performance by making certain that activity areas are well lighted and the contrast between an object of attention (perhaps a ball) and its background are maximized. Environments that invite glare should be avoided in working with anyone, but in particular with older adults. Performers should be encouraged to wear any corrective lenses prescribed for them, even though they often prefer not to wear their glasses for activities (Haywood & Trick, 1983). Since vision provides so much of the perceptual information needed to perform skills successfully, efforts to enhance the visual information delivered to the central nervous system should also enhance skill performance.

Kinesthetic Development

Types of Kinesthetic Receptors

The kinesthetic (proprioceptive or somato-sensory) system is important to skill performance because it yields information regarding the relative position of the body parts to each other, the position of the body in space, an awareness of the body's movements, and the nature of objects with which the body comes in contact. Unlike the visual system, which relies on the eyes as sensory receptors, kinesthetic information is derived from various types of receptors throughout the body. *Muscle spindles*, one type of receptor, are located among the muscle cells and gauge the degree of tension in a muscle. *Golgi tendon organs* function similarly to muscle spindles by responding to changes in muscle tension but are found at the muscle-tendon junctions. The three types of *joint receptors* in the tissues of the joint capsule or the joint ligaments include the spray-type *Ruffini endings, Golgi-type receptors*, and *Modified Pacinian Corpuscles*. The spray endings signal direction, rate, and extent of joint movement plus steady position. The latter joint receptors give information about stationary joint position.

In the inner ear, the *vestibular semicircular canals* register head movements to maintain or regain body balance. The canals are located in three planes. Head movements cause hair cells at the base of each canal to deflect and send sensory nerve impulses to the brain. The *utricle* and *saccule* provide information about body position in relation to gravity. Movement of the head in a straight line also causes hair cells to deflect in these structures and send sensory impulses to the brain. And finally, the *cutaneous receptors* in the skin and underlying tissues provide information about touch, temperature, pain, and pressure (Dickinson, 1974). Some of the cutaneous receptors respond to mechanical stimulation, some to thermal and pain stimulation, and others to bending of the hair or pressure on the skin. When a gymnast walks along a balance beam, the kinesthetic receptors throughout her body provide constant information on limb position and movement and on balance to enable the gymnast to accurately judge her spatial position while performing specific skills.

Development of Kinesthetic Receptors

Recall from chapter 3 that many reflexes are stimulated through kinesthetic receptors. Hence, the onset of a reflex indicates that the kinesthetic receptor involved is functioning. The first prenatal reflex that can be elicited is opposite-side neck flexion through tactile stimulation around the mouth at just 7.5 weeks after conception. Thus we know that cutaneous receptors are present and functioning around the mouth at this early prenatal age. Tactile stimulation to other body parts has been used to determine that cutaneous receptor development proceeds in an oral, genital-anal, palmar, and plantar (sole of foot) sequence. Note that this developmental sequence follows the cephalocaudal and proximodistal growth directions discussed earlier in chapter 2. By 12.5 prenatal weeks, cutaneous receptors are developing in the hand, as are the muscle spindle receptors in the biceps brachii muscle of the upper arm. We know, too, that the vestibular apparatus is anatomically complete at approximately 9 to 12 weeks of life. During the 4th to 6th prenatal months, cutaneous receptors for touch and pressure continue to develop, as do muscle spindles, Golgi tendon organs, and joint receptors. Perhaps these receptors function long before birth, but sensitivity to temperature via cutaneous receptors is unrefined and pain sensitivity is poorly developed. The functional status of the vestibular system before birth is unclear, but we have seen that the righting reflexes appear around the second postnatal month (Timaras, 1972). Hence, the system for kinesthetic sensation is functional early in life.

Kinesthetic Perception

As was the case with vision, kinesthetic sensations are able to be processed early in life, but improvements in kinesthetic perception are made throughout childhood. The major aspects of kinesthetic perception are perception of tactile location, of multiple tactile points, of objects, of the body itself, of limb movements, of spatial orientation, and of direction. Balance, too, relies on kinesthetic (as well as visual) sensation. We will discuss how these aspects of kinesthetic perception develop, noting that knowledge in some areas remains limited.

Tactile Location. Tactile localization is the ability to identify (without vision) a spot on the body that has just been touched. Four-year-olds are less accurate than 6- to 8-year-olds in locating a touch on the hands and forearms. Performance on this type of task does not improve significantly between 6 and 8 years of age (Ayres, 1972; Temple et al., 1979). Based on this limited data, then, the perception of tactile locations on the hands and arms seems relatively mature by age 5.

Multiple Tactile Points. One type of tactile point perception involves discriminating between two points touching the skin in close proximity. Threshold discriminations vary with different areas of the body, but it is not known if they vary with age (Van Duyne, 1973; Williams, 1983). Ayres (1966), however, reported that only half of a group of 5-year-olds could consistently discriminate a touch on different fingers, though average performance improved through 7.5 years of age (the oldest age tested).

Perception of Objects. Recognition of unseen objects and their characteristics by manipulation is another aspect of kinesthetic perception. In infants such manipulation is often more accidental than purposeful. By age 4 an average child can handle objects purposefully and can explore the object's major features by age 5. Manual exploration becomes systematic at about age 6 (Van Duyne, 1973) and in the next two years, haptic (cutaneous) memory and object recognition also improve (Northman & Black, 1976). Research by Temple et al. (1979) indicates that children also increase their speed of tactile recognition during this age span.

Perception of the Body (Body Awareness). To carry out everyday activities as well as perform complex skills, a sense of the body, its various parts, and its dimensions is needed. One aspect of body awareness is the *identification of body parts*. As children get older, more of them can label correctly the major body parts (DeOreo & Williams, 1980), and they can name more detailed body parts (Cratty, 1979). The rate at which an individual child learns body part labels is largely a function of the amount of time parents or other adults practice with the child. Probably two thirds of the 6-year-olds can identify the major body parts, and mistakes are rare in all normally developing children after age 9.

Children also need a sense of the body's *spatial dimensions*, such as up and down. The "up-down" dimension is usually the first mastered, followed by "front-back," and finally "side." A high percentage of 2.5- to 3-year-olds can place an object in front of or behind their body, but more of them have difficulty placing the object in front of or behind something else. By about 4 years, most children can do the latter task as well as place an object "to the side" (Kuczaj & Maratsos, 1975). Although up-down and front-back typically are mastered before age 3, an understanding that the body has two distinct sides is developed at approximately 4 or 5 years of age (Hecaen & de Ajuriaguerra, 1964). This side awareness is termed *laterality*. The child comes to realize that, despite the two hands, two legs, and so on, being the same size and shape, they can be positioned differently and move independently. Eventually, the child is able to discriminate right and left sides, that is, to label or identify these dimensions. An age-related improvement in the ability to make right-left discriminations occurs between 4 or 5 years and 10 years of age, with most children responding almost perfectly by age 10 (Ayres, 1969; Swanson & Benton, 1955; Williams, 1973). But children can be taught to label right-left at younger ages too, even as young as 5 years of age (Hecaen & de Ajuriaguerra, 1964). Young children also have difficulty executing a task when a limb must cross the midline of the body. This ability improves between 4 years and 10 years, but some 10-year-olds still have difficulty with cross-midline tasks (Ayres, 1969; Williams, 1973).

Lateral dominance is the preferential use of one of the hands, feet, or eyes. If the favored hand, foot, and eye are on the same side of the body, the dominance is termed *pure*; otherwise, it is *mixed*. Lateral dominance emerges sometime during early childhood, but the exact age of emergence is not established. Hand dominance is evident in most children by age 4, although there are some indications that it can occur earlier, and that the preference remains stable during childhood (Sinclair, 1971).

Several theories have been forwarded to explain the emergence of lateral dominance. The most popular of these links lateral dominance to cerebral dominance of the brain; that is, a right-sided person has a dominant left hemisphere and vice versa. The perceptual-motor theory of Doman and Delacato suggests that pure lateral dominance is necessary for proper "neurological organization" (Delacato, 1966). Further, individuals with mixed dominance could anticipate problems in perceptual-motor performance, reading, speech, and other cognitive abilities. This theory has been criticized, however, because several other investigators failed to find a similar significant relationship between lateral dominance and perceptual-motor performance, perceptual judgments, or cognitive performance (Sabatino & Becker, 1971; Horine, 1968; Williams, 1973).

Limb Movements.   Perception of the extent of movement at a joint is often assessed by asking a child to accurately reproduce a limb movement or relocate a limb position without the assistance of vision. Children improve in this task over the 5- to 8-year age span, with little improvement noted after age 8 (Ayres, 1972; Williams, 1983).

Spatial Orientation.   Kinesthetic spatial orientation involves perception of the body's location and orientation in space independent of vision. Temple et al. (1979) tested this perception by asking children to walk a straight line while blindfolded, and then measured their deviation from the straight path. Performance improved between 6 and 8 years of age, the latter being the oldest age-group included in the study. Inasmuch as this was the only age-group tested, investigations of spatial orientation over a wider age range are needed.

Perception of Direction.   *Directionality*, the ability to project the body's spatial dimensions into surrounding space, is often linked to laterality. Children with a poor sense of laterality typically have poor directionality as well. Although this relationship seems intuitively logical, deficiencies in laterality are not known to cause deficiencies in directionality (Kephart, 1964). Note that information for these latter judgments is obtained through vision, so judgments of directionality rely on integration of visual and kinesthetic information. Long and Looft (1972) suggest that improvements in the sense of directionality are made between 6 and 12 years of age. By age 8, children typically can use body reference for directional reference. They are able to say correctly "the ball is on my right" and "the ball is to the right of the bat." At age 9 years, children can change the latter statement to "the ball is to the left of the bat" when they walk around to the opposite side of the objects. Children can identify right and left for a person opposite them and continue to improve in directional references such as these through age 12. Long and Looft note that refinement of directionality must take place after 12 years of age since many adolescents at this age could not transpose left-right from a new perspective, such as looking into a mirror.

Balance.   Although balance can be simply defined as stability or body equilibrium, balance tasks are complex in nature. The characteristics of balance tasks can vary widely to include components such as the base of support and number of supporting limbs or surfaces, the elevation and position of the body, movement of the body (stationary or static vs. moving or dynamic), and the use of vision (eyes open vs. eyes closed). Performance on a balance task with one set of characteristics has little relation to performance on a task with other characteristics (Drowatzky & Zuccato, 1967). So, the assessment of balance ability at any age is related to the assessment task. Before we consider age-related changes in balance, we should recognize that balance is arbitrarily included in our discussion of kinesthesis. Much of the information needed to perform a balance task is obtained from the vestibular system and other kinesthetic receptors, but visual information is critical to balance, too.

Strong evidence indicates that balance performance improves as children advance from 3 to 19 years of age (Bachman, 1961; DeOreo & Wade, 1971; Espenschade, 1947; Espenschade, Dable, & Schoendube, 1953; Seils, 1951; Winterhalter, 1974). The exact pattern of improvement depends largely on the assessment task. On some balance tasks, the average performance of a group of children does not change significantly from year to year, but improvement is steady over a number of years (DeOreo & Wade, 1971); on others, there is significant improvement each year. Despite this general trend to improve balance ability with increasing age, instances of no improvement or even decline in performance scores have been noted (Bachman, 1961; Espenschade, 1947; Espenschade, Dable, & Schoendube, 1953).

No definitive explanation is available for these findings, but a partial explanation may rest in the predominant use of quantitative rather than qualitative assessments of balance. It is possible that at certain ages and on certain tasks children attempt a more mature performance pattern with a resulting, presumably temporary, decline in quantitative score. For example, DeOreo (1971) noted that young children could attempt to walk a balance beam with either a shuffle step, mark time pattern, or a more mature alternate step pattern. When a child first changes from an easier shuffle step to a more difficult alternate step pattern, he or she may lose balance and step off the beam sooner than when using a shuffle step. With more practice, though, the child will travel the beam longer and faster. Children then can be expected to make both qualitative and quantitative improvements in balance performance.

Kinesthetic Changes With Aging

Very little is known about how aging affects the kinesthetic receptors themselves, but changes in kinesthetic perception are known. Some, but not all, older adults lose cutaneous sensitivity, vibratory sensitivity, temperature sensitivity, and pain sensitivity (Kenshalo, 1977). Older adults experience some impairment in judging the direction and amount of passive lower limb movements (Laidlaw & Hamilton, 1937). However, they remain fairly accurate in judging muscle tension produced by differing weights (Landahl & Birren, 1959). A decline in the ability to balance is experienced among older adults, as indicated by studies on postural sway (Hellebrandt & Braun, 1939; Hasselkus & Shambes, 1975). Whether the decrements noted result from increased perceptual thresholds, changes in the peripheral nerves, or changes within the central nervous system remains unclear (Timiras, 1972).

Auditory Development

Although not as important to performance as vision or kinesthesis, auditory information is still valuable for accurate skill performance. Sounds are often critical cues to initiate or time movements. Just as with the other senses, we must distinguish between *auditory sensation*, merely hearing sound, and *auditory perception*, actually judging sound. Auditory sensation is considered first, beginning with the prenatal development of the ear.

Auditory Sensation

The external ear, the middle ear, and the cochlea of the inner ear are involved in hearing. The inner ear develops first and is close to adult form by the third prenatal month. The external ear and middle ear are formed by midfetal life (Timiras, 1972). Fetuses reportedly respond to loud sounds, but perhaps this response is actually to tactile stimuli, that is, vibrations (Kidd & Kidd, 1966). In the newborn, hearing is imperfect, partly because of the gelatinous tissue filling the inner ear. This material is reabsorbed during the first postnatal week so that hearing improves rapidly (Timiras, 1972). Improvements are noted in auditory acuity through childhood and adolescence, but these might be attributed, at least in part, to improvements in attentional level and ability to follow directions (Kidd & Kidd, 1966).

Auditory Perception

In addition to hearing sound, children must learn to judge the characteristics of the various sounds they hear. Some aspects of auditory perception are perception of auditory location, of differences in similar sounds, and of auditory figure-and-ground. These are similar to aspects of perception in the other senses.

Location.   Children must perceive the direction from which a sound comes so that they can connect the sound with its source (see Figure 6.6). As early as 4 to 6 months, infants are able to turn their heads in the general direction of a sound. They can localize distant noises at 11 to 12 months and continue to improve so that by the age of 3 years, they can localize sounds for their

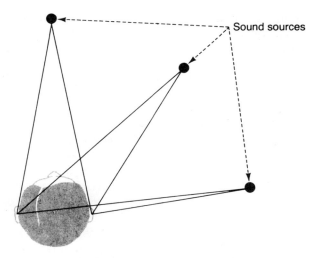

Figure 6.6 Sound localization. The more a sound deviates from the straight-ahead position, the greater is the time difference in the arrival of the sound at each ear. From *A Primer of Infant Development* by T.G.R. Bower, 1977, San Francisco: W.H. Freeman. Copyright 1977 by W.H. Freeman. Reprinted by permission.

general direction (Dekaban, 1970). However, more detailed aspects of localization, such as threshold levels and localization of multiple sources, have not been examined in children.

Perception of Differences.   Tasks requiring children to distinguish two sounds similar in pitch, loudness, or speech sound (for example "d" and "t" or "b" and "p") are termed discrimination tasks. Infants as young as 1 to 4 months can discriminate basic speech sounds (Doty, 1974), but the period from 3 to 5 years brings increasing accuracy in recognizing differences in sounds (DiSimoni, 1975). Temple et al. (1979) found a further improvement in auditory discrimination between 6 and 8 years, as did Birch (1976) between 7 and 10 years with an auditory matching task. A similar trend apparently exists for discrimination of pitch (Kidd & Kidd, 1966). In general it appears that by 8 to 10 years of age, children have greatly improved their ability to detect differences in similar sounds, but they continue to refine auditory discrimination skills through at least 13 years of age.

Auditory Figure-and-Ground.   Often, certain sounds must be attended to while ignoring other, irrelevant sounds in the background. For example, try listening to someone on the telephone ("figure" sounds) while a stereo is playing and several people in the room are talking ("ground" sounds). It is known that this is an important aspect of auditory perception and that some children have more difficulty than others separating auditory "figure" from the background; unfortunately, little else is known about age-related changes in this perceptual process.

Auditory Changes With Aging

More older adults than younger adults suffer a loss of hearing sensitivity, but the source of this loss is not clear. Some auditory decrement might be due to physiologic degeneration, but lifelong exposure to environmental causes may also contribute to a loss of hearing (Timiras, 1972). In fact, extreme environmental noise, such as listening to loud music on stereo headsets can lead to early hearing loss. The absolute threshold (i.e., loudness of sound) for hearing pure tones and speech increases in older adulthood, as do the differential thresholds for pitch and speech discrimination (Corso, 1977). Older adults are at a distinct disadvantage in adverse listening conditions, too. Beyond these changes in hearing we know little about changes in auditory perception with advancing age, but as with vision, the perceptual process relies on clear and accurate sensations. Whatever factors affect hearing might also affect auditory perception.

Summary 6.1—Visual, Kinesthetic, and Auditory Development

From our discussions, it is clear that the visual, kinesthetic, and auditory systems function at an early age and continue to improve throughout infancy and childhood. By 8 to 12 years of age, aspects of visual perception have developed to near-adult levels. Kinesthetic perception typically develops to near-adult levels by about age 8, somewhat earlier than visual perception, although this generalization is based on limited research. Young children can perceive the location of sound, and by age 10 perform at near-adult levels on many auditory discrimination tasks. Refinement of auditory skills continues through the early teens. Some aspects of auditory perception have not been studied with children. In general, though, children between the ages of 8 and 12 approach adult levels of performance on many perceptual tasks, with only small refinements in perceptual skills yet to be made. It is clear that some aspects of perceptual development are not well documented, and further research is needed. Little is known, too, about the cause of changes in the perceptual processes with advancing age, but results of these decremental changes in the sensory systems are known to reduce the quality of the sensory information reaching the central nervous system, thereby affecting motor skill performance.

Concept 6.2   Intersensory integration improves in childhood.

Think for a moment about the softball infielder mentioned earlier in this chapter. Remember that the player *saw* and *heard* the bat hitting the ball. These perceptions were made with two separate sensory systems, vision and audition. Concept 6.1 focused on the developmental improvements made within such individual sensory systems, that is, on *intrasensory* functioning. But the game of softball requires the infielder to combine the perceptions from individual sensory systems in order to make more complex judgments. This aspect of perception is termed *intersensory* integration. The player integrates information from two or more senses to make an accurate judgment of the ball's path. Examples of intersensory integration in skilled performance are many. The gymnast on a narrow balance beam integrates visual and kinesthetic information to perform stunts. A dancer integrates musical sounds with visual and kinesthetic information to present a dance, and so on. Intersensory integration is necessary for nearly all skilled performances.

If you have ever watched a young child's first attempts to hop and clap his or her hands in time with music, you know that intersensory integration is not fully functional in early life. The kinesthetic input from clapping is not well integrated with the beat of the music to assist the timing of the hop! How does the ability to use information from many senses simultaneously develop?

Integration of the Senses

It is generally accepted that intersensory integration is partially functional at birth and improves as a child grows and develops. This developmental process of intersensory integration can be described in three levels. The first level is the automatic integration of basic sensory stimuli, a process inherent to the functioning of the subcortical brain. Automatic integration is probably functional at birth or very early in infancy. The second level involves the integration of a particular stimulus or the features of a stimulus when it is experienced in two different senses. For example, an object first manipulated but not seen is later recognized when seen as being one and the same object. The highest level involves the transfer of concepts across sense modalities

(Williams, 1983). These two levels of integration are attained through the experiences of childhood.

It is tempting to think that intersensory integration follows intrasensory development, that visual or kinesthetic sensation and perception improve first, then sensory integration follows. In fact, the development of intra- and inter-sensory integration is simultaneous. Some evidence suggests that even very young infants can interact with their environment through two senses concurrently. For example, Aronson and Rosenbloom (1971) had infants 30 to 55 days of age watch their mother while her voice was projected normally or from a displaced location. The infants became visibly agitated when their mother's voice came from a displaced location. Spelke's (1979) research also demonstrated that 3- to 4-month-old infants, when shown two side-by-side movies, spent more of their time watching the movie for which the proper soundtrack was played. At a young age, then, children are uncomfortable with discrepancies between two senses, such as vision and audition, indicating they must be capable of the first level of integration, the automatic integration of basic sensory stimuli.

It is misleading to emphasize the perceptual development of one sense system independent of other systems. Auerbach and Sperling (1974) argue that a single common dimension underlies perception when two or more sensory systems are used. For example, we can localize an object through vision and through audition. Rather than possessing a "visual direction" or an "auditory direction," we judge direction via a common directional dimension, independent of the two senses that provided the information. The many experiences that contribute to a child's perceptual development are typically intersensory; thus, it is more accurate to view intrasensory refinement and intersensory integration as interrelated processes.

The Development of Sensory Integration

Visual-Kinesthetic Integration. Because sensory refinement and integration are interrelated processes, the discussion of the course of development in sensory integration is based on visual-kinesthetic, visual-auditory, and auditory-kinesthetic integration. Goodnow (1971a) conducted a series of experimental studies of sensory integration in children. In an initial study involving visual and kinesthetic integration, Goodnow presented five shapes (Greek and Russian letters) by either sight or feel to three age-groups (5.0 to 5.5-year-olds, 5.6- to 6.8-year-olds, and 9.0- to 10.0-year-olds). She then presented these five shapes with five new ones, again by sight or feel, and challenged the children to identify the familiar shapes. The four presentation patterns possible were: (a) visual presentation-visual recognition (V-V), (b) kinesthetic presentation-kinesthetic recognition (K-K), (c) visual presentation-kinesthetic recognition (V-K), and (d) kinesthetic presentation-visual recognition (K-V). The judgments required of the children represent the second level of sensory integration, that is, the integration of the features of stimulus information. Goodnow found that children, especially the youngest ones, had more difficulty in the K-K pattern than in the V-V pattern. This performance discrepancy narrowed in the older age-groups. The K-V task proved more difficult for the children than the V-K task. Goodnow noted that scores of the youngest group in the kinesthetic conditions were extremely variable. This study and others, using similar tasks and different age-groups, lead us to the conclusion that visual-kinesthetic integration improves with age. When the kinesthetic task involves active manipulation of an object, recognition is relatively good in 5-year-olds, but slight improvement continues until age 8. If passive movements are involved, performance is not as advanced and improvements continue through age 11 (Williams, 1983).

Visual-Auditory Integration. Goodnow (1971b) also examined visual-auditory integration. She presented an auditory-visual task by tapping out a sequence (∗ ∗∗∗) and then asking children to write the sequence, using dots to picture "where the taps came." This auditory-visual (A-V) task could be reversed by asking children to tap out a pictured sequence (V-A). Children around age 5 did not perform the A-V sequence as well as children at age 7. A trend toward improved performance on the V-A sequence was also found between the ages of 6.9 and 8.5 years. The result of this experiment and similar studies with other groups indicates that visual and auditory integration improves over the age span of 5 to 12 (Williams, 1983), with young children finding A-V tasks more difficult than V-A tasks. Performance differences due to order of sensory presentation, however, diminish after age 7 (Rudel & Teuber, 1971).

Auditory-Kinesthetic Integration. The amount of research conducted on auditory-kinesthetic integration is small compared with the amount involving vision. Temple et al. (1979) included the Witeba Test of Auditory-Tactile Integration in a test battery administered to 6- and 8-year-olds. In this test, an experimenter twice says the name of an object or shape to a child. The child then feels a number of objects or shapes, attempting to select the one that matches the auditory label. The investigators found that 8-year-olds were much better than 6-year-olds. Based on limited data, then, auditory-kinesthetic integration improves in childhood. In summary, then, sensory integration improves in childhood, and the accuracy of children's performance depends upon the order of sensory presentation, with vision-first presentation yielding better performance than auditory-first presentation.

Spatial-Temporal Integration. Another aspect of integration involves the spatial-temporal characteristics of the task to be performed. Recall Goodnow's second experiment. When children viewed the dot pattern, they were dealing with a spatial stimulus. When they listened to an auditory pattern, they were attending to a temporal (time) stimulus. Sterritt, Martin, and Rudnick (1971) devised nine tasks that varied not only the number of sensory integrations to be made, but the type of integration, including spatial-temporal characteristics. That is, a short pause between two tones (temporal) must be integrated with a short space between two dots (spatial). The nine tasks were presented to 6-year-olds. The easiest task for the children was the V-V spatial (intrasensory) task. Intermediate in difficulty were those tasks requiring the integration of visual spatial stimuli and visual *or* auditory temporal stimuli. The children found integration of two temporal patterns difficult, whether the task was intra- or intersensory. While progressing in intersensory integration, then, children also improve their ability to integrate spatial and temporal stimuli as well as improve the ability to integrate two sets of temporal stimuli.

Summary 6.2—Intersensory Integration

Infants have a limited ability to integrate basic sensory stimuli, but during childhood higher levels of sensory integration are attained. Improvements in intersensory integration occur simultaneously with, rather than after, improvements in intrasensory development. Children also learn to integrate sensory stimuli along a spatial-temporal dimension. Spatial-spatial integration tasks are mastered first, followed by mixed spatial and temporal tasks, and finally temporal-temporal tasks. Hence, we generally know the course of intersensory and intrasensory development.

Concept 6.3   Assessment of perceptual-motor development can detect deficiencies that directly affect skill performance.

Our discussions of intra- and intersensory development stressed the importance of perception to motor skill performance. But, consider a child learning to read or to add two-digit numbers. The form of letters and numbers, their orientation in space (such as "d" or "b"), and the direction of their processing (left-to-right in reading, but right-to-left in adding) are just a few aspects of perception that must be mastered before a child can perform these cognitive activities. Obviously, perception is important to cognition. Is there a link then between perceptual-motor functioning and cognitive functioning?

Several theories were proposed during the late 1950s and 1960s that suggested the two are directly linked. One assumption was that deficiencies in cognitive functioning (typically reading) due to faulty perceptual judgments could be identified by perceptual-motor test batteries and remedied by training a child on perceptual-motor activities requiring those perceptual judgments. Among these theories is the neurological organization theory of Delacato (1959, 1966), the physiological optics program of Getman (1952, 1963) (see Cratty, 1979, for a review of these two programs), the visual perception tests and the program of Frostig, Lefever, and Whittlesey (1966), the sensory-integration tests of Ayres (1972), the movigenics theory of Barsch (1965), and the perceptual-motor theory of Kephart (1971). Of course, the value of such programs rests on the assumption that perceptual-motor functioning and cognitive functioning are linked. Before we can accurately assess the value of perceptual-motor activity programs we must examine this proposed perceptual-motor/cognitive link more closely. We will do this, first, by examining one of the most popular theories, that of Kephart, as well as its accompanying test battery and program. Although each of the theories varies in its strengths and weaknesses, the Kephart theory represents the basic tenets of most such theories.

Kephart's Theory

Newell C. Kephart, a clinical psychologist, proposed one of the better-known and most popular perceptual-motor programs. The basis of Kephart's theory is that perception and cognition develop from a motor base, in that a child must establish motor "generalizations" to reach full intellectual growth. Kephart emphasized the generalizations of posture and balance, laterality, locomotion, contact, receipt and propulsion, and body image. He outlined seven developmental stages that represent increasingly efficient information-processing strategies. A child must learn the stages sequentially and completely, or later learning at higher levels will be deficient.

Stages of Perceptual-Motor Development

The first of these stages is the Motor Stage, during which an infant gains control of bodily experiences through kinesthetic information and begins to learn laterality, the internal sense of sidedness. This stage is achieved in late infancy. In the next stage, Motor-Perceptual, both visual and auditory information become more important, and perceptual data is matched with motor data. A sense of directionality, the projection of laterality into space, is developed in this stage, which spans early childhood up to approximately 4 years of age. The Perceptual-Motor Stage is next. Vision plays a larger role in exploration of the environment; hence, perception now takes the lead in perceptual-motor matches, while hand movement confirms visual information. At approximately 5 years of age the child enters the Perceptual Stage, when he or she can compare objects in the environment without motor involvement. In the Perceptual-Conceptual Stage, the child of 7 to 10 years of age is capable of abstracting the common properties of a class of things, such as dogs or automobiles. Subsequently, the child can integrate present and past perceptual information and reaches the Conceptual Stage. In the final stage, Conceptual-Perceptual, conception dominates the perceptual process. This stage is achieved after age 11 (Ball, 1971).

In Kephart's view, normal children proceed automatically through these sequences, but a slowly learning child either does not progress through the sequences or is markedly delayed (Kephart, 1971). Any child who skipped a stage or left it uncompleted must be returned to that stage, and by training, subsequently moved through the remaining stages. Supplementary experiences, then, are needed to enhance the development of children who are developmentally delayed. Kephart further suggested that providing perceptual-motor activities for all children, especially in the preschool years, decreases the likelihood that a stage would be left incomplete or skipped entirely.

The Purdue Perceptual-Motor Survey

Kephart and a colleague, Eugene C. Roach, proposed the Purdue Perceptual-Motor Survey (PMS) to help educators identify children whose perceptual-motor abilities are insufficient for the acquisition of academic skills (Roach & Kephart, 1966). The Purdue PMS is intended for boys and girls 6 to 10 years of age and includes 22 items, each scored on a 4-point scale for a maximum score of 88. The survey items are divided into five categories: (a) balance and posture, (b) body image and differentiation, (c) perceptual-motor match, (d) ocular control, and (e) form perception. For survey scores to be meaningful to educators, average scores or "norms" are needed. Roach and Kephart gathered and reported normative data based on 200 children, but all were from one school. Although the children were divided into six socioeconomic groups, it is not clear that the range available in this one school represented all of the socioeconomic groups that might be given the survey. Any test or survey of this type also should yield a *reliable* score, that is, a score that is essentially the same for the same child regardless of the particular day the survey is taken. This test characteristic is estimated by retesting a number of participants and correlating their two scores. The test-retest reliability reported for the Purdue PMS is .946, a high correlation. The authors also correlated the scores of the normative group with their teachers' ratings to establish validity, the ability of a test to measure what it is intended to measure, and obtained an estimated concurrent validity of .654. This moderate correlation was considered acceptable by the authors.

Kephart (1971) proposed a training program for those identified as "slow learners" by poor performance on the Purdue PMS. The types of activities included are perceptual-motor, perceptual-motor matching, ocular control, chalkboard training, and form perception. Some are similar to test items in the Purdue PMS. The skills are presented in a hierarchy, with the gross motor activities trained first, followed by fine motor skills. Eye-hand coordination, eye movement control, and perceptual monitoring of motor activities are highlighted.

To summarize Kephart's program, we might outline the assumptions made in his theory, survey, and training program. First, Kephart assumes that perception and cognition are linked by a common motor base. Certain motor generalizations are necessary for attainment of full intellectual functioning. Slow learners are those who have not proceeded through the developmental stages in the proper time frame. These children may be identified by the Purdue Perceptual-Motor Survey and restored to the normal course of development by a training program of perceptual-motor activities. Kephart also assumed that developmental problems may be forestalled by early (preschool) training in perceptual-motor activities.

Critiques of Kephart's Theory

The foundation of Kephart's theory is the perception-cognition link through a motor base. Is there evidence that such a link exists? Well, there is evidence that *perceptual-motor* development and *perception* are linked in early development. Held and Hein (1963) conducted a study in which they eliminated motor activity for some newborn kittens while providing them with visual experiences identical to other kittens who were allowed to move freely (see Figure 6.7). The restricted kittens later failed to make accurate depth perception judgments and to exhibit paw placing or eye blinking to an approaching object. Evidently, self-produced movement is related to the development of behavior requiring visual perception. The feedback produced by such movements is used to modify perceptual processes, implying a perceptual-motor/perceptual link, but *not* cognitive link.

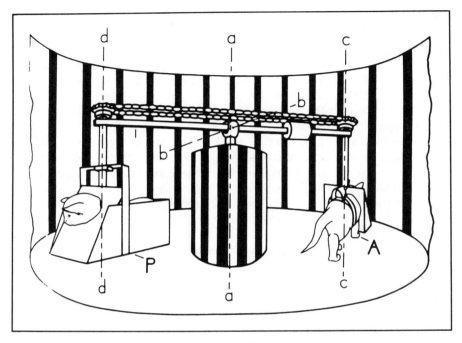

Figure 6.7 The apparatus used by Held and Hein for equating motion and consequent visual feedback for an actively moving (A) and a passively moved (P) animal. From "Movement-produced stimulation in the development of visually guided behavior," by R. Held and A. Hein, 1963, *Journal of Comparative and Physiological Psychology*, **56**, 873. Copyright 1963 by the American Psychological Association. Reprinted by permission.

Strong evidence of a perceptual-motor/cognitive link is lacking. Most studies have reported little or no relationship among *perceptual-motor* development, *perception*, and *cognition* (Williams, 1983). The behavioral study undertaken by Belka and Williams (cited in Williams, 1983) is an example. These investigators tested two subdomains of perceptual-motor behavior, gross and fine, on 63 children, age 5, 6, and 7 years. They included two subdomains of perception, vision, and audition. A standardized test appropriate for each age level measured cognitive behavior. Belka and Williams found perceptual-motor behavior and perceptual behavior to be related only in the younger groups, indicating that the close link between the two domains might diminish with age. Perception and cognition were related at all ages. In contrast, relationships between *perceptual-motor* and *cognitive* behavior were low and only significant at age 6. This and similar studies indicate that the perceptual-motor/cognitive link is indirect, if it exists at all. Hence, Kephart's basic theoretical assumption of a perceptual-motor/cognitive link has no strong experimental support.

Slow Learners

Kephart advocated a perceptual-motor training program for slow learners who are of normal intelligence but a year or more behind in achievement, that is, delayed in cognitive development. Slow learners often display sensory-perceptual judgments appropriate for children at a younger age (Williams, 1983). The same is true of performance on perceptual-motor tasks. Although this may indicate that delayed development in several domains is related, it is still not strong evidence of a direct link between perceptual-motor and cognitive functioning. Without such evidence there is little reason to assume that perceptual-motor training would improve cognitive functioning. Indeed, little research evidence shows that visual-motor training like that recommended by Kephart improves performance. Goodman and Hamill (1973) reviewed 16 well-designed experimental studies on this topic and found that the overwhelming majority failed to show that children improved on readiness skills, intelligence, achievement, language, or the visual-motor skills themselves with training on visual-motor skills.

Perceptual-Motor Deficiencies Versus Cognitive Deficiencies

Kephart's assessment tool, the Purdue Perceptual-Motor Survey, should be considered. It is doubtful that the survey is the best method of identifying children with academic deficiencies, because the perceptual-motor/cognitive link cannot be substantiated. On the other hand, the Purdue PMS may be useful in identifying children with *perceptual-motor* deficiencies. Adequate directions and scoring criteria are given for the survey, and a minimum of special equipment is necessary. It is easy to administer, but the tester should be trained to give the tests. The survey does need further standardization and cross-validation (Buros, 1972). So, the Purdue PMS can be used to screen children for perceptual-motor deficiencies. Kephart's training activities may be helpful to children with such deficiencies, providing a variety of experiences that can help children refine their perceptual-motor skills. However, its usefulness as a means for cognitive development in children remains questionable.

Summary 6.3—Perceptual-Motor Assessment and Uses

We reviewed Kephart's theory, survey, and training program as an example of the many perceptual-motor theories and programs. Each theory is slightly different and stresses certain aspects of perceptual-motor development more than other aspects, and each should be thoroughly reviewed and critiqued before use. But many of the basic assumptions are similar. Generally, they propose that perceptual-motor and cognitive functioning are directly linked, that perceptual-motor assessments can identify slow learners, and that the slow learners can improve their cognitive functioning by participating in perceptual-motor activity programs. In fact, little evidence currently exists for anything but a weak link between the two domains, leaving the assessments and training programs inappropriate for their intended purpose. Despite this, perceptual-motor surveys can be used to assess perceptual-motor skills, and programs can provide practice experiences for all children and remedial opportunities for those whose perceptual-motor development is delayed. The importance of perceptual-motor responses in skilled performance has been firmly established. Because childhood is a time of perceptual improvement and refinement, perceptual-motor programs may help provide children with the opportunity to reach their full potential for perceptual-motor performance.

Concept 6.4   Children refine their perceptual-motor skills through practice of perceptual-motor activities.

We have established that the sensory systems of infants are at least minimally functional. Infants can differentiate the facial features of a nearby person, right their heads and bodies reflexively, and localize sound. But beyond this, perceptual judgments and perceptual-motor responses must be refined during early childhood so that children can undertake both complex motor skills and higher-order thought processes. Recall that all physical skills are, to some extent, perceptual-motor skills, and that early childhood is certainly a time when children acquire the skills to function in their physical environment. What would happen if a child were confined to a hospital bed throughout these early years? The Held and Hein (1963) study on kittens discussed earlier would lead us to conclude that movement experiences are vital to normal perceptual-motor development. Although this study involved animals, it seems readily apparent that children also require experience in perceptual-motor responses to truly master their environment. The studies of Dennis (1940, 1963) discussed in concept 3.3 also demonstrated the negative effects on motor skill of prolonged sensory and motor deprivation in infancy. Most children acquire basic perceptual-motor skills naturally by engaging in numerous activities during their early years. Will these unplanned, chance experiences be broad enough to involve every aspect of perception? Will they sufficiently optimize perceptual-motor skills? Are perceptual-motor opportunities adequate for every child? Most educators think not and thus include perceptual-motor activities in the regular physical education, music, and early childhood curricula. These activities expose children to a wide range of stimuli and provide opportunities to explore and practice perceptual-motor responses. As a result, children gradually master their physical environment and become increasingly confident in their abilities. We will review the aspects of perception as they would be required in the performance of a motor skill. In some physical education and early childhood programs, educators prefer to teach these aspects of perceptual-motor development as a self-standing, supplementary program. Other educators incorporate these experiences into everyday curricular activities.

Benefits of Perceptual-Motor Activities

A comprehensive activities program includes skills requiring visual, kinesthetic, and auditory perception so that children acquire experience in all three areas. Recall that children must refine their ability to *integrate* information from two or more perceptual systems, too. Activities requiring intersensory integration, then, are also desirable. Those aspects of perceptual-motor development that provide experiences for intersensory development and intrasensory integration are presented now.

Visual Perception

Form Perception. One aspect of visual space orientation is form perception, that is, the ability to recognize forms and shapes regardless of their orientation, size, color, etc. Many teachers use geometric shapes as targets for a beanbag or ball toss or challenge children to travel along various geometric shapes taped to the floor. In this way children experience the shapes in many orientations and sizes and learn to match a name to the shape.

Figure-Ground Perception. In many catching and striking skills, the performer must attend to a ball approaching from a confusing, multicolored background. Children eventually need practice with such perceptual displays, but early in learning they will benefit from a simpler display. For example, balls and backgrounds of contrasting solid colors should be provided when possible. The contrast between ball and background can be gradually lessened or the background made more complex as a child acquires skill.

Distance and Depth Perception. Distance and depth perception should also be refined in childhood. Recall that depth perception is related to visual acuity.

Children who have great difficulty judging depth should be referred to an eye care specialist for examination. Fine judgments of depth and distance are practiced in many ways. You might set up a throwing task with targets at varying distances, challenging the children to judge the distance to each target and gauge their throw accordingly. This activity involves kinesthesis, too, because children must learn to vary the force of the throw.

Spatial Awareness. It is often necessary to make judgments about space based on visual information. A simple form of this perception is to locate objects in space. A more difficult task is to view a space and judge whether the body can fit through it. Children practice this visual-kinesthetic task when they climb on playground apparatus. Openings in the apparatus can be made in geometric shapes to involve form perception.

Kinesthetic Perception

Body Awareness. Body awareness or body image is an important aspect of kinesthesis. Recall that body awareness involves perception of the locations and names of the body parts, their relation to one another (including joint position), and movement of specific body parts. Children can practice touching and naming body parts on cue ("touch your wrist," "touch your heel to your knee"), forming various shapes such as letters and numbers with their bodies, and moving a body part on cue ("shake your foot").

Laterality. Laterality is an awareness that the body has two distinct sides. A popular activity for practicing left-and-right side movements is "Angels in the Snow." Lying on his or her back, a child is asked to move two limbs in an arc along the floor. Combinations are varied to include same-side and opposite-side pairs. When done in the snow or sand, the outline of an angel is traced, hence the name. Children can also be challenged to make symmetrical and nonsymmetrical shapes. Left-right discriminations are practiced in many ways. Simple rhythmic activities often require steps or hops to be taken on a particular foot.

Spatial Dimensions. Much attention is often focused on laterality and left-right discrimination in perceptual-motor programs, but awareness of other body dimensions is equally important. These dimensions include up-down, front-back, and side. Many activities involve spatial dimensions. One of the most enjoyable activities for children is a lummi stick routine to music wherein sticks are tapped in front of the body, in back, to the side, and so forth in rhythmical patterns.

Crossing the Body's Midline. Many motor skills require alternate patterns of movement on the right and left sides (skipping, swimming) or movements of the limbs from one side, across the body's midline, to the other side (batting). Simple activities that practice crossing the midline include chalkboard drawings such as connecting dots placed on the child's right and left. Basic skills, such as skipping and striking skills, also demand alternate patterns or crossing the midline.

Lateral Dominance. Most of us prefer the primary use of one of our hands, feet, and eyes and the other as secondary, or supportive. In most activity programs, teachers allow children to learn skills first with their preferred limb. Eventually children are prompted to attempt skills with the other limb. In many sports, it is desirable to master some skills with both limbs. Soccer kicking and basketball dribbling are two examples.

Tactile Discrimination. Touch is an important aspect of kinesthetic perception and is related to accurate body awareness. Children need experience in localizing touches, and discriminating multiple touches and varied surfaces. Teachers often vary the texture of the surfaces that children contact. It is also fun and valuable to play games in which children are blindfolded and challenged to identify or match objects and textures.

Directionality. Directionality is an aspect of directional awareness that is often linked to laterality. It refers to the ability to project the body's spatial dimensions into surrounding space. Teachers can guide practice of directionality by cueing children to place objects in relation to their body (i.e., "put the hoop in front of you, now over you, now to your left side"). Eventually, relationships between objects can be practiced ("place the hoop behind the chair"). Cueing children to move in a particular direction gives them practice as well. When children are still unsure of left and right, they can be reminded of the appropriate label by identifying their right or left hand or foot. Marching and other rhythmic activities offer many opportunities to move in various directions.

Balance. Among the elements of the kinesthetic system are the vestibular apparatus and receptors in the head and neck muscles, tendons, and joints. Sensations from these receptors provide information important to our sense of balance, an integral part of most skill performance. Balance is specific to the environmental situation (i.e., whether one is stationary or moving, elevated or on the ground, has eyes open or closed, is supported by one, two, or more body parts, etc.) rather than general for all balance tasks. For this reason it is important for children to experience a wide range of balancing tasks. Activities should be variable, including stationary and moving skills, experiences at different elevations (on the floor and on apparatus), balances on different body parts, and experiences with the eyes open and closed.

Auditory Perception

Auditory Localization. The ability to listen for auditory cues and identify the source of a sound is important for everyday life as well as motor performance. For example, in crossing a busy street, sound is used to help locate traffic. Many traditional games have a "listening" component, such as "Mother May I?" "Red Light," and "Simon Says." Children can practice locating a sound by playing games such as "Where Is the Bell?" (Gallahue, 1982). One child leaves the room while another child is given a jingle bell small enough to conceal in his or her hand. The group forms a circle and shakes their fists above their heads when the child returns. The child must locate the classmate with the bell.

Auditory Discrimination and Figure-Ground Perception. Discrimination and auditory figure-ground perception involve attention to one specific sound amidst a background of varied sounds. Children enjoy practicing sound discrimination when they are challenged to change movement directions on a sound cue. The teacher may tap a beat softly on a drum, but the children must change the direction they are traveling every time they hear a loud sound. The teacher could also play music and periodically sound a bell as a signal. Note that this activity also involves directionality.

Summary 6.4—Perceptual-Motor Activities

Practice with activities requiring a response based on perception of a stimulus helps children improve their level of skill performance. The aspects of perception involved in skill performance are many and varied. Therefore, comprehensive physical education and early childhood programs should include a variety of tasks requiring visual, kinesthetic, and auditory perceptual-motor responses as well as tasks requiring intersensory integration.

Suggested Readings

Corbin, C.B. (1980). *A textbook of motor development* (2nd ed.). Dubuque, IA: William C. Brown.

Williams, H. (1983). *Perceptual and motor development*. Englewood Cliffs, NJ: Prentice Hall.

Physiological Changes and Exercise Over the Life Span

Physical fitness is multifaceted. It is comprised of several factors, or components, such as endurance and strength. Fitness in one component does not guarantee fitness in another. For example, an individual may be very strong but not very flexible. The components of fitness that we will discuss in detail are endurance, strength, flexibility, and body composition. Some writers describe additional components of fitness, such as agility and power, but the first four are the essential components. Potentially, physical fitness can be improved through a systematic program of exercise aimed at these four components. Our discussion of the fitness components begins with endurance for vigorous activity, or *working capacity*.

Concept 7.1   Working capacity increases with physical growth and with training.

Of all the fitness components, working capacity has the greatest implications for lifelong health, but at the same time its development in children is surrounded by many myths. It was thought for many years that the cardiovascular-respiratory system of children limited their capacity for extended work. Despite the fact that a misinterpretation of blood vessel size, as mentioned in chapter 2, contributed to this view and was discovered soon after, the myth persisted for decades (Karpovich, 1937). Too, many parents and teachers feel that children automatically get enough exercise to become and remain fit, and consequently, they do not believe that it is necessary to promote physical fitness for children. Recent studies (Bailey, 1976; Gilliam, Katch, Thorland, & Weltman, 1977) tend to counter this view by showing that the sedentary lifestyle adopted by many adults in modern society has spilled over to the lives of their children. A high percentage of children and teens already exhibit one or more of the risk factors for coronary heart disease. Concern is rising that children in poor physical condition are likely to remain so throughout their adult lives. Educators and exercise leaders must thoroughly understand working capacity development and potential so that children can be challenged to attain an appropriate level of fitness for vigorous activity.

Our discussion of working capacity begins with the basic physiologic adaptations to whole-body exercise that requires endurance. But keep in mind that performance on endurance tests reflects a variety of factors. People with good neuromuscular coordination can move more efficiently and are likely to perform longer than those less coordinated. Cultural factors, too, influence performance because cultural norms sometimes dictate whether vigorous physical activity for endurance and all-out effort is socially acceptable or not. Realizing that factors such as these play a role in endurance capacity, we now focus on those factors that directly influence working capacity. Basic physiological responses of the body to increased demand of vigorous activity and changes in these responses that occur throughout growth will be reviewed. Lastly, we will discuss the changes that tend to occur with aging and how they affect an older adult's capacity for prolonged activity.

Physiologic Responses to Short-Term Exercise

Vigorous physical activity can be a short burst of intense activity, a long period of submaximal or maximal work, or a combination of these. Our bodies meet the demands of brief, intense activity and longer, more moderate activity with different physiologic responses. During a brief period of intense activity the body responds by depleting local reserves of oxygen and phosphate compounds and by breaking down glycogen (energy reserves) to lactic acid. This creates a deficit of oxygen that must eventually be replenished. The rate at which the body can meet this demand for short-term, intense activity is called *anaerobic power*, and the maximum oxygen deficit that can be tolerated is called *anaerobic capacity*. Adaptation to the demands of short-term, intense activity is much the same in children as it is in adults. A major difference may be that children possess a smaller absolute quantity of energy reserves because they have less muscle mass (Eriksson, 1978; Shephard, 1982). Measures of anaerobic power, such as 50-yd dash performance, show a steady improvement in children with increasing age, and consequently, body size. Remember that increased coordination and skill are partially responsible for some of this anaerobic power improvement, too.

Anaerobic capacity is also smaller in children than adults, again because of their smaller body size and their lower concentrations of some of the enzymes involved in the breakdown of glycogen (Shephard, 1982). As body size increases, increased anaerobic capacity (oxygen deficit tolerance) is a natural outcome. Beyond the natural change accompanying children's growth, evidence indicates that anaerobic capacity can be improved through training on anaerobic activities (Grodjinovsky, Inbar, Dotan, & Bar-Or, 1980).

Once adult body size is attained, improvement in anaerobic power and capacity is achieved through training alone. It is not clear, however, whether anaerobic power and capacity necessarily decline with advancing age. Indications that anaerobic power and capacity are significantly lower in 65-year-olds than 25-year-olds should be viewed with caution, because such results could reflect in part the reluctance or inability of older adults to undertake an all-out effort in anaerobic tests such as sprinting up a flight of stairs (Shephard, 1978b).

Physiologic Responses to Prolonged Exercise

How do our bodies sustain submaximal physical activity for prolonged periods? Unlike short-term exercise, the energy for prolonged exercise is derived from the oxidative breakdown of food stores in addition to the local reserves depleted in the first few minutes of exercise. The rate at which we meet this long-term oxygen demand is termed *aerobic power*. Sustained, prolonged activity then depends on the transportation of sufficient oxygen to the working muscles for longer periods of time. Heart and respiration rates, cardiac output, and oxygen use increase to deliver the oxygen needed for prolonged activity. Increased respiration rate brings more oxygen to the lungs, making it available for diffusion into the bloodstream. Cardiac output, the amount of blood pumped into the circulatory system, increases, allowing more oxygen to reach the muscles. For the most part, increased cardiac output is achieved by increased heart rate and increased stroke volume. Changes in stroke volume during exercise are relatively small, but one of the benefits of training is greater initial stroke volume. The limiting factor to continued vigorous activity is the heart's ability to pump enough blood to meet the oxygen needs of the working muscles. In very heavy activity the heart rate rises throughout the session until exhaustion ends the activity. When vigorous activity is stopped, the heart rate drops quickly for 2 to 3 min, then more gradually for a time span related to the duration and intensity of the activity. This description is necessarily a brief summary of the physiological responses to exercise. A more detailed treatment is available in exercise physiology textbooks (c.f. DeVries, 1980; Fox & Mathews, 1981; Sharkey, 1984).

Assessment

There are several methods of assessing the physiological responses to sustained activity. A common measure of fitness for endurance activities is "maximum oxygen consumption" (Heyward, 1984). The more efficiently the body uses oxygen, that is, consumes less oxygen for the same amount of work performed, the more fit the individual. In a test of maximum oxygen consumption, the actual amount of oxygen consumed during activity is measured or estimated. This score is typically expressed as oxygen consumed per minute per kilogram of body weight. Maximum oxygen consumption is a common measure of endurance in studies of children and older adults because it can be estimated from an exercise period of limited length and intensity (a submaximal test), thus avoiding the need for an exercise bout to exhaustion (a maximal test). Too, direct measures of oxygen use require more sophisticated and expensive equipment than that needed for estimates from submaximal tests.

Another measure of physiologic response to prolonged exercise is that of maximal "working capacity," which means the highest work load that can be tolerated before exhaustion is reached (Adams, 1973). Because maximal effort is required, it may be difficult to motivate individuals to work to exhaustion, and the rare possibility of heart attack exists during such a test. For this reason it may not be advisable to ask children to exercise to exhaustion. Estimates of working capacity from submaximal working capacity tests remain the preferred procedure for testing children and older adults.

Other measures of endurance fitness are less common. For example, maximal cardiac output can be measured directly, but this test is difficult to administer because it requires intubation. Measurement of electrocardiograph changes during exercise is of interest when studying adults (Heyward, 1984), but not very applicable for most children because its main purpose is to identify impaired heart function. Hence, the most applicable measures of endurance fitness in children and older adults for research purposes remain maximum oxygen consumption and working capacity based on submaximal exercise efforts. Recently, several investigators attempted to identify field tests for children that estimate endurance nearly as reliably as measured in a laboratory. Maximum oxygen consumption scores from laboratory tests were compared with performance in 800-m, 1,200-m, and 1,600-m runs for 83 children in grades 1, 2, and 3. The 1,600-m run was the best predictor of maximum oxygen consumption for both boys and girls. An average velocity score on the 1,600-m run had a slightly higher correlation with maximum oxygen consumption than a total time score. It can be concluded that a 1,600-m run is a useful field test of endurance in children. This test also proved to have a high test-retest reliability (Krahenbuhl, Pangrazi, Petersen, Burkett, & Schneider, 1978).

Development

How do children respond physiologically to prolonged activity? Children tend to have "hypokinetic" circulation (Bar-Or, Shephard, & Allen, 1971); that is, their cardiac output is less than an adult's. This smaller cardiac output reflects children's: (a) smaller body size and, consequently, smaller demand for oxygen; (b) advantage in dissipating heat from a small body with a relatively large surface area; and (c) ability to readily extract oxygen within the muscles (Shephard, 1982). The tendency of hypokinetic circulation is gradually reduced with growth and training. Children also have a lower blood hemoglobin concentration than adults. Hemoglobin concentration is related to the blood's ability to carry oxygen. You might assume that these two factors, the hypokinetic circulation and low hemoglobin concentration, result in an oxygen transport system that is less efficient in children than in adults. However, children's ability to extract relatively more of the oxygen circulating to the active muscles seems to compensate for the first two limiting factors, which results in a comparatively effective oxygen transport system. Children do have a lower tolerance for extended periods of exercise than adults, ostensibly the result of smaller glycogen stores. When glycogen stores are exhausted, performance is limited.

Children exhibit comparable values of oxygen consumption to adults *if* consumption is measured relative to units of body weight. When *absolute* amounts of oxygen consumption are considered, children have smaller values than adults because absolute maximum oxygen consumption increases with growth in body size. Values of oxygen consumption measured across different age groups are shown in Table 7.1.

It is important to recognize the relationship between increasing body size and improving ability to sustain work during growth. With body growth comes increased heart and stroke volume, increased total hemoglobin, and increased lean body mass. These factors foster improved cardiac output, and subsequently, working capacity and absolute maximum oxygen consumption. Recalling how variable children are in size, despite their chronological age, you can see that evaluations of working capacity among children should be related to body size rather than age alone. In the past, evaluation has frequently

Table 7.1 Average Maximum Oxygen Consumption Over Ages 4 to 33

Variable	Sex	Age-Groups (yrs)						
		4 to 6	7 to 9	10 to 11	12 to 13	14 to 15	16 to 18 (M) 16 to 17 (F)	20 to 33 (M) 20 to 25 (F)
N	M	10	12	13	19	10	9	42
	F	7	14	13	13	11	10	44
Maximum oxygen consumption	M	1.01	1.75	2.04	2.46	3.53	3.68	4.11
	F	0.88	1.50	1.70	2.31	2.58	2.71	2.90
Maximum oxygen consumption/ kg body weight (ml/min)	M	49.1	56.9	56.1	56.5	59.5	57.6	58.6
	F	47.9	55.1	52.4	49.8	46.0	47.2	48.4

Note. Adapted from *Experimental Studies of Working Capacity in Relation to Sex and Age* by P. Åstrand, 1952, Copenhagen: Munksgoard.

been based only on age. Although one expects average working capacity and average body size to increase throughout childhood and adolescence, individual working capacity follows the spurts and plateaus of growth and must be considered independently.

Adulthood

Peak maximum oxygen consumption is reached in young adulthood. How well is it maintained into middle and older adulthood? Some information on this topic is available, but it remains difficult to separate the inevitable consequences of aging from those brought about by decreased activity levels. Accordingly, the available data sketch the norm for older adult groups who have gradually decreased their level of activity during middle and older adulthood, rather than indicating the limits of performance for those who remain active. Keeping this in mind, we now review the structural and functional changes in the cardiovascular and respiratory systems with aging.

Structural Cardiorespiratory Changes. The major structural changes in the nondiseased heart with advanced aging include a progressive loss of cardiac muscle, loss of elasticity in cardiac muscle fibers (Harrison, Dixon, Russell, Bidwai, & Coleman, 1964), and fibrotic changes in the heart valves (Pomerance, 1965). The major blood vessels also lose elasticity. Whether these changes are an unavoidable consequence of aging or a reflection of a chronic lack of oxygen is unclear. Heart volumes are well maintained in active older adults (Davies, 1972), and a few case histories of very active older adults indicate that excellent physiological functioning is maintained. For example, Clarence DeMar ran 12 miles per day throughout his lifetime and competed in marathons at age 65. The autopsy following his death from cancer at age 70 showed well developed cardiac muscle, normal valves, and coronary arteries 2 to 3 times the size normally seen (Brandfonbrener, Landowne, & Shock, 1955).

The consequences of these structural changes in the heart and blood vessels are numerous. The maximum achievable heart rate gradually declines with aging, although the decline is not as great as once thought. A 65-year-old man can attain a maximum rate of 170 beats/minute, for example, compared with 200+ beats/minute for children and young adults (Shephard, 1978a, 1981). Resting heart rate values for older adults are comparable to those of young adults. Similarly, the stroke volume of older adults is comparable to the young during *light* work loads but is reduced by 10% to 20% during *vigorous* activity (Becklake, Frank, Dagenais, Ostiguy, & Guzman, 1965; Grimby, Nilsson, & Saltin, 1966; Shephard, 1981). Since cardiac output is the product of heart rate and stroke volume—and neither of these is greatly reduced in older adults during light work—there is little difference between young and old adults in cardiac output under these conditions.

Functional Cardiorespiratory Changes. Older adults reach their *peak* cardiac output at a lower intensity of work than do younger adults (Brandfonbrener et al., 1955; Shephard, 1978a). The more rigid arteries of the older adult resist the volume of blood pumped into them by the heart. In turn, this resistance raises resting pulse pressure and systolic blood pressure. Whether blood pressure increases or decreases during exercise depends on the health of the cardiac muscle fibers and their ability to tolerate increased work load. During vigorous activity the blood pressure is typically higher in older adults than younger adults (Julius, Amery, Whitlock, & Conway, 1967; Sheffield & Roitman, 1973), but some postcoronary patients cannot sustain their systolic blood pressure as their work load increases (Shephard, 1979).

Pulmonary function may also impose limitations on older adults' physiologic responses to vigorous exercise. One of the important pulmonary function measurements is *vital capacity*, the maximum volume of air expelled from the lungs following maximal inspiration. A large vital capacity reflects a large inspiratory capacity of the lungs and results in better alveolar ventilation. Because the greatest part of oxygen diffusion to the capillaries takes place at the alveoli, better alveolar ventilation contributes to increased amounts of oxygen circulating in the blood and reaching the working muscles (see Figure 7.1). Vital capacity tends to increase with training. A sufficient number of capillaries in the lungs optimizes oxygen diffusion as well. Hence, a decreased vital capacity or decreased number of lung capillaries would detract from vigorous physical performance. A decreased vital capacity with aging is well established (Norris, Shock, Landowne, & Falzone, 1956; Shephard, 1978b) as is a reduced number of capillaries in the lungs (Reid, 1967). The change in vital capacity is probably related to a loss of elasticity in tissues of the lungs and chest wall (Turner, Mead, & Wohl, 1968). These pulmonary changes, though, are more dramatic in smokers than nonsmokers.

The result of all these changes is that maximum working capacity and maximum oxygen consumption (whether absolute or relative to body weight) decline with advancing age, and the recovery period following vigorous activity lengthens. Yet, there is evidence (Dehn & Bruce, 1972; Drinkwater, Horvath, & Wells, 1975; Kasch & Wallace, 1976; Shephard, 1978b; Smith & Serfass, 1981) that these changes are not as dramatic in older adults who remain active compared with those who become sedentary. Environmental factors contribute to many of the declines. A lifetime of negative environmental factors such as smoking or poor nutrition can be responsible for or accelerate the changes. In contrast, a lifetime of exposure to positive environmental factors such as healthful exercise can better maintain endurance levels. People who would like to maintain as much endurance as possible over their life

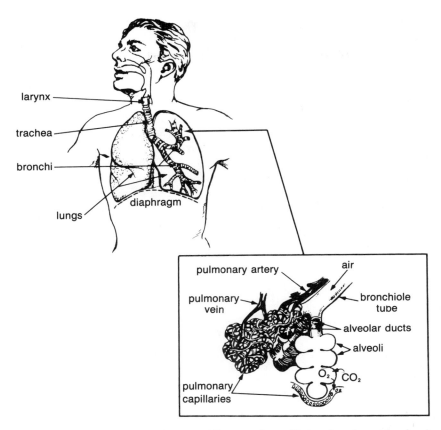

Figure 7.1 The respiratory system. Oxygen diffusion to the capillaries takes place at the alveoli, enlarged on the right. From *Physiology of Fitness* (2nd ed.) (p. 244) by B.J. Sharkey, 1984, Champaign, IL: Human Kinetics Publishers. Copyright 1984 by B.J. Sharkey. Reprinted by permission.

span are encouraged to stop smoking, eat properly, and follow an appropriate exercise program designed for endurance.

Gender Differences

Differences between boys and girls in maximum oxygen consumption and working capacity are mimimal before the adolescent growth spurt. During childhood, body size is a far better predictor of endurance than sex of the child. After puberty, though, boys on the average attain a considerable edge over girls in working capacity and absolute maximum oxygen consumption. Several factors contribute to this gender difference. One is body composition. The average man has more lean body mass and a smaller percentage of fat or adipose tissue than does the average woman. Interestingly, women are about equal to men in maximum oxygen consumption per kilogram of *fat-free* body mass, but when adipose tissue is included, women have a lower maximum oxygen consumption. Another factor in gender differences in oxygen consumption is the tendency for women to have lower hemoglobin concentrations than men (Åstrand, 1976). The average adolescent or adult man, then, has an edge over the average woman in both oxygen consumption and working capacity (see Table 7.2). This advantage is maintained through adulthood. Keep in mind that environmental factors influence the endurance capacities of individual men and women over the remainder of the life span. So it would not be surprising to find that an active woman has a higher maximum oxygen consumption than a sedentary man.

Table 7.2 The Physical Working Capacity at Heart Rate of 170 of Canadian School Children

Age (Year)	Boys		Girls	
	Absolute Value (Watts)	Relative Value (Watts·kg⁻¹)	Absolute Value (Watts)	Relative Value (Watts·kg⁻¹)
7	50	1.96	39	1.57
8	57	2.08	47	1.74
9	63	2.08	50	1.68
10	70	2.09	55	1.66
11	81	2.16	59	1.65
12	90	2.18	68	1.62
13	107	2.28	74	1.50
14	119	2.26	71	1.39
15	121	2.10	73	1.35
16	139	2.20	75	1.39
17	143	2.18	78	1.39

Note. Based on data of Howell & MacNab (1966). Measurements made in school classrooms, without habituation of subjects. Readings would probably be up to 10% higher, given climatic control (20 to 22° C) and some familiarization with experimental procedures. Measurements are in watts (1 watt = 6 kg m/min) and watts per kilogram of body weight. Reproduced with permission from Shephard, R.J.: *Physical Activity and Growth* (p. 70). Copyright 1982 by Yearbook Medical Publishers, Inc., Chicago.

Training

You may already know that adults who engage in vigorous activity 20 min or longer, at least 3 times per week, can improve their cardiovascular endurance. Such training results in a decrease in heart rate for a given exercise intensity (as the body becomes more efficient in transporting oxygen), increased heart volume, increased stroke volume, increased blood volume, and increased total hemoglobin. The result is greater working capacity (Adams, 1973).

Training Effect in Children.   Does the same training effect occur in children as in adults? Educators are interested in whether endurance in children can be improved with proper training. The answer is not as easily determined as you might think because of the confounding variable of continuous growth while studying children. Hence, no matter what their level of training, working capacity increases as a normal function of growth. Researchers must attempt to determine the influence of training above and beyond this increase due to growth. It is insufficient to point out that children and teens engaged in regular swimming or running programs have higher working capacities than their less-active peers. Such specialized programs might attract children who are big for their age, hence their greater working capacity. It is always difficult to compare active and nonactive children. Children in a nonactive group may not participate in specialized training programs but could be just as active as those who do through participation in less structured activities. All factors must be considered when examining the value of endurance training to children.

Consider two studies that are representative of the research conducted on children's training. The first examined training responses in untrained children 9 to 11 years old (Vaccaro & Clarke, 1978). These children were put on a training schedule in which they swam 3,000 to 10,000 yd per day, 4 days per week. After training 7 months, they had increased their average maximum oxygen consumption by 15%, while a control group increased only 5%. The swimmers similarly showed greater improvement in their working capacity than the control group (see Table 7.3). So this study indicated that children benefit from training. In the second study (Stewart & Gutin, 1976), 10- to 12-year-olds were randomly divided into two groups. One group was given interval training four times per week, while the other group participated in nonendurance activities (stretching and low intensity games). After 2 months no differences in maximum oxygen consumption between the two groups were evident. How can we account for the disparate findings of these two studies?

Table 7.3 Average Endurance Measures and Their Standard Deviations in Children Before and After Training

Study	Measure	Group	Pretraining M	SD	Posttraining M	SD
Stewart & Gutin (1976)	Maximum oxygen consumption (ml/kg/min)	Trained	49.8 ±	6.07	49.5 ±	6.12
		Control	48.4 ±	4.26	49.2 ±	5.16
Vaccaro & Clarke (1978)	Maximum oxygen consumption (ml/kg/min)	Trained	47.3 ±	8.20	55.4 ±	6.96
		Control	46.8 ±	6.58	49.0 ±	6.34
	Physical working capacity at HR = 170 (kgm/min)	Trained	400 ±	92.58	480 ±	116.18
		Control	380 ±	77.45	410 ±	68.66

Note. Data compiled from Stewart & Gutin (1976) and Vaccaro & Clarke (1978).

Critical research design differences exist between the two studies cited. First, Vaccaro and Clark's subjects were untrained before starting their relatively intensive training program. The interval training program used in the Stewart and Gutin study may not have been significantly more active in intensity than the ordinary activity level of the control group children. Another difference was the length of the respective training programs: 7 months versus 2 months. It may be that more than 2 months of training is necessary before significant improvements in the physiologic responses to training occur. When considered along with other similar investigations, indications are that children can improve their endurance beyond that occurring with normal growth if they engage in training programs *of sufficient intensity and duration*.

Training Programs for Children. It is not possible here to discuss training methods in detail, but some training concerns regarding children should be kept in mind. Training programs must be sufficiently intense and long enough to show improved endurance, but they could be so demanding that they are harmful to young children. What is a safe level of training intensity and duration for children? One of the principles followed in training is that of progressively "overloading" the body, meaning that the intensity/duration of each exercise bout is gradually increased over a period of weeks and months. This principle is valuable in programming for children. Teachers should begin by asking their students to exercise at a level comfortable for them. With this level as a baseline, an individualized program that gradually increases the exercise challenge for the child can be designed. A constant threat to a well-planned training program is the pressure that can be placed on children by adults. Children might attempt an exercise intensity above a reasonable level just to please a parent, win a valuable prize, or gain prestige among classmates. Such pressures must be minimized, enabling children to stop activity if they become overly fatigued.

Training Programs for Older Adults. Appropriate training results in improved endurance in children and young adults, but is the same effect true for older adults in light of the structural and functional changes discussed earlier? In fact, older adults can significantly increase their maximum oxygen consumption with a sufficient training program (Shephard, 1978b). Training also results in other improvements, including a faster recovery rate, increased stroke volume, decreased systolic blood pressure, and increased vital capacity. The guiding principle in design of training programs for older adults as well as for children is the *gradual* increase in the intensity and duration of exercise. A more extensive discussion of these improvements and training regimes for older adults is available in Shephard (1978b).

Long-Term Training Effects. Despite the favorable response of the body to training at any age, the question arises whether active youths have an advantage over sedentary ones in maintaining endurance into older adulthood. This aspect of fitness is ideally assessed through long-term longitudinal studies; however, difficulties in obtaining longitudinal data (expense and subject attrition) make such research nearly nonexistent. In the absence of such studies, consider a cross-sectional study conducted by Saltin and Grimby (1968), which measured the maximal oxygen consumption of three groups of men between 50 and 59 years of age. The first group was comprised of those who were nonathletes in their youth, the second of men formerly athletes but now sedentary, and the third of men who had been athletes and maintained an active lifestyle throughout adulthood. The investigators had to rely on self-reports (rather than laboratory data) to determine activity level. Even so, measures of maximum oxygen consumption yielded average values of 30, 38, and 53 ml/min/kg body weight for the nonathletes, sedentary former athletes, and active adults, respectively. Despite the limitations of this single study, the evidence suggests that regular activity in childhood has positive lifelong benefits. Nevertheless, the most important factor in endurance remains the *present* activity level. At all ages, the capacity for prolonged, vigorous work tends to be transitory. Endurance is maintained (or improved), if an individual is *currently* training for endurance; conversely, endurance capacity decreases when an individual discontinues his or her training program.

Effect of Diseases on Working Capacity

Teachers and coaches must keep in mind that some diseases reduce working capacity. These diseases fall into the categories of cardiovascular, pulmonary, infectious, and neuromuscular disease, although not all the diseases in these categories reduce working capacity. The cardiovascular diseases that reduce working capacity of children include cyanotic congenital heart disease (affecting oxygenation of the blood) and valvular disease (affecting the valves in the heart). However, children with congenital heart disease who survive infancy eventually demonstrate near-normal exercise performance. Whether a child with a cardiovascular disease must refrain from physical activity depends upon the particular disease involved (Shephard, 1982).

There are also a number of cardiovascular diseases that may affect the exercise performance of older adults. Among them are arteriosclerosis (hardening of the arteries), atherosclerosis (formation of lipid deposits in the arteries), ischemic heart disease (affecting the blood supply to the heart), and peripheral vascular disease (affecting circulation). Persons suffering from such diseases must be carefully monitored during physical activity. Although inactivity is a probable contributor to onset of these diseases, overly stressful activity after the disease is established could lead to cardiac failure. While the role of exercise in prevention and treatment of heart attack is still controversial, exercise is often used in rehabilitation programs following a heart attack. The major result is increased cardiac output. To be effective, rehabilitative exercise programs must be vigorous enough to create improvement without placing the participant at risk. Among the important guidelines for designing rehabilitative programs are establishment of a safe entry level into the program, gradual increase of intensity, and individual monitoring. Exercise leaders should work closely with a physician or exercise physiologist when designing or leading such programs.

Two pulmonary diseases that reduce working capacity in children are severe asthma (breathing difficulty due to temporary bronchial constriction) and cystic fibrosis (an exocrine gland disorder resulting in pancreatic insufficiency, chronic pulmonary disease, and excessive loss of salt). The amount of functional impairment in asthmatic children is variable. Some children show little effect, especially during periods of remission. In fact, some asthmatics who are placed on training programs demonstrate improved lung function, improved working capacity, and reduced amounts of adipose tissue (Walker, 1965). In other children, however, even light exercise induces bronchospasm (Shephard, 1982). Cystic fibrosis affects response to exercise as well as normal growth and development through a secondary lack of nutrients (Shephard, 1982).

Among the respiratory diseases that affect older adults are chronic bronchitis and emphysema. Chronic bronchitis is characterized by a recurrent cough, lasting at least 3 months in 2 successive years. Emphysema involves abnormal enlargement of the terminal air spaces in the lungs. In both of these obstructive lung diseases much of the oxygen breathed in during exercise is used by the respiratory muscles themselves. As a result, an unusually high portion of muscular effort is carried out anaerobically.

Infectious diseases, such as influenza, infectious mononucleosis, and chicken pox have variable effects on working capacity (Adams, 1973). It is important for a teacher or coach to keep this in mind when monitoring performance. Athletes desiring to maintain peak efficiency may expect to adhere to training schedules and performance levels during illness, but this is an impractical goal. Neuromuscular diseases do not affect physiologic responses to exercise directly, but they contribute to inefficient and uncoordinated performance. Inefficient movement can reduce working capacity because energy is expended on unnecessary movements.

Clearly, diseases have a variable effect on exercise performance, making cooperation and communication imperative among teachers and coaches, medical personnel, parents (in the case of children), and the participant. Activity may be beneficial in many cases, yet it should never place the participant at increased risk. The limits of activity, then, must be planned carefully, expectations set accordingly, and the participant monitored closely.

Summary 7.1—Working Capacity and Training

Endurance for vigorous activities improves as the body grows. In addition, endurance is increased at any age by training, although the effects are transitory. Training must be maintained to preserve higher levels of endurance. After the adolescent growth spurt, gender differences in working capacity are apparent. While the cause of these differences is still open to discussion, body size, body composition, and hemoglobin levels are at least partially involved. Societal norms and expectations often communicate to individuals, especially women, that all-out endurance efforts are inappropriate. These attitudes are changing, but complete acceptance takes many years, because the adults of today are products of their upbringing and they in turn tend to raise their children in the same manner they were raised. Some cardiovascular, pulmonary, infectious, and neuromuscular diseases reduce working capacity, so educators must work closely with the affected individual, parents (if appropriate), and medical personnel to plan appropriate endurance activities.

Concept 7.2   Muscle strength improves with age and with training, but muscle hypertrophy is linked to hormonal influence.

Keep in mind the earlier discussion of muscle growth in concept 2.3, as the improvement in muscle strength with training is reviewed. For example, consider a pair of twins, a boy and a girl, age 10. We know their muscle mass follows a sigmoid growth pattern and that this growth is largely due to an increase in muscle fiber diameter. But what about gains in muscle strength, that is, the ability to exert force? Strength tends to improve with increased muscle mass. Do strength gains simply follow the gains in muscle mass, or can the twins improve strength beyond that which accompanies muscle growth? First, consider that the amount of isometric force exerted by a muscle group depends on the fibers activated and on leverage. Further, the fibers activated depend on both the cross-sectional area of the muscle and the degree of coordination in activating the fibers. The cross-sectional area of muscle increases with growth so that strength increases with muscle growth. But does coordination of contractile effort improve at the same pace as muscle mass increases?

This question must be answered before the development of muscle strength in the twins can be described. We know from our earlier discussion that there are gender differences in the growth of muscle mass. What implications do these differences have for strength development in the twins? Could the twins be given an appropriate training program to improve their strength beyond that typically acquired with growth, and what implications might this have for maintenance or improvement of strength in their adult years?

Strength Development

If strength development directly followed muscle mass development, the peak gain in strength during childhood would coincide with the peak gain in muscle mass (see Table 7.4). Teachers and coaches then could predict chil-

Table 7.4 Development of Isometric Muscle Force (Newtons) in Selected Urban Populations

Sample	8	10	12	Age 14	16	18
Handgrip force						
Boys	146	192	240	348	491	527
Girls	134	168	226	291	343	343
Elbow flexion force (right arm)				*†		
Boys	128	164	216	301	344	—
Girls	114	149	192	176	217	—
Elbow extension force (right arm)				*†		
Boys	113	142	173	253	292	—
Girls	97	123	164	160	178	—
Knee extension force (right leg)				*†		
Boys	235	310	375	504	535	—
Girls	228	308	372	363	383	—
Leg lift force (dynamometer)				*†		
Boys	649	952	1275	1627	1906	—
Girls	577	903	1158	1014	1173	—
Back lift force (dyamometer)				*†		
Boys	360	476	644	889	959	—
Girls	318	421	574	607	633	—

*Based on data accumulated by Shephard (1978b) for handgrip and on unpublished results of Howell et al. (1968) for other muscle groups.
†In the sample of Howell et al. (1966), final column is for children one year older than the previous category (i.e., 15.6 years). Reproduced with permission from Shephard, R.J., *Physical Activity and Growth* (p. 104). Copyright 1982 by Yearbook Medical Publishers, Inc., Chicago.

dren's strength levels by measuring their muscle mass, which in turn could be estimated from weight measurements or calculations from both weight and skinfold measurements. In chapter 2 we noted that peak gain or velocity indicates the time of fastest growth. Several studies indicate that these peak gains do not coincide with one another. For example, Stolz and Stolz (1951) found that boys on the average reach their peak gain in strength approximately 6 to 9 months *after* their peak weight velocity and 1.6 years after their peak height velocity. Carron and Bailey (1974) generally confirmed this trend in finding that maximum gains in overall, upper body, and lower body strength occurred about 1 year after peak height and peak weight velocity in boys. Only one study examined strength development in girls with this method. Jones (1947) concluded that girls reach their peak growth rate at 12.5 years, on the average, but their near-adult levels of strength in a thrusting movement are reached at 13.5 to 14.0 years. Hence, this limited data on girls agree with the findings for boys.

Keep in mind that peak weight velocity is not necessarily equivalent to peak growth in muscle mass, because increasing body weight could reflect increasing fat weight as well as muscle weight. Tanner (1962), however, indicates that if peak weight and peak muscle mass velocity do not coincide, peak muscle mass velocity occurs *before* peak weight velocity. This widens the gap between peak muscle mass velocity and peak strength gain and lends support to the theory that muscles grow first in size and then in strength. Tanner (1962) suggests that this sequence probably results from the effects of adrenocortical and testicular hormones on the protein structure and enzyme systems of the muscle fibers.

Another way to examine muscle growth and strength development is to relate measures of muscle strength to various body sizes in children and determine whether or not strength increases at the same rate as body size. Asmussen and Heeboll-Nielsen (1955, 1956) took this approach in studying Danish children between 7 and 16 years of age. It was assumed that body height could represent changes in body size, including body weight; that is, body weight is proportional to the body height raised to the third power in this age-group. In fact, Asmussen and Heeboll-Nielsen showed this was approximately true for their Danish sample of boys and girls. The children then were grouped into height classes with 10 cm intervals and measured for isometric strength (exertion of force against immovable resistance). Successive height groups demonstrated increasing muscle strength, but at a rate greater than that of their height.

Asmussen and Heeboll-Nielsen also grouped boys of the same height into two age-groups, a younger group and an older group. The age difference was approximately 1½ years. Arm and leg strength were greater in the older subgroups than the younger by approximately 5% to 10% per year of age. The experimental work of Asmussen and Heeboll-Nielsen, then, also demonstrates that strength is not related to muscle size alone. As children mature, some factor other than muscle growth contributes to improved strength. This factor most likely is improved coordination of muscle fiber recruitment, that is, increased skill in using the muscles to exert force.

The studies mentioned thus far typically measured isometric strength directly, that is, with a cable tensiometer or a dynamometer. The benefit of measuring strength with this equipment is minimization of the effects of skill, practice, and experience. Yet, factors such as these are involved in the performance of sport skills. For this reason studies of *functional* muscle strength development are also important. Two skills that involve functional muscle strength are vertical jumping and sprinting. Performance on both is influenced by practice or experience but also leg strength. Asmussen and Heeboll-Nielsen (1955, 1956) also measured performance on these two skills in successive height groups of their Danish children. They found that functional muscle strength, like isometric strength, increased at a faster rate than would be anticipated from muscle growth alone. Further, the rate of functional muscle strength gain was even greater than that of isometric strength, emphasizing again the role of improved coordination and skill in improved muscle strength with advancing maturity.

Maximal levels of strength are recorded by men in young adulthood, on the average, and by women in adolescence, although cultural norms may influence the latter generalization. Recall from chapter 2 that there is a loss of muscle mass in advanced old age, a loss that can be as dramatic as 50% of the young adult level. This decrease of muscle mass is by loss of both muscle fiber number and size (atrophy), but the molecular mechanism of this loss is presently unclear. The loss is particularly noticeable in the muscles of the upper leg. It is not surprising, then, to find that strength losses of 18% to 20% are typical in old age (Shephard, 1978b), although they tend to be significant only after age 60 (Shock & Norris, 1970). Both isometric strength, the ability to exert force against immovable resistance, and dynamic strength, the ability to exert force against movable resistance, decline. As with so many other aspects of aging, it is impossible to distinguish with present information whether the loss of muscle mass and strength in old age is inevitable or a reflection of reduced activity levels.

Gender Differences

Boys and girls are similar in strength levels until about 13 years of age, although boys are slightly stronger than girls of the same height (Asmussen, 1973). Remember from chapter 2 that boys gain more muscle mass in adolescence than girls as a result of higher secretion levels of androgens. In fact, boys have a spurt of increased strength at approximately 13 years of age that corresponds to increased secretion of androgens. It is not surprising, then, that men are stronger on the average than women. In fact, women can produce only 60% to 80% of the force that men can exert, although most of these differences are attributable to differences in arm and shoulder strength rather than trunk or leg strength (Asmussen, 1973).

Only half of the difference in strength between men and women can be accounted for by the average difference in body or muscle size, so other factors must contribute to the difference. Cultural norms probably play a role in the sex differences in strength. For example, Shephard (1982) noted the effect of repeating strength measures on boys and girls. While the boys showed no tendency to improve over three visits, the girls improved on each subsequent visit in almost every case and improved significantly on two of the eight strength measures taken (see Table 7.5). While this effect could be attributed to learning, it is possible that the task gained acceptability to the girls as they became more familiar with it. Motivation should not be discounted as a major factor in strength measurement. Certainly, Shephard would have concluded

Table 7.5 Effect of Test Repetition on Measurements of Isometric Muscle Force (Results for 52 "Naive" Children Aged 9 Years, Tested at Intervals of 2 to 3 Days)

| | Muscle Force (Newtons) | | | | | |
| | Boys | | | Girls | | |
Measurement	Visit 1	Visit 2	Visit 3	Visit 1	Visit 2	Visit 3
Tensiometer technique (Clarke, 1966)						
Elbow flexion	195	192	201	174	177	186
Shoulder flexion	120	120	120	101	101	104
Hip flexion	218	219	206	187	204	208
Knee flexion	174	180	172	158	159	164
Knee extension	209	203	191	208	213	214
Dynamometer readings						
Handgrip (Stoelting)	159	148	150	131	124	130
Leg extension (Mathews)	1330	1490	1410	967	1380	1484†
Back extension (Mathews)	529	598	602	378	521	547†

Note. Based on data of Shephard et al. (1977).
†A statistically significant and important learning effect was observed in the two tests using the dynamometer of Mathews (1963). Reproduced with permission from Shephard, R.J., Physical Activity and Growth (p. 80). Copyright 1982 by Yearbook Medical Publishers, Inc., Chicago, IL.

that gender differences in strength are much greater if they had recorded only the first set of scores.

Recent research has hinted that there are gender differences in muscle fiber composition; that is, the proportions of Type I (slow-twitch) and Type II (fast-twitch) muscle fibers are not the same in men and women. If so, part of the gender differences in strength might be attributed to muscle fiber composition, because indications from animal studies show that muscle composition is related to isometric strength (see Komi, 1984, for a review). Such research is limited, and continued investigation is necessary to confirm any relationship between sex differences in strength and muscle composition.

Strength Training

It is well known that an adult's muscle strength increases with strength training. Strength training also brings about muscle hypertrophy, but this process is related to hormonal levels. As we discussed in chapter 2, only post-pubescent men have sufficient adrenal androgen and testosterone levels to yield significant increases in the size of muscles trained through progressive resistance exercise. In light of this, can prepubescent youngsters increase their strength with training?

Children. Let's consider Rohmert's (1968; cited in Bailey, Malina, & Rasmussen, 1978) examination of strength training effects in 8-year-old boys and girls. The children were divided into two groups. One group executed a 1-second maximal isometric contraction every day with several different muscle groups. The other did the same but with a 6-second contraction. By the end of the study, the children's strength had increased, especially that of the 6-second group. The children improved at about the same rate as that expected of adults. When Rohmert expressed the strength scores as a function of final strength, he found that the children had begun at a relatively lower level of strength, so they made relatively more progress in training than adults would. Some of the strength improvement in Rohmert's children could be attributed to muscle growth, since Rohmert did not measure muscle size, but the study was of short duration (10 weeks), so training obviously played a role in the increase and the more extensive training yielded greater improvement. Ikai (1967) demonstrated an improvement in muscle *endurance* with training in adolescents 12 to 15 years old. In this study, the criterion for muscle endurance (ability to exert submaximal force for extended periods) was the number of contractions completed at one-third maximal strength, performed at 1-second intervals. Results indicated that the adolescents' gains in muscle endurance also were greater than those expected with adults.

It is often found that children and adolescents who participate regularly in sports are stronger than those who do not (Bailey et al., 1978). This could be taken as proof of strength development through the training obtained by sport participation. Keep in mind, though, that young athletes are often maturationally advanced compared with nonathletes, perhaps reflecting a self-selection process. Bigger, more mature children may experience more success in physical activities than their counterparts and consequently pursue regular sport participation. With this limitation in mind, we can recognize that some sports provide sufficient resistive exercise to improve strength in children, at least in the muscle groups used for that sport activity.

Methods.   If training can improve strength in young athletes, would it be wise to encourage these young athletes to weight train? For adults, strength programs often take the form of weight training, wherein progressively heavier weights are used to provide resistance for body movements. But an important difference exists between children and adults. Children's bones are still growing at sites called epiphyseal growth plates. These areas are subject to injury, either by trauma or the stress of repeated use. Injury is significant when it comes at an early age and causes cessation of growth at an epiphyseal growth plate, especially one located in a weight-bearing bone. Such injuries are rare in young athletes, but the risk is present in an activity requiring a youngster to repeatedly lift or push heavy weights. Any activity that could ultimately limit an individual's ability to be active throughout life is of doubtful benefit to youths. A safer approach is to work against light resistance, such as the body weight, in push-ups, sit-ups, or rope-climbing, at least until skeletal growth is nearly complete.

Older Adults.   Earlier, we recognized that the typical adult loses muscle mass and strength in older age. Could this process be forestalled or reversed by training? It appears that older adults can benefit by specific weight training programs. Chapman, DeVries, and Swezey (1972) demonstrated a strength increase in older adults with training, although they trained only index finger strength. Moritani and DeVries (1980) compared five younger (average age about 22) and five older men (average age about 70) on their potential for muscle hypertrophy with training. The participants trained three times per week for 8 weeks on two sets of 10 repetitions of elbow flexion against a weight level representing two thirds of their maximum force. The investigators found that both groups increased in strength after the 8 weeks of training. Neural factors, that is, a gain in muscle activation level, seemed to be responsible for the increase in older men. The younger men improved both by improved muscle activation level and by hypertrophy of the muscle. Many questions regarding strength training in older adults remain, especially with regard to forestalling the loss of muscle mass, but it does seem that strength training yields improvement in strength at any age. However, older adults with osteoporosis (skeletal atrophy) should begin training with light resistance.

Prediction of Strength

It would be useful to predict which children would be capable of success in tasks requiring strength when they reached late adolescence or early adulthood. This prediction is only possible if strength is stable throughout childhood and adolescence, that is, if the strongest children are the strongest adolescents, the weakest children are the weakest adolescents, and so on. The stability of any factor such as strength can be demonstrated by measuring that factor in childhood, then again in adolescence, and correlating the two scores. A high correlation, .80 to 1.0, indicates that children tend to retain their relative position in the group over the age span tested. Lower correlations indicate some adolescents are relatively stronger or weaker than they were as children, hence their strength could not be predicted accurately by their childhood score. This procedure was used in two research studies. As early as 1920, Baldwin showed that measures of grip strength at 9 to 10 years of age were correlated with scores at 15 to 16 years of age by coefficients of only .65 for boys and .45 for girls. Rarick and Smoll (1967) confirmed low correlation coefficients for strength stability in the Wisconsin Growth Study by recording strength measures on some 25 boys and 24 girls every year from 7 to 12 years and then again at age 17. Although correlations between measures 1 or 2 years apart were sometimes high, only a few measures across the full 10-year span, 7 to 17 years, were above .50 (see Table 7.6). Strength in adolescence cannot be predicted accurately by childhood scores. Several factors probably contribute to the futility of attempting to predict strength across the growing years. Motivation is one factor, and the extent and intensity of participation in activities are others. Undoubtedly, another factor is the variability in rate of maturation among individuals. A late maturing, relatively weak 7-year-old might be among the strongest individuals as a 17-year-old!

Summary 7.2—Strength Development

We can now say that the twins mentioned earlier will become stronger as they grow, reflecting in part their growth in muscle mass, but that their strength will increase at a rate faster than that accounted for by muscle growth alone. This additional increase in strength is largely due to improved coordination in recruiting the muscle units needed to exert force. Before the age of 13, the twins will follow a similar pattern of strength development, but

Table 7.6 Age-to-Age Correlations of Strength Measures

Measures	Childhood					Childhood to Adolescence					
	7 to 12	8 to 12	9 to 12	10 to 12	11 to 12	7 to 17	8 to 17	9 to 17	10 to 17	11 to 17	12 to 17
Boys											
Wrist flexion	.375	.550	.163	.486	.533	.378	.493	.327	.434	.244	.419
Elbow flexion	.279	.628	.825	.807	.733	.235	.193	.602	.446	.618	.634
Shoulder med. rot.	.202	.372	.605	.625	.702	.258	.307	.568	.612	.505	.674
Shoulder adduction	.523	.491	.315	.550	.676	.491	.418	.485	.566	.681	.662
Hip flexion	.353	.406	.668	.682	.813	.334	.393	.355	.682	.402	.515
Hip extension	.706	.481	.614	.674	.861	.344	.076	.430	.117	.426	.488
Knee extension	.430	.465	.277	.668	.732	.429	.503	.483	.721	.735	.797
Ankle extension	−.020	.634	.737	.794	.763	.209	.416	.413	.640	.480	.590
Girls											
Wrist flexion	.361	.406	.553	.640	.655	.387	.013	.454	.473	.436	.457
Elbow flexion	.367	.627	.592	.763	.770	.566	.308	.336	.473	.350	.114
Shoulder med. rot.	.184	.300	.751	.774	.758	.156	−.152	.327	.276	.496	.372
Shoulder adduction	.133	.608	.302	.597	.740	.260	.360	.622	.309	.499	.185
Hip flexion	.477	.512	.774	.898	.890	.506	.366	.530	.655	.666	.712
Hip extension	.636	.512	.665	.769	.796	.336	.394	.595	.523	.378	.575
Knee extension	.763	.722	.661	.651	.754	.673	.508	.730	.756	.641	.646
Ankle extension	.035	.276	.533	.770	.670	.267	.306	.523	.520	.275	.265

Note. From "Stability of Growth in Strength in Motor Performance From Childhood to Adolescence" by G.L. Rarick and F.L. Smoll, 1967, *Human Biology*, **39**, pp. 299, 301, 302. Copyright 1967 by Wayne State University Press. Reprinted by permission.

then the male twin is likely to make rapid gains over his sister. This gender difference results in part from the large increase in muscle mass promoted in males by increased secretion of the androgen hormones. At the same time, cultural norms may prevent an adolescent girl from both participating in activities that build strength and from giving an all-out effort on strength tests.

The twins could improve their strength beyond those increases accompanying muscle growth and improved coordination by appropriate training. Light-weight resistance exercise is preferable in childhood and early adolescence to heavy-weight resistance. After approximately 13 years of age, the adolescent boy can promote significant muscle hypertrophy by heavier resistance training. Yet we are likely to have limited success in predicting the strength level of our adolescent twins from childhood strength measures.

Whether or not a lifelong exercise program promoting strength could forestall any loss of muscle tissue in old age for the twins is yet to be thoroughly researched. But people of any age can improve their muscle strength with training. Muscle strength is important to the performance of many everyday skills as well as sport skills. Flexibility, too, is important in motor skill performance and is the topic to which we now turn.

Concept 7.3   Flexibility decreases without training, even during childhood and adolescence.

Flexibility, the ability to move joints through a full range of motion, is often beneficial to maximal performance, while limited flexibility is a factor in sports injuries. Yet, this important aspect of physical fitness is sometimes overlooked in young athletes. Endurance and strength are often emphasized at the expense of flexibility. Exceptions to this generalization are dancers and gymnasts who have long realized the importance of flexibility to their activities. One reason for the casual, indifferent attitude toward flexibility is the assumption that young people are naturally supple and need no further flexibility training. Additionally, lack of flexibility is typically viewed as a problem only with older adults when resulting limitations upon movement are more readily apparent. The scientific investigations summarized in the following discussion yield some surprising information concerning these misconceptions about flexibility.

Development of Flexibility

An important characteristic of flexibility is its specificity; that is, a certain degree of flexibility is specific to each particular joint. For example, you can be relatively flexible at one joint and inflexible at another. This means that one or two flexibility measures cannot accurately represent your overall flexibility.

The range of motion undertaken at any joint depends on that joint's anatomical structure and the extent of its habitual use. To improve poor flexibility, the joint must be regularly and systematically moved through an increasingly larger range of motion. Athletes, then, tend to increase the flexibility of joints used in their sport, while laborers who spend much of their time in one posture may lose flexibility in some joints. It is likely that persons who do not exercise fully lose flexibility because everyday activities rarely require movements through a full range of motion. The belief that flexibility is related to the length of one's limbs is incorrect. So at any age, flexibility reflects the normal range of movement to which specific joints are subjected.

Early Decline of Flexibility

The improvement of endurance and strength with age was discussed earlier. Does this trend hold for flexibility? Some improvement in flexibility with age has been noted in young children, but unfortunately, most studies show a decline in flexibility beginning in the early teens. After reviewing the information available in 1975, Clarke concluded that boys tend to lose flexibility after age 10 and girls after age 12. For example, Hupprich and Sigerseth (1950) administered 12 flexibility measures to 300 girls, ages 6, 9, 12, 15, and 18 years. Most of the flexibility measures improved across the 6-, 9-, and 12-year-old groups, but declined in the older groups (see Table 7.7). More

Table 7.7 Average Range and Standard Deviations of Flexibility Measures (Degrees) of Girls

Age Group (Years)	N	Hip Flexion-Extension	Side Trunk Flexion-Extension	Elbow Flexion-Extension	Shoulder
6	50	121.3 ± 16.7	92.0 ± 14.0	156.0 ± 6.0	228.4 ± 12.9
9	50	126.5 ± 19.9	107.2 ± 18.1	157.3 ± 6.9	219.7 ± 11.0
12	50	139.1 ± 18.2	118.3 ± 20.4	157.4 ± 8.1	215.5 ± 12.0
15	50	126.9 ± 17.8	110.4 ± 18.8	155.7 ± 7.5	213.0 ± 11.9
18	100	128.6 ± 11.1	104.4 ± 18.0	151.3 ± 7.8	212.8 ± 12.0

Note. Adapted from "The Specificity of Flexibility in Girls" by F.L. Hupprich & P.O. Sigerseth, 1950, Research Quarterly, **39**, 30-32.

recent studies noted even younger turnaround ages. Krahenbuhl and Martin (1977) found that both boys and girls declined over the age range of 10 to 14, while Milne, Seefeldt, and Reuschlein (1976) reported that second graders in their study already had poorer flexibility than kindergarteners. Research, then, has identified a trend toward declining flexibility, which begins at least by the early teens and sometimes earlier. Girls as a group are usually more flexible than boys (DiNucci, 1976; Phillips et al., 1955). This probably reflects the social acceptability of stretching exercises over more vigorous exercises for girls and higher proportions of girls than boys participating in gymnastics and dance, where flexibility is emphasized. These trends may be changing, so that neither forms of exercise nor specific activities are viewed as more appropriate for one gender than the other.

Unfortunately, adolescence does not mark the end of the trend toward reduced flexibility. Boone and Azen (1979) obtained 28 flexibility measures on 109 males in age-groups from 18 months to 54 years and found a steady decline throughout each time period. For example, hip rotation range declined 15° to 20° in the early years and about 5° per decade of life thereafter. The greatest losses occurred in movements not habitually performed. Undoubtedly, one factor in the loss of flexibility is the limited range of motion required in everyday life. Those individuals not engaged in sports, dance, or a regular exercise routine for flexibility seldom move through a full range of motion. Even those who participate in sports and dance may not move joints their full extent, or they may exercise some, but not all, of the body's joints. This trend toward declining flexibility after childhood represents the average state of fitness among representative groups of people. It does not indicate that everyone automatically will lose flexibility. In fact, athletes, dancers, and others engaged in flexibility training usually maintain or improve their range of motion as they age.

Gains in Flexibility With Training

It is generally accepted that a loss of flexibility is a characteristic of old age. Changes in the cartilage, ligaments, and tendons of the joints occur with aging, but there is no evidence that these changes are the *cause* of decreased flexibility (Adrian, 1981). In fact, most research links loss of flexibility in older adults to degenerative diseases of the tissues. It is generally agreed that flexibility training can improve range of motion in the joints of the young, and Munns (1981) demonstrated that older adults, too, can improve the range of motion in their joints with training. She formed two groups of 65- to 88-year-olds. One group served as a control, while the other participated in a 1-hour program of exercise and dance, three times per week for 12 weeks. The exercised group improved significantly over the control group in all six flexibility measures. Inactivity is certainly a major factor of many that may contribute to flexibility decline in old age. Fortunately, a loss of flexibility can be reversed by specific training, even in old age.

Summary 7.3—Changes in Flexibility

The possible range of motion in a joint reflects activity and training more than one's age, per se. Flexibility declines in the average adolescent and adult as a result of limited daily activity and lack of exercise. Flexibility training can bring about an improvement in range of motion at any age.

Concept 7.4 Body composition is affected by genetic and environmental factors, especially diet and exercise.

Your body mass can be divided into two types of tissues: lean tissues that include muscle, bone, and organs, and the fat or adipose tissue. The relative percentages of lean body mass and fat tissue that comprise the body mass give a measure of *body composition*. Body composition is important for at least two reasons. First, it is related to physical fitness. Higher proportions of lean body mass are positively linked, and higher proportions of fat tissue are negatively linked to working capacity. Excess fat weight adds to the work load when the body is moved, propelled, or lifted. Excess fat can also limit range of motion. Furthermore, obesity places a person at risk of suffering coronary heart and artery disease, stroke, and hypertension.

Body composition is also important because it can influence feelings about oneself. A lean body appearance is valued in many societies. Obesity may contribute to a negative body concept and self-concept, thus decreasing the ease with which an obese person relates to others. Remember that everyone has some fat tissue, which is needed for insulation, protection, and energy storage. In women, a minimal level of fat tissue (approximately 12% of body weight) is necessary to support functions of pregnancy. It is only *excess* fat weight that is negatively related to fitness and health.

Two major environmental factors can be used to manage the relative amounts of lean and adipose body tissue. One is diet. For example, an individual can consume too much foodstuff, resulting in excess fat storage. The second environmental factor is exercise. Since physical activity requires energy, calories from food are used for the activity and not stored as adipose tissue. Maintenance of body composition is, in part, a matter of balancing the calories consumed in the diet against the individual's metabolic rate and the amount of physical exertion. The relationship between body composition and exercise, especially during the growing years, is the focus of the following discussion.

Body Composition

Body Composition and Exercise—The Parizkova Studies

Fat tissue increases rapidly during two periods: the first 6 months after birth and again in early adolescence. In girls this increase continues throughout adolescence, while in boys the gain stops and may even reverse for a time. Muscle tissue also grows rapidly in the early postnatal months, followed by a steady period of increase during childhood, and it again increases rapidly during the adolescent growth spurt, more dramatically for boys than girls. Two environmental factors may alter this typical pattern: diet and exercise. Overeating results in excess fat weight, while starvation can lead to levels of fat so low that energy is obtained by muscle wasting. Exercise also affects body composition, and this relationship deserves close attention.

Both cross-sectional and longitudinal studies have been conducted on the relationship between exercise and body composition. Cross-sectional studies generally show that young athletes have lower proportions of body fat than children who are more sedentary (Parizkova, 1973). However, it is impossible to determine from a cross-sectional study whether an active lifestyle results in leanness. (It may be that leaner children find activity easier and adopt an active lifestyle.) Longitudinal studies, then, are more valuable in the study of the interrelationships between activity levels and body composition, and wherever possible, longitudinal information is discussed.

Parizkova conducted a series of studies on body composition and activity level of boys and girls in Czechoslovakia. The first study was cross-sectional and one of the few studies to examine very young children; the remainder of the studies were longitudinal. In the cross-sectional study, Wolanski and Parizkova (1976; cited in Parizkova, 1977) compared skinfold measures in two groups of children aged 2 to 5 years. One group of children attended special physical education classes with their parents, while the other group did not participate in any type of physical training program. Even at this young age children in the physical education group had lower levels of subcutaneous fat. The following discussion focuses upon Parizkova's longitudinal studies as some of the only work of this type available.

Teenage Boys. An extensive longitudinal study of teenage boys (Parizkova, 1968, 1977) examined the same issue. Nearly 100 boys were divided into four groups by activity level. The most-active group of boys were involved in basketball or track at least 6 hr per week. The least-active group only participated in unorganized and unsystematic activity. The remaining two groups were intermediate in activity level. The boys were first tested at an average age of 10.7 years and followed successively until 14.7 years of age. Over the 4 years, the children in the most-active group significantly increased in body mass, while their absolute level of fat weight remained the same; hence, the fat proportion of total weight decreased. The inactive group, in contrast, increased significantly in absolute fat weight. Interestingly, the two groups did not differ in amount of fat weight at the beginning of the study, but did by the end of the study. In the active group the increased lean body mass alone accounted for the increase of body weight with growth (see Table 7.8). Physical activity had a beneficial effect on body composition in these boys.

Parizkova (1972) followed 41 of these boys for another 3 years, until 17.7 years of age. The body composition trends of the first 4 years continued. The most-active and least-active groups differed in total weight by the time they reached age 16.7. The active group was heavier because of the boys' greater lean body mass, although they had less fat weight than the inactive boys. In

Table 7.8 Average Values and Standard Deviations (*M* and *SD*) of Relative Fat (%) and Absolute Lean Body Mass (kg LBM) of Groups With Different Activity Regimes

Group		1 1961 *M*	*SD*	2 1962 *M*	*SD*	3 1963 *M*	*SD*	4 1964 *M*	*SD*	5 1965 *M*	*SD*
I	% fat	15.7	5.4	14.1	5.7	12.7	1.5	9.7	3.3	9.9	4.6
	kg LBM	31.6	3.3	35.0	3.8	40.4	5.4	45.5	6.8	54.4	7.1
II	% fat	15.5	5.6	13.5	5.9	12.4	4.7	11.4	4.1	12.5	4.1
	kg LBM	30.2	4.3	33.8	4.5	37.9	5.3	44.1	7.2	49.1	8.3
III	% fat	14.7	6.4	14.5	7.5	14.8	5.7	12.5	5.9	13.6	4.2
	kg LBM	31.0	3.1	34.1	3.4	37.3	3.6	43.9	5.1	49.7	5.4
IV	% fat	17.2	6.2	19.1	6.0	16.6	5.9	14.7	4.4	15.9	5.4
	kg LBM	31.4	3.3	33.8	3.9	37.8	4.6	43.8	6.3	49.6	6.6

Note. Subjects were groups of boys followed longitudinally during five years (from 10.7 to 14.7 years of age, 1961 to 1965, n = 96). Group I was most active and Group IV was least active. Data are from Parizkova (1968a,b). From *Body Fat and Physical Fitness* (p. 130) by J. Parizkova, 1977, The Hague, The Netherlands: Martinus Nijhoff B.V., Publishers. Copyright 1977 by Martinus Nijhoff B.V. Reprinted by permission.

some years the active group actually gained more lean body mass than total body weight because their fat weight declined. Parizkova determined that the groups did not differ in average skeletal age, so the body composition differences noted cannot be attributed to maturational differences, but rather to activity level. It was noted, too, that the boys kept their relative position within the group in both distribution and absolute amount of subcutaneous fat. That is, the relative amount of fat weight and its pattern of distribution in the body was relatively stable over the years of the study. Sixteen of these 41 men were followed for another 6 years. Although this number was too small for a reliable analysis by activity level, Parizkova (1977) noted that percent body fat declined in the group until 21.7 years of age, then varied widely among individuals, probably reflecting changes in lifestyle. The Parizkova studies, then, indicate that physical activity has a favorable influence on boys' body composition during the growing years.

Teenage Girls. The growth of adipose and lean muscle tissue differs dramatically between the sexes during adolescence when girls have proportionately greater fat to muscle gains than boys. Even so, the beneficial activity effect on body composition found in boys also occurs among active girls. Over a span of 5 years Parizkova (1963, 1977) studied 32 girls who belonged to a gymnastics school and 45 girls who were not engaged in any type of training. The girls were first measured at the age of 12 or 13. The gymnasts had a regular, yearly cycle of training in which they attended a rigorous camp in the summer, discontinued training in the fall, and resumed a heavy training schedule from October to December. Measures of the girls' fat weight paralleled Parizkova's findings with boys: The gymnasts remained at the same level of subcutaneous fat during the 5 years, while the control group gained a significant amount of fat weight (see Figure 7.2). Height and body weight trends in the two groups were similar over the 5 years, so the differences were truly in body composition.

The cyclic nature of the gymnasts' training schedule provided information about their weight and skinfold thicknesses as they went through the various training cycles. During periods of inactivity, the gymnasts gained both total body weight and skinfold (including subcutaneous fat tissue) thickness, but during training, the gymnasts increased in total body weight, while their skinfold thicknesses declined. Hence, the weight increments during the various activity periods resulted from different ratios of fat and lean body weight. Parizkova also recorded caloric intake of the gymnasts and found that more calories were consumed during periods of intense training, but fat deposition *declined* and lean body mass increased.

Direct Comparison of Boys and Girls. Parizkova's longitudinal studies show the same general relationship between body composition and activity among

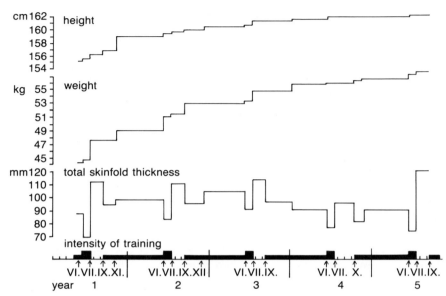

Figure 7.2 Changes in height, weight, and subcutaneous fat (sum of ten skinfold measurements) in a group of regularly training girl gymnasts (n = 11) during a five year period of varying intensity of training (see bottom scale). Data are from Parizkova (1963a, 1965). From *Body Fat and Physical Fitness* (p. 154) by J. Parizkova, 1977, The Hague, The Netherlands: Martinus Nijhoff B.V. Publishers. Copyright 1977 by Martinus Nijhoff B.V. Publishers. Reprinted by permission.

both boys and girls, but they do not allow direct comparison of the sexes. So, Parizkova (1973, 1977) simultaneously followed 12 boys and 12 girls engaged in swimming training from age 12 to age 16. At 12, the average height, weight, lean body mass, and fat weight of the two groups were about the same. Lean body mass values were higher for the swimmers than the average levels for teens not in training, probably reflecting the swimmers' previous training. By the age of 15, the boys were significantly taller, heavier, and leaner than the girls, but both sexes showed an increased proportion of lean body mass at the expense of fat weight over the 2 years of training. Although higher in percent fat than the boys, the girls did not gain as much fat as the typical nontraining, adolescent girl.

In summary, the Parizkova investigations show that involvement in training programs has a favorable effect on the body composition of adolescents. Limited information also suggests that the body composition of preschool children benefits from activity. While children and adolescents engaged in active training adhere to the general growth trend of increased weight, this increase represents the addition of relatively more lean body mass and less fat weight than in their nontraining peers. Higher caloric intake during train-ing is evidently used to increase lean body mass rather than fat stores. It may be possible to carry training to an extreme, so that the energy required for continued growth cannot be met. Relatively little scientific information is avail-able on this issue; yet in theory, this condition mimics that of starvation and presumably has similar negative effects.

Exercise and Obese Children

It is commonly recognized that the incidence of obesity in all industrial-ized countries is high, even among children, and that more people become obese as they age. As noted earlier, obesity is unfortunate from both medical and social viewpoints. This is particularly true for children. Obese children are likely to be obese adults and therefore at risk of heart disease, stroke, and hypertension. Too, the economy of work done by obese children is poor: Their working capacity is low, because they require more energy just to move their bodies burdened with excess fat weight (Vamberova et al., 1971; cited in Parizkova, 1977). During the years when an obese child is forming a self-concept, he or she must deal with negative feedback and evaluation from adults and peers alike (Allon, 1973; Dwyer & Mayer, 1973; Stunkard & Mendelson, 1967). It is desirable for educators to intervene, when possible, and positively influence the factors contributing to the child's obesity.

Lowering Caloric Intake. Obesity may be reduced over a period of time by lowering caloric intake, increasing activity to burn more calories, or a com-bination of the two. Adopting an increased activity approach alone yields slow progress, because a 2-mile jog, for example, burns approximately 150 calories, and a deficit of 3,500 calories is needed to lose 1 lb of fat weight. Which approach is best for obese children? Overeating in young children is proba-bly rare (Mayer, 1968), but reduced motor activity is a common characteris-tic of obese children. For example, Stafanik, Heald, and Mayer (1959) noted that among 14 obese and 14 thin boys attending a summer camp, the obese boys consumed fewer calories but were also less active than the thin boys. So, inactivity probably does not result from obesity, but rather precedes it (Parizkova, 1977). Once children are overweight, they are trapped in a vicious cycle: Activity requires relatively greater effort by an obese child, activity is less pleasurable, and vigor of participation is reduced (even when the child is engaged in games or exercise); hence, fewer excess calories are burned, and the child remains overweight.

Adults who significantly reduce their caloric intake without exercising may lose lean body mass as well as fat weight (Parizkova, 1977). To prevent this loss of lean body tissue, simultaneous exercise and reduced caloric intake are most effective. In children, a reduction of caloric intake to the 1,000 calorie-per-day level can temporarily slow down or even arrest growth (Vamberova, 1961; cited in Parizkova, 1977). The increased number of calories expended by increased activity permits weight reduction while maintaining caloric intake at safe levels. Exercise, then, plays an important role in weight reduction at any age, but particularly in children. The goal should be both avoidance of lean muscle tissue loss by engaging in vigorous exercise and control of caloric intake, rather than calorie control alone.

Effects of Increased Activity. Parizkova, Stankova, Sprynarova, and Vamberova (1963; cited in Parizkova, 1977) demonstrated the effect of increasing activity level in obese children. Seven boys with an average age of 11.8 years were studied during 7 weeks of a summer camp that provided increased activity levels but also controlled caloric intake (1,700 calories per day). Over the summer the boys reduced their body weight an average of 11.4%, lost about 5 kg of fat weight, and raised their percentage of lean body mass from 69.9% to 75.9%. At the beginning of the summer, the boys' free fatty acid level (the usable fuel form of the triglyceride molecule, which must be broken down to metabolize fat) tended to decline during exercise and remain low during the subsequent rest period. By the end of the summer, the free fatty acid level increased significantly during the rest period. This change was probably due to the boys' improved ability to mobilize fat from its storage locations. The exercise program was thus effective in increasing the metabolic activity of adipose tissue. While Parizkova was able to report favorable results from such a summer program, follow-up studies (Parizkova, 1977) revealed a common problem. Most boys gained back much of the fat weight lost over the summer when they returned to their home environment. The success of most intervention techniques is tied to continued participation by the child and family support.

Some research indicates that new adipose tissue cells are formed only during the prenatal and early postnatal months, and during adolescence (Knittle & Hirsch, 1968; Hirsch & Knittle, 1970). After adolescence, only the *size* of fat cells is variable. Research on this topic is limited, but if it is accurate, diet and exercise are particularly important for young persons. Animal studies suggest that regular vigorous exercise prevents the addition of excess fat cells during growth, perhaps making weight control easier for the remainder of life (Oscai, Babirak, Dubach, McGarr, & Spirakis, 1974).

Body Composition, Exercise, and Aging

As noted in chapter 2, total body weight among average individuals usually declines after age 50, reflecting a decline in lean body weight rather than fat weight. Other evidence suggests such changes in body composition are not an inevitable consequence of aging. For example, Shephard (1978) compiled data collected by Kavanagh and Shepard (1977), Pollock (1974), and Asano, Ogawa, and Furuta (1978) on older track participants, ages 40 to 70 and older. No tendency for increasing weight or body fat with advancing age was found. Further, those older adults still running 30 to 40 miles per week showed no significant loss of lean body mass. Saltin and Grimby (1968) similarly found no tendency among orienteerers to gain fat weight in adulthood, although they did lose body weight after age 45, presumably reflecting a decline in lean body mass. Apparently, the maintenance of endurance training throughout adulthood has a favorable effect on body composition, although questions remain about the extent of lean body mass loss after the late 40s.

Can exercise programs *begun* in older adulthood bring about beneficial changes in body composition? Research conducted to answer this question is equivocal. In some cases little or no change in body weight, fat weight, or lean body mass was found in older adults who began training (Parizkova & Eiselt, 1968; DeVries, 1970; Adams & DeVries, 1973). On the contrary, Sidney, Shephard, and Harrison (1977) recorded significant losses of estimated percent body fat and subcutaneous fat in older adults after 14 weeks of endurance training. A smaller number of older subjects in this study who continued to train for 1 year lost additional fat weight, but not body weight, which implies an offsetting increase of lean body mass occurred. Obviously, further research is needed to resolve these conflicting findings.

Summary 7.4—Factors Affecting Body Composition

Body composition is important for several health and social reasons, including its relation to physical fitness. Although body composition is controlled to an extent by genetic factors, the environmental factors of diet and exercise can greatly affect the relative levels of fat and lean body mass. Both diet and exercise can be manipulated by someone who wishes to change his or her body composition. Favorable changes in body composition result from regular, vigorous exercise at any age: Specifically, lean body mass increases at the expense of fat weight. Because dramatic reductions in caloric intake alone can result in a loss of lean body mass in adults or in cessation of growth in children, exercise should be an important aspect of any weight reduction program.

Research indicates that physical activity is beneficial throughout the life span. Activities promoting endurance, strength, flexibility, and low body fat improve fitness at any age, while inactivity leads to a loss of fitness and tendency to increased fat tissue at any age. Some questions regarding the impact of an active lifestyle on the length of life remain to be answered by research, but there is little doubt that good physical health and fitness improve the quality of life. Several myths about fitness—for example, that children are naturally fit, and that older adults necessarily lose fitness—are incorrect. In their place now is the view that an active lifestyle is desirable throughout the life span.

Suggested Readings

Bailey, D.A., Malina, R.M., & Rasmussen, R.L. (1978). The influence of exercise, physical activity, and athletic performance on the dynamics of human growth. In F. Falkner & J.M. Tanner (Eds.), *Human growth* (Vol. 2) (pp. 475-505). New York, NY: Plenum Press.

Parizkova, J. (1977). *Body fat and physical fitness*. The Hague, The Netherlands: Martinus Nijhoff B.V.

Rarick, G.L. (Ed.) (1973). *Physical activity: Human growth and development*. New York, NY: Academic Press.

Shephard, R.J. (1978). *Physical activity and aging*. Chicago, IL: Year Book Medical Publishers.

Shephard, R.J. (1982). *Physical activity and growth*. Chicago, IL: Year Book Medical Publishers.

Smith, E.L., & Serfass, R.C. (Eds.) (1981). *Exercise and aging: The scientific basis*. Hillside, NJ: Enslow Publishers.

8

Information Processing, Memory, and Mental Capacity

An important aspect of motor development is the ability to process the information provided by the sensory systems discussed earlier in chapter 6. Models of how information is processed have greatly facilitated the study of motor skill learning and performance. Information processing *models* generally show the components of the information processing system in their proposed relationship to one another. One such model is pictured in Figure 8.1. The components are functional rather than structural; that is, they represent processes that appear to be involved in skill performance, based on either logical assessment of what must precede a skilled response or on research investigations of these processes. They do not necessarily represent locations or centers in the nervous system.

Following a single motor response through the model in Figure 8.1 will help you to understand the components of an information processing model. Imagine a basketball player who wants to pass to a teammate sprinting down the court. The passer's sensory receptors receive stimuli and transduce (convert) them to neural information: kinesthetic stimuli regarding body orientation and limb position, light waves indicating the position

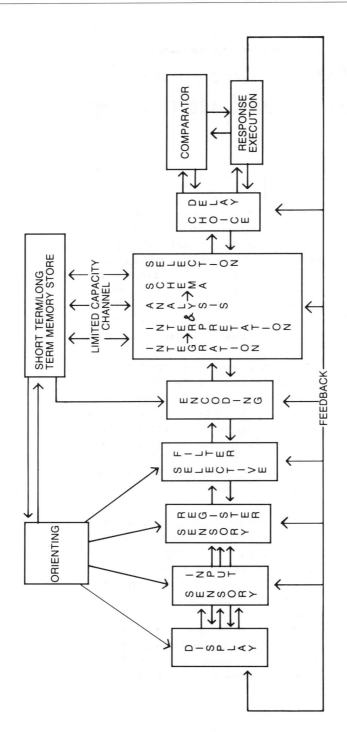

Figure 8.1 An information processing model. Adapted from "Information processing in children's skill acquisition" in *Psychology of Motor Behavior and Sport* (p. 219) by A.L. Rothstein in R.W. Christina and D.M. Landers (Eds.), 1977, Champaign, IL: Human Kinetics Publishers. Copyright 1977 by Human Kinetics Publishers. Adapted by permission.

and movement of the other players, and sound waves generated by those in the environment. This *sensory input* is held briefly in the *sensory register* component of memory. The player has the ability to *selectively filter* the sensory input and attend only to the information critical for the response. He or she need not be passive, but can *orient* the eyes, ears, and body to better receive relevant stimuli. The neural signals must be *encoded*, that is, transformed into signals that can be further processed in the brain and stored in memory. This may involve organizing and grouping the signals. Next, the signals from the various sensory systems must be *integrated*. For example, the sound of a player running down the court must be matched to the visual image of this event. This new perceptual information must now be *interpreted* and *analyzed*, in part by comparing it with stored *memories* of similar experiences. Based on this analysis, a response *schema* is selected. A schema is theorized to be a set of rules governing a class of situations. It is unlikely that humans store a motor response for each set of unique stimulus situations. Rather, the system generalizes. The basketball player will select a response and its timing based on a set of rules developed from previous experiences about passing to a person who is moving. The schema will allow the player to adjust for the teammate's speed, path, and height, the nearness of opponents, and so on. These latter phases of processing take place in a channel or path of *limited capacity*.

A limited amount of information can be dealt with at one time by the passer. Once the player's response is selected, it may be held in *choice delay*, if necessary, until the appropriate time for execution. As the response is executed it is *compared* with the intended response. If the response is not being carried out as planned, some immediate correction of responses longer than 500 msec is possible. This internal *feedback* about the response and the external feedback generated during and after the response are further input to the system. The response and its feedback are then used to improve the schema for this class of skills. The basketball player will benefit from this experience when a similar situation arises in the future.

This brief example of information processing serves as the background for an analysis of developmental factors in information processing. Although little is known about the development of some components in the model, information available on others contributes to an understanding of the development and stability of skill learning and performance. A discussion of memory development is reserved for the last section of this chapter.

Concept 8.1   The amount of useful information that can be processed increases during childhood to an optimal level in adulthood, but some decline is apparent in older adulthood.

Information Processing Ability

Childhood

Age differences exist in the *selective filtering* and *attention* component of information processing. It seems that young children are less capable than adults of identifying relevant stimuli in the visual field and attending to them exclusive of irrelevant stimuli. For example, Smith, Kemler, and Aronfried (1975) found that young children at ages 5 and 6 attended to *both* relevant and irrelevant stimuli in a display. In contrast, older children, ages 7 and 8 years and 10 and 11 years, attended to more of the relevant stimuli, picking up irrelevant stimuli incidentally. Children up to age 12 also seem to weigh auditory stimuli too heavily compared with visual stimuli, diverting some of their attention away from critical visual information (Perelle, 1975). Ross (1976) proposed that the development of attention occurs in three stages. During the infant and early childhood years, children attend to one stimulus in the display exclusive of all others, termed the *overexclusive* mode. The next stage, *overinclusive*, spans the late childhood and preadolescent years. Children in this mode attend to many stimuli in the display, some of them irrelevant to the task at hand, as did the 5- and 6-year-olds of Smith et al. (1975). Transition to the third stage, *selective* attention, is typically complete by age 12, so that adolescents can focus on the relevant stimuli, even in complex displays.

Age differences in attention are probably related to age differences in experience. Whereas adolescents and adults know from past experience which stimuli are relevant to a particular response and which are not, children are more limited in past experiences. Educators can assist children by pointing out the relevant stimuli in a task. Patterson and Mischel (1975) demonstrated that children can be taught to resist irrelevant cues, and Stratton (1978b) noted that children can acquire selective attention strategies. Is it helpful to have children learn in a sterile environment? Probably not, since children can actually benefit by learning a skill in the presence of irrelevant stimuli *if* the latter will be present during performance. As long as the irrelevant cues do not prevent learning of the skill, children can learn to attend to the relevant stimuli and filter out irrelevant stimuli (Stratton, 1978a).

Children obviously become more efficient in processing increasingly larger amounts of information as they mature. This could be attributed to an increase in the child's limited capacity channel, but a variety of other factors can be involved as well (Rothstein, 1977). One factor might be the improving ability of children to integrate information from the different sensory systems as discussed in concept 6.2. Improved memory control processes, which are discussed later in this chapter, might also contribute to improved information processing. The development of improved schemata and perhaps the development of "subroutines" for basic parts of complex tasks could be involved. Subroutines could be executed automatically, thus requiring little of the performer's attention and freeing it for attention to other factors. Whether an increased channel capacity or some of these other factors are involved, children can be expected to handle more information as they mature.

The Use of Schemata.   The earlier sketch of an information processing model included *schemata*, or generalized programs for executing a response. We can think of performers as having programs consisting of commands for carrying out the many muscle contractions needed to make a motor response. A schema can be applied in many ways, depending upon the exact environmental conditions. A program based on the schema would designate which muscles contract, their order, force, and temporal pattern (Schmidt, 1977). When this response is executed, the initial conditions, intended response, feedback from this response, and movement outcome are related to one another. And as many such responses are made over time, the performer abstracts a relationship between the intended response (based on the initial conditions) and the movement outcome. Children have had few experiences from which to develop this relationship. Their schemata, then, are not as accurate nor as powerful as those of adults in adapting to a variety of initial conditions.

It follows that children benefit from practicing to form a better schema in a *variety* of conditions, rather than in a restricted setting where initial conditions are relatively constant. This reasoning is supported by two research teams. The first, Kerr and Booth (1977), divided children into two groups, both of which learned an underhand tossing task with their eyes closed. One group only practiced at a distance of 3 ft, while the other group practiced at both 2 ft and 4 ft. Hence, one group was able to practice under more variable conditions than the other. The test was to execute the task at 3 ft. The variable-practice group outperformed the restricted-practice group, despite the fact that the latter practiced at the test distance. Carson and Wiegand (1979) further demonstrated an advantage of variable practice: better remembrance of a motor skill. In this investigation preschoolers practiced a bean bag toss for accuracy under variable or restricted conditions. After 2 weeks the children were tested on the task to determine how well they had retained their skill. The children who practiced in the highly variable situation retained their skill better than the others. Both of these studies indicate that children are able to form schemata for motor responses through practice in variable conditions. In summary, though young children have less refined schemata than adolescents or adults, they benefit from practice in a variety of settings.

Feedback.   It is widely recognized that *feedback* is one of the most influential factors in skill performance. This is particularly true for children who are in the early stages of forming schemata for various skills. At the same time, it is clear that children often do not recognize the relevant stimuli amidst the perceptual display presented to them. You might expect, then, that children benefit from *augmented* feedback provided by a teacher, such as, "You swung too late," and from hints on which aspects of the available feedback are particularly relevant, such as reminding children to feel for a level swing. Yet, too much information cannot be effectively used by children. For example, the teacher who says, "You stepped to the left instead of straight ahead, dropped your rear shoulder, swung too late, and did not follow through," probably has overwhelmed the child. So, in teaching children, educators should provide informational feedback but in limited quantity on any single performance.

Neuromuscular Control. Another aspect of performance that undergoes development is *neuromuscular control*, that is, the execution of muscular contractions in the proper pattern, sequence, and timing. Williams (1981) identified two age-related changes in neuromuscular control. The first change is refinement of force production. Shambes (1976) found that when young children tried to maintain certain balance positions, they used more force than necessary and sometimes more muscle groups than necessary, compared with skilled adults. Because training is known to produce changes in the timing of motor unit firing (contraction of a muscle fiber group), children probably learn to refine force production through practice. Simard (1969) demonstrated that children as young as 3 years and as old as 12 years could be taught some degree of control in maintaining the activity of a motor unit. In addition, there is an age-related improvement in the ability to inhibit a muscle contraction, also a necessary aspect of skilled movement, because an opposing muscle group must be inhibited just prior to the execution of a movement by the prime muscles. Gatev (1972) observed that infants up to 9 months of age executed movements without well-defined inhibitory processes. Two- and 3-year-olds demonstrated improved but still immature inhibitory processes. Hence, it appears that the neuromuscular control phase of movement is not fully operational at birth but also undergoes a developmental process. It is likely this aspect of performance is related to the development of improved response schemata. A variety of motor experiences, then, are of great value for the refinement of neuromuscular control in children.

Speed of Processing Information. In addition to these developments in information processing, the *speed* of processing increases as children mature. This is apparent even in the simplest of motor responses, a reaction time task. *Reaction time* is the time span between the onset of a stimulus (such as a light or buzzer) and the beginning of a movement (such as lifting the finger from a button). The maximum speed of this response increases from 3 years of age through adolescence (Wickens, 1974). An improvement with age also occurs in the time required to process input to produce a response in a continuous tracking task (Pew & Rupp, 1971). Factors considered to be central processes (processes of the central nervous system) appear responsible for the slower processing speed exhibited by children (Elliott, 1972). Attention is one such central process, and another (discussed later in this chapter) is speed of the memory processes. In addition, the speed with which motor responses can be selected is a function of age (Wickens, 1974). Clark (1982) demonstrated this by manipulating the spatial stimulus-response compatibility of a reaction time task when testing 6-year-olds, 10-year-olds, and adults. In the compatible condition, participants pressed a key on the right if the right stimulus light came on and a key on the left if the left light came on. In the incompatible condition, the participants pressed a key opposite the direction of the light. Spatial compatibility then affects the participant's response selection. Clark found that processing time decreased with advancing age in the incompatible condition. While these central factors of attention, memory, and response selection are involved in the slower processing speeds of children, peripheral factors are not. For example, nerve impulse conduction speed in the peripheral nerves does not contribute substantially to the speed differences between children and adults. Thus, young children are able to process information faster as they mature because of improvements in central factors such as response selection and speed of the memory processes.

Older Adulthood

Older adults, similar to young children, exhibit limitations in the processing of information. These limitations, too, are apparently related to central processes. But important differences are found between performers at opposite ends of the life span. For example, older adults do not exhibit declining performance in all types of skill. There is little change in the performance of single, discrete actions that can be planned in advance (Welford, 1977b) or on simple, continuous, and repetitive actions, such as alternately tapping two targets (Welford, Norris, & Shock, 1969). However, performance decrement is large among older adults on actions requiring a *series* of different movements, especially when speed is important (Welford, 1977c). The major limitations on older adults, then, seem to involve the decisions based on perceptual information and the programming of movement sequences (Welford, 1980b). These are central rather than peripheral factors. Let's consider some of the central components of information processing that are affected by aging in more detail.

Older adults apparently learn new tasks more slowly than younger adults whether they are cognitive or motor tasks. For example, rote learning of cognitive material is slower in older adults, because they need more repetitions to "reach criterion," that is, learn the material at a predesignated level. This may reflect the need for more time in which to register the information in the long-term memory store. Similarly, older adults improve more slowly than younger adults in new motor skills, although skills learned early in life are well maintained (Szafran, 1951; Welford, 1980b).

Attentional factors also play a role in the performance limitations of older adults. Older adults perform their fastest on a reaction time task when a warning signal is given a consistent time before the stimulus, but their slowest when the warning signal interval is variable from trial to trial. This suggests that a fixed interval minimizes distraction by irrelevant associations (Birren, 1964b). Rabbitt (1965) also demonstrated that older adults are hampered more than younger adults by the presence of irrelevant stimuli in a card-sorting task. In this task, participants are challenged to sort a stack of cards based on information given on the card face, such as the shape of a symbol or its color. If information is placed on the card face that is not relevant to the sorting task, the performance of older adults suffers compared with younger adults. So, many older adults do not attend to critical stimuli as well as they did in their younger years and are more easily distracted. The cause of this decline in performance might be a lowered *signal-to-noise* ratio in the central nervous system. The neural impulses of the central nervous system take place against a background of random "neural noise" such that the effectiveness of a neural signal depends on the ratio between the signal strength and the background noise, that is, the signal-to-noise ratio. With aging, signal levels decrease because of changes in the sense organs, loss of brain cells, and factors affecting brain cell functioning, while at the same time, noise level increases (Crossman & Szafran, 1956; Welford, 1977a). Older adults can compensate for this lower signal-to-noise ratio if given extra time to complete a task, but if they must perform a series of movements or make a series of decisions rapidly, they are at a disadvantage.

Central factors are also implicated in slower *speed* of information processing among older adults. A slowing of reaction time with aging has been consistently documented in the research literature. Although a slight slowing of neural impulse conduction velocity is associated with aging, it is not great enough to account for the magnitude of lengthened reaction times. Movement time, too, shows a very slight slowing (Singleton, 1955), but the speed of planned, repetitive movements such as tapping is maintained (Fieandt, Huhtala, Kullberg, & Saari, 1956). Because almost all behaviors mediated by the central nervous system are slowed with aging, central factors are assumed to be largely responsible for slower information processing speed (Birren, 1964b). Recognize, though, that the schemata of older adults can be particularly complete and refined for skills with which the adult has had a lifetime of experience. Provided that time factors do not limit performance, older adults can demonstrate very accurate performance on well-practiced tasks.

Summary 8.1—Information Processing

The learning and performance of cognitive and motor tasks is described by information processing models that outline the components involved in these processes. These components are ways we can explain the functions carried out by the brain, rather than physical structures in the central nervous system. Many of the components develop over the course of childhood. Among them are attention and selective filtering, response schemata, and neuromuscular control. The speed of information processing also increases during childhood, which in turn contributes to improved motor performance.

At the opposite end of the life span, older adults demonstrate limitations in information processing. Attentional factors and speed of processing play a role in declining performance, perhaps reflecting changes in the signal-to-noise ratio within the central nervous system. Repetitive, self-paced tasks are not affected as much as tasks requiring a series of rapid movements.

An important aspect of motor performance is the ability of an individual to relate present conditions for performance to memories of past experiences. This aspect of information processing is discussed next.

> **Concept 8.2   Children use their memory systems more effectively as they mature, whereas older adults experience memory deficits.**

Memory plays a role in the improved performance of both motor skills and cognitive skills in children. For a young batter to hit a pitched ball, a large influx of perceptual information received must be combined with memories of previous experiences before a response is made. Evidence suggests that children do not use their memory systems as effectively as adults, and this could account for some of the performance differences between children and adults. Memory might play a role, too, in performance differences between young adults and older adults. Differences in effective usage of the memory system could be due to the *capacity* of available mental space, the *strategies* of memory use, or perhaps a combination of both. Members of the Piagetian school of thought propose that mental space increases with age (Pascual-Leone, 1970; Case, 1972a, 1972b, 1974b), but other developmentalists favor the view that processing strategies are deficient in, or unavailable to, children. Both groups present supporting evidence, but the current research leans toward the view that strategies of memory use best explain age-group motor performance differences (Chi, 1976; Thomas, 1980). These strategies, or control processes, refer to the handling of information and include the development and use of remembering strategies, rehearsal strategies, and the labeling, grouping, and coding of information to be remembered. The evidence supporting the assertion that control processing strategies rather than memory capacity are the key to memory development are now examined. We will also discuss the development of memory strategies and their persistence throughout adulthood.

Memory

Models of Memory

Before discussing the development of memory, it is valuable to recognize some of the models of memory that explain the recall and recognition of information used by adults. Many such models are suggested, but most fall into one of two categories, multistore models or levels of processing models. Neither type of model was originally proposed to explain the development of memory in children, but they provide the context and terminology for much of the developmental research. A basic knowledge of these two frameworks is, therefore, helpful to an understanding of the developmental work on memory.

The multistore models of memory have in common the notion of three memory storage components: the sensory store, the short-term store, and the long-term store. The first holds sensory information for a brief time, perhaps only a second. The short-term store holds information for a matter of seconds but is limited in its capacity for information. The capacity of the long-term store is thought to be unlimited. Children undoubtedly have a smaller "data base" than adults because they have had fewer experiences. Once information is placed in long-term store it can remain there throughout life, although one can have difficulty retrieving it from memory storage. Control processes or strategies are used to move information through the three storage components.

In the levels of processing models, remembering is related to the depth that information is processed. In other words, the more completely information is learned, the better it is remembered. If information is originally processed in a superficial or shallow manner, it is not well remembered. The control processes are critical to this model in that use of these processes moves information to a deeper level of memory. However, both of the memory frameworks, multistore and levels of processing models, consider control processes to be important aspects of memory.

Memory Capacity

Although the importance of control processes to memory is established, we should consider whether the capacity of the mental space increases with age, either instead of or in addition to better usage of the control processes. Chi (1976) examined this point in a review of research studies that analyzed the capacity of children's short-term store. She found several studies that examined what is termed the *recency effect* (see Figure 8.2). In these studies subjects were presented lists of information to remember. The tendency on such a task is to remember more items from the end of the list (the more recent) than from the middle of the list. Although children make more errors than adults, the shape of the "forgetting curve" is relatively stable across age-groups. Hence, children evidently do not run out of short-term memory space when they get to the end of the list. Chi also found no evidence that children lose the information in short-term store faster than adults. Thus, the view that children have limited short-term storage capacity is not strongly supported by research on the topic.

Memory Control Processes

Now consider the various control processes and their development. One of the most important is *rehearsal*, in which the information to be remembered is rehearsed in a serial fashion and continually attended to in the short-

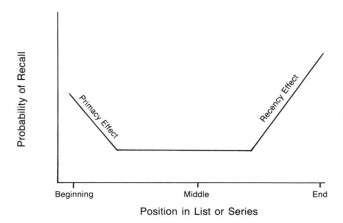

Figure 8.2   The "forgetting curve." Note that the probability of recall is highest for the beginning and end of a list.

term memory store (Chi, 1976). This process is similar to repeating a phone number, but need not be overt. Rehearsal is under an individual's control, and it takes time. This strategy is not widely used by children under 5 years of age (Chi, 1976; Daehler, Horowitz, Wynns, & Flavell, 1969). Children of 4 and 5 years can be instructed to use verbal rehearsal in motor performance, such as saying "jump" when one jumps, to better remember a sequence of motor tasks. However, this verbal rehearsal fails to assist children so young, because they do not realize it is a strategy for recalling the task (Weiss, 1983). After 5 years of age children begin to use rehearsal strategies, and the strategies become more sophisticated, at least through the age of 11 years (Ornstein & Naus, 1978). This improvement is illustrated in part by observing the pause time between items to be learned. Young children do not pause to rehearse between items, in contrast to adolescents and adults. Chi (1976) proposes that children learn to rehearse in three stages. They first assemble the rehearsal process, then learn when to execute the process, and finally learn to execute it correctly. Teaching children a rehearsal strategy in addition to the skill itself will enhance their skill acquisition (Thomas, Thomas, & Gallagher, 1981).

The control process termed *naming* or *labeling* refers to the attachment of a verbal label to a stimulus. It is likely that children remember less than adults because of a deficient naming process. That is, very young children might label information to be remembered, but they fail to *use* the labels to help themselves remember. Instructing children to use labels improves their recall, although it is important that the label be meaningful. Another memory strategy is *grouping* or *chunking*, wherein information to be remembered is placed into subgroups. Adults demonstrate grouping, but young children do not (Belmont & Butterfield, 1971). Yet, when children over 7 are taught to use adult grouping strategies, their performance improves (Harris & Burke, 1972; Liberty & Ornstein, 1973; McCarver, 1972). Gallagher and Thomas (1980a) also demonstrated that presentation of arm movements in an *organized* order facilitated recall of the movements by children 7 and older. Another process that is not used by young children is *recoding*. This involves searching the short-term store for two or more items that can be combined, based on some similarity, and then reentering the new code into the long-term store as a single item. For example, a tennis player experiences many balls with backspin during a practice session. The player then combines the knowledge gained from these occurrences and recodes them as information about balls with backspin.

Speed of Memory Functions

In addition to the differences in the control processes themselves, there is a difference in the speed with which memory functions are performed between young children and adults. Children take longer than adults to process information to be remembered. As children get older, they eventually can process either the same amount of information faster or more information in the same amount of time. Because speed is so important in many skills, memory processing speed influences motor performance. Age-related differences in memory processing speed are apparent when encoding and knowledge of results (KR) are studied in memory processing. For example, Chi (1977a, 1977b) found that speed encoding is slower in children than adults. Her 5-year-old subjects required more than twice as much time to identify pictures of classmates, implying that the adults encoded information to be remembered twice as fast as children. This permitted more time for further processing of the information in the adults' short-term store. Other evidence of slower processing speeds required by children is found in studies where KR is provided for the performer. The preciseness of information given verbally to a performer upon completion of a motor task is also important in processing speed. For example, we could say to a batter "you missed," "you swung ahead of it," "you missed by 2 cm," or "you missed by 2.4 cm." When the period of time between KR and the next attempt at the task is held constant, adults typically perform better with more precise KR (unless the information is so precise as to be meaningless). However, this is not the case with young children. Thomas, Mitchell, and Solomon (1979) gave both 2nd and 4th graders either no KR, general KR (you were short or long), or precise KR (how far short or long) after they performed trials of an arm positioning task. As seen in Figure 8.3, the precision of KR was associated with reduced positioning error only at the older age level. The younger children performed more poorly when given precise KR. Presumably, the more precise the information, the greater the information load that must be processed by the performer during this fixed time span. The younger children could not process the increased information load of the precise KR in the time span allotted, although it is possible that the precise KR was too complex for the younger children. To clarify this issue, in a follow-up study Gallagher and Thomas (1980b) systematically varied the time span following KR (see Figure 8.4). Children at age 7 performed far worse than 11-year-olds or adults when the time span was 3 sec. They performed just a little better with 6 sec, but did as well as the older groups only when they were given 12 sec to process the KR. Children, then, move information through their memory systems at a slower rate than adults, and this can affect their performance on tasks when speed is important.

Changes in Memory During Older Adulthood

Older adults are generally able to recall less information than younger adults (Craik, 1977). There are two plausible explanations for this memory

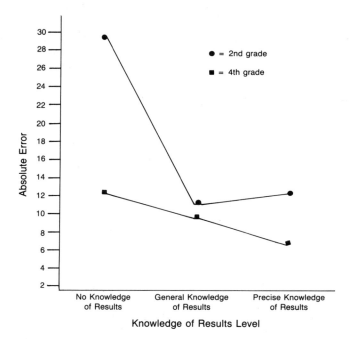

Figure 8.3 The interaction of grade level (age) and precision of knowledge of results for retention. From "Precision Knowledge of Results and Motor Performance: Relationship to Age" by J.R. Thomas, B. Mitchell, & M.A. Solomon, 1979, *Research Quarterly*, **50**, p. 696. Copyright 1979 by the American Alliance for Health, Physical Education, Recreation, and Dance. Reprinted by permission.

deficit. On the one hand, the loss of neurons in the brain that occurs with aging could involve a change in the *structure* of the brain. The other possibility is a change in the *functioning* of the memory processes. For example, the control processes may not be as efficient in older adults as in younger adults, or perhaps the speed of processing slows in old age. Because there is some research support for each explanation, both must be considered. It has even been suggested that a structural change is responsible for memory deficits in some older adults, while a functional change is responsible in others (Arenberg, 1980). Some aspects of memory are affected in older adulthood, but others do not change. Smith (1980), for example, found little evidence that a storage deficit is involved in poorer memory. The memory span, that is, the number of information items that can be held in short-term store, remains constant at least until the 60s. However, items that exceed the span in number are not as well remembered by older adults (Welford, 1980a).

Processing deficits involving *encoding* items into memory are characteristic of old age. Spontaneous organization of material to be remembered is par-

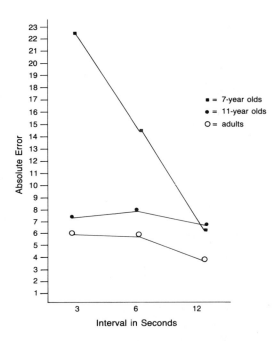

Figure 8.4 The interaction of age level and post-knowledge of results interval during performance of a ballistic movement. From "Effects of Varying Post-KR Intervals Upon Children's Motor Performance" by J.D. Gallagher and J.R. Thomas, 1980, *Journal of Motor Behavior*, **12**, p. 44. Copyright 1980 by J.D. Gallagher and J.R. Thomas. Reprinted by permission.

ticularly affected. Younger adults regularly organize material in anticipation of recalling the information, while older adults do so less often. Older adults may also be deficient in retrieving the information encoded into memory, but this is difficult to assess. When an older adult fails to recall information, it may be either that the information was not encoded properly or that it was encoded but cannot be retrieved (Smith, 1980). Persons who study memory using the levels of processing models alternately propose that memory deficits are a matter of shallower (more superficial) processing by older adults, rather than encoding or retrieval deficits (Craik & Simon, 1980). Some evidence indicates that memory loss is due to the slowing of mental functions. That is, older adults employ the same control processes as younger adults, but simply carry them out at a slower rate. For example, older adults rehearse more slowly than younger adults (Salthouse, 1980). The several plausible explanations of memory loss in older adults will be a research frontier for some time to come as investigators attempt to find the best explanation for such memory losses.

Summary 8.2—Memory Processes and Deficits

Memory plays a role in the performance of motor skills, because the information that is associated with skill performance is matched to the memories of previous experiences on similar tasks. For skills involving a speedy response to events in the environment, the memory process must operate efficiently to allow a response within the imposed time frame. Hence, memory deficits at any age can limit performance and are exhibited by both the young and the old. Evidence shows that the control processes that move information through the memory system are not as efficient at either end of the life span. The ability to rehearse, label, organize, and recode information to be remembered generally advances in late childhood. Older adults also have more difficulty getting information into memory as well as retrieving it from memory storage, but structural changes in the brain could be involved in their memory loss. The speed of processing information into memory, too, might be involved in the performance of both the young and old. Depending on the source of the memory deficit, though, it is possible for educators to assist performers of any age in remembering information. To do this, a teacher should allow sufficient time for rehearsal or suggest strategies to organize information and movements to be remembered.

At the beginning of this discussion of memory, we recognized that either memory stategies, memory capacity, or both could be involved in the development of memory. Here, we have discussed the development of memory strategies. Next, we will discuss developmental changes in memory capacity.

Concept 8.3   Children's mental capacity increases with age.

Thus far we have examined learning and performance from an information-processing viewpoint that stresses the functional components of cognitive processing in motor performance. We considered the development of information processing by examining the development of the many functional units in our information-processing model. Piaget (1952) took another view of cognitive development by proposing a temporal sequence of development in which change in mental capacity with maturation was emphasized. He suggested that children move through a sequence of stages, each stage characterized by observable behaviors. Piaget's stage model was appealing but was criticized because of the lack of a functional mechanism by which learning occurred (Thomas & Bender, 1977). In light of such criticism, a neo-

Piagetian model was proposed (Pascual-Leone, 1970; Pascual-Leone & Smith, 1969) that conceptualized Piaget's cognitive-developmental variable as a quantitative parameter called the central computing or *mental space* (M-space). M-space is assumed to grow as a function of age, and it explains how a child moves through the Piagetian stages (Pascual-Leone, 1970). Neo-Piagetian theory is of particular interest as it is applied to children's skill acquisition.

Neo-Piagetian Theory

Neo-Piagetian theory explains children's skill development through the general stages proposed by Piaget. A brief description of these stages is given in Table 8.1. The first stage, the Sensorimotor Stage, is a period when motor activities are coordinated with perceptions. The real beginning of cognition comes in the Preoperational Stage as the child starts to use symbols, and thinking is expressed by speech rather than movement. During the Concrete Operations Stage, the child acquires the use of elementary logic and reason and hierarchical classification. Alternative solutions to problems are recognized as the child becomes less egocentric. In the final Formal Operations Stage, the teenager reaches the highest level of cognitive functioning. Laws can be formulated and applied, symbols can be manipulated to solve problems, and deductions can be reached by hypothesis.

Table 8.1 Piaget's Stages of Cognitive Development

Stage	Age (yr)	Characteristics
Sensorimotor	Birth to 2	Infant is learning simple motor behavior and sensory perception; infant is learning to coordinate perception and movement.
Preoperational	2 to 7	Child is egocentric; language begins to replace sensorimotor activity; thinking is expressed by speech.
Concrete operations	7 to 11	Child is aware of alternate solutions; examines parts for knowledge of whole; expresses self in intellectual experimentation.
Formal operations	11–	Child deduces by hypothesis; approaches problems systematically; formulates laws.

Schemes

Neo-Piagetian theory combines the notion of these general stages with a quantitative factor to explain a child's development. The psychological system of the child is proposed to consist of: (a) a repertoire of schemes, and (b) the M-space in which the schemes are integrated with task demands (environmental conditions). The Piagetian *scheme* is conceptualized as a subjective unit of thought or set of reactions, functioning as a "mental blueprint" (Case, 1974b). A scheme can be transferred from one situation to another by assimilation of the situations. The three types of schemes in neo-Piagetian theory (see Figure 8.5) are: a *figurative* scheme that assigns meaning, an *operative* scheme that provides a blueprint for internal or external action, and an *executive* scheme that contains task instructions and solution plans (Pascual-Leone, 1976; Todor, 1978). A set of conditions termed the *releasing component* (rc) increases the likelihood that a scheme will be applied, *if* these conditions match favorably with reality. The *effecting component* (ec) of a scheme represents the consequences of applying that scheme to a situation. Case (1974a, 1974b) suggests that children expand their repertoire of schemes with increasing age. This expansion is achieved partly by incorporating new information into existing figurative schemes, thus forming new schemes. This

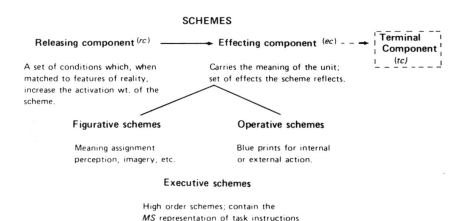

Figure 8.5 Schemes and their constituents. From "A Neo-Piagetian Theory of Constructive Operators: Applications to Perceptual-Motor Development and Learning" by J.I. Todor in *Psychology of Motor Behavior and Sport—1977* (p. 510) by D.M. Landers & R.W. Christina (Eds.) (pp. 507-521), 1978, Champaign, IL: Human Kinetics Publishers. Copyright 1978 by Human Kinetics Publishers. Reprinted by permission.

process is termed *Content-* or *C-learning.* New schemes are also acquired by consolidating two or more figurative and/or operative schemes, a process known as *Logical-* or *L-learning.*

M-Space

The second component of the child's psychological system is the M-space, of which there are two forms. *Structural* M-space is the maximum number of schemes that can be used by a child in a single act. It is associated with Piaget's general stages (see Table 8.2). The size of the structural M-space is taken to be an unknown but constant space, *e*, plus an age-related number of schemes, *k*, that can be used in a single task. This M-space construct was validated for cognitive tasks in a number of studies (Case, 1972a, 1972b, 1974b; Pascual-Leone, 1970; Pascual-Leone & Smith, 1969). It is obvious from observing children that not all of them perform similarly at a given age, as would be predicted from structural M-space alone. The variability in children's performance arises from the second form of M-space, *functional* M-space. This represents children's tendency to use the structural M-space available to them. Pascual-Leone (1970) suggests that functional M-space is mediated by a number of variables, including Witkin's cognitive style. The dimensions of cognitive style are *field dependence*, characterized by a reliance on irrelevant contextual stimuli, and *field independence*, characterized by an ability to differentiate self and an object (Haywood, Teeple, Givens, & Patterson, 1977). Field-dependent children are classified as low functional M-processors, be-

Table 8.2 M-Space Development

Developmental Substage	Age (yr)	M-Space
Early preoperational	3 to 4	$e + 1$
Late preoperational	5 to 6	$e + 2$
Early concrete	7 to 8	$e + 3$
Late concrete	9 to 10	$e + 4$
Early formal	11 to 12	$e + 5$
Middle formal	13 to 14	$e + 6$
Late formal	15 to 16	$e + 7$

Note. From "Learning and Development: A Neo-Piagetian Interpretation" by R. Case, 1972, *Human Development,* **15**, 342. Copyright 1972 by S. Karger AG, Basel. Reprinted by permission.

cause they assign higher weight than desirable to irrelevant cues. In contrast, field-independent children are high M-processors, capable of carrying out a task via the instructions given and ignoring conflicting perceptual cues. High and low M-processors can be identified by performance on such tasks as the Children's Embedded Figures Test (Witkin, Oltman, Rasben, & Karp, 1971). (Figure 6.3, p. 174, illustrates a similar test item.) This interpretation of functional M-space is empirically supported (Case, 1974b; Case & Globerson, 1974; Pascual-Leone, 1970).

Motor Skill Acquisition. Aspects of neo-Piagetian theory, then, have the support of research investigations utilizing *cognitive* tasks. Several investigators applied the theory to children's *skill* acquisition. Todor (1978) sought to test the theory's ability to predict and explain between- and within-group differences in motor performance. He used a modified Rho Task (see Figure 8.6) as the skill measure. In this task children were required, upon a stimulus, to rotate a handle once around to a stop, let go, then knock down a distant target as fast as possible. Reaction time, the time to circle, pause time in hitting the stop, and linear time to move to the target were recorded. Todor suggested that efficient performance of this task has an M demand of three, since three schemes would have to be integrated. These are (a) an operative scheme for

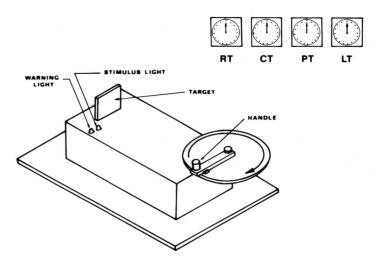

Figure 8.6 The Rho Task From "A Neo-Piagetian Theory of Constructive Operators: Applications to Perceptual-Motor Development and Learning" by J.I. Todor in *Psychology of Motor Behavior and Sport—1977* (p. 515) by D.M. Landers & R.W. Christina (Eds.) (pp. 507-521), 1978, Champaign, IL: Human Kinetics Publishers. Copyright 1978 by Human Kinetics Publishers. Reprinted by permission.

movement to the target, (b) a scheme for knowledge of the hand opening (leaving the handle), and (c) a scheme for target location. Inefficient performance would be characterized by movement under three separate schemes. An intermediate level of performance would be the integration of two of the three schemes.

Todor tested children between 5 and 12 years of age. A profile of the time scores representing the most efficient performance was identified and the results confirmed the suggestion that M capacity limited motor performance. Only 9% of the 5- to 6-year-olds were efficient, showing that most of them lacked the M capacity to integrate this task. Of the 7- to 8-year-olds, 42% and 79% of the 9- to 10-year-olds were efficient. All of the 11- to 12-year-olds were efficient, demonstrating not only that they had the capacity to integrate the task, but that cognitive style limitations diminished with increasing age. Thus, Todor demonstrated that both the M capacity and utilization of functional M-space increased for motor performance with increasing age.

Thomas and Bender (1977) also tested the applicability of neo-Piagetian theory to children's skill acquisition. Of particular concern to Thomas and Bender was the performance of high and low M-processors from various Piagetian stages. High and low M-processors from the late Pre-Operational Stage (6 years old) and the Early Concrete Stage (8 years old) were identified by their performance on an embedded figures test. Each age-group was given an age-appropriate form (e + k) and a more difficult form (e +k + 1) of a curvilinear arm positioning task. In this task subjects hand-controlled a pointer that swept a 180° arc. The number of stops to the arm movement presented on each trial was taken to represent the number of schemes required by the task. Two experiments were conducted, one with sight of the stops permitted and one without. Consistent with neo-Piagetian theory, high M-processors in both age-groups performed better than low M-processors. Thus, functional M-space accounted for the variability of children's performance within a Piagetian stage. Performance level was similar between the 6-year-olds on a two-scheme task and the 8-year-olds on a three-scheme task, demonstrating increased processing capacity for a motor task over age. Neo-Piagetian theory appears to be, on the basis of the Todor and the Thomas and Bender investigations, a useful viewpoint from which to examine children's skill acquisition.

Extensions of Piagetian Theory to Adulthood

At least two proposals have attempted to extend Piagetian theory into adulthood by focusing upon continued development and maintenance of concrete and formal operational abilities. Arlin (1975, 1977) proposed a fifth stage of cognitive development termed *problem-finding*. Creative thinking in finding problems to tackle and discovering questions to ask, rather than answering questions, characterize this stage. Adults, according to this view, may seek out challenges. In a different line of thought, Riegel (1976) hypothesized that adults do not remain in the stable equilibrium of formal operations as proposed by Piaget but rather are in constant flux or disequilibrium between internal forces and the social environment. Hence, adults update their identity in response to their experiences.

The fifth stage of cognitive development is controversial, because the major characteristics of the proposed fifth stage tend to be gradual modifications in existing thought structures rather than structural changes taking place after adolescence (Fakouri, 1976). Experiences stimulate adult cognitive growth, making the social environment an important feature of adult development and involving both cognition and personality. In the adult, then, cognitive growth involves both cognitive change and personality change.

Proposals for a fifth stage of cognitive development extend only into young adulthood. One of the hypotheses tested with middle and old adults is *cognitive regression*. It is hypothesized that mental abilities are lost in old age in an order opposite that of acquisition in childhood, such that an old adult eventually becomes similar in thought process to a child in the preoperational stage. Some studies have supported cognitive regression. For example, Papalia (1972) challenged 6- to 74-year-olds to perform tasks involving the conservation of number, substance, weight (success indicating concrete operations), and volume (success indicating formal operations). For example, in a conservation of volume task, the person is challenged to recognize that the volume of water poured from a tall, thin glass to a short, wide glass is conserved even if the water level appears different. Old adults between 65 and 74 years of age did remarkably poorer on the substance, weight, and volume tasks than 55- to 64-year-olds, and in fact, performed at a level similar to adolescents 11 to 13 years of age. Other studies (Rubin, 1976) have challenged cognitive regression. Rubin found no difference between middle-aged and older adults in their conservation judgments, even following false, disconfirming examples. How can we explain these contradictory findings? Several explanations have been advanced.

One reason for the findings is that the studies testing the cognitive regression hypothesis have been cross-sectional. The older adults in such studies may not have had as much formal education as younger subjects, or their education may have stressed memorization more than logical reasoning. The conservation tasks used in the Piagetian studies also may have been irrelevant to the older adults, and thus they were not motivated to perform well. Younger subjects may have been exposed to such tasks in their formal education. Greater familiarity with a task could influence the strategy used to solve it. Some of the tasks seem childlike, perhaps causing older adults to feel insulted or confused by such an apparently simple task. The conservation tasks themselves yield inconsistent results among individuals of any age. Poor performance on a single conservation problem does not predict poor performance on all such problems. In some studies even young adults did not consistently solve tasks at the formal or concrete ability level. Consequently, no study thus far has shown a regression to concrete operations by adults who previously used formal operations. We know then that older adults perform cognitive tasks differently than young adults, but this difference is not necessarily indicative of a *loss* in mental function. Attempts to analyze adult motor development from a Piagetian viewpoint have yet to be reported in the literature.

Summary 8.3—Mental Capacity

Information processing models are useful in examining many components of children's skill acquisition, but increased capacity for processing is not addressed by such models. In contrast, neo-Piagetian theory suggests that children's repertoire of schemes expands with age such that children can perform increasingly more demanding tasks. A task can be more demanding because it requires attention to more schemes or because it requires the integration of more movements. Neo-Piagetian theory also explains variable performance among children in the same Piagetian stage by proposing that children vary in their usage of the mental capacity available to them. Applications of neo-Piagetian theory to children's *motor* performance indicate the theory is a helpful viewpoint of skill development. Educators, by analyzing a given motor task for its processing demands, can predict the age at which children have the capacity to perform the task. Children can be expected to handle increasingly more demanding tasks with advancing age. Within any stage, children whose cognitive style is influenced by irrelevant cues can be expected to perform more poorly than children who are capable of following through on task instructions by ignoring irrelevant perceptual cues.

Cognitive development continues into adulthood, although the changes may be modifications of thought processes rather than structural changes. Some evidence indicates cognitive regression in older adulthood, but performance differences may reflect different educational experiences and motivations among older adults rather than a loss of mental ability. It has not been shown that older adults stop using mental operations previously demonstrated. Hence, it is more accurate to recognize older adult performance as different from rather than poorer than that of young adults.

An awareness of the information processing levels, mental capacity, and memory levels characteristic of an age-group and the way such characteristics affect motor skill performance is valuable when programming physical activities. At the same time we should remember that no individual behaves in isolation, but rather in a social environment.

The social context in which individuals grow and mature can be a powerful influence on their interest and participation in physical activities. These influences are discussed in the next chapter.

Suggested Readings

Chi, M. (1976). Short-term memory limitations in children: Capacity or processing deficits? *Memory and Cognition*, **4**, 559-572.

Poon, L.W., Fozard, J.L., Cermak, L.S., Arenberg, D., & Thompson, L.W. (Eds.). (1980). *New directions in memory and aging*. Hillsdale, NJ: Lawrence Erlbaum Associates.

Rothstein, A.L. (1977). Information processing in children's skill acquisition. In R.W. Christina & D.M. Landers (Eds.), *Psychology of motor behavior and sport—1976* (pp. 218-227). Champaign, IL: Human Kinetics.

Thomas, J.R., & Bender, P.R. (1977). A developmental explanation for children's motor behavior: A neo-Piagetian interpretation. *Journal of Motor Behavior*, **9**, 81-93.

Todor, J.I. (1978). A neo-Piagetian theory of constructive operators: Applications to perceptual-motor development and learning. In D.M. Landers & R.W. Christina (Eds.), *Psychology of motor behavior and sport—1977* (pp. 507-521). Champaign, IL: Human Kinetics.

Welford, A.T. (1980). Motor skill and aging. In C.H. Nadeau, W.R. Halliwell, K.M. Newell, & G.C. Roberts (Eds.), *Psychology of motor behavior and sport—1979* (pp. 253-268). Champaign, IL: Human Kinetics.

Wickens, C.D. (1974). Temporal limits of human information processing: A developmental study. *Psychological Bulletin*, **81**, 739-755.

9

Sociocultural Influences on Motor Development

Social learning is one of the most potent environmental factors in development. Children learn certain behaviors by observing others, who serve as models, and by internalizing these behaviors (Bandura & Walters, 1963; Bandura, 1969). Models, especially those significant to the child, can encourage or discourage behaviors by whether or not they engage in them or by how they label them. For example, saying "only girls cry" to a young boy influences him to believe it is inappropriate for him to cry. Learners need not reproduce behaviors outwardly to internalize them or receive direct encouragement from models, although encouragement strengthens the chances that the learner will reproduce the behaviors.

The toys and furnishings provided children are also a part of the socialization process, because they stimulate particular kinds of play. Thus beginning at a very young age, children are socialized for participation as a functioning member of society, both broadly and for a specific social role (Loy, McPherson, & Kenyon, 1978). This process of social learning, however, extends through the life span as other people and situations influence individuals.

Socialization involves many types of

behavior, including social skills, physical skills, traits, values, knowledge, attitudes, norms, and dispositions. Socialization is critical for motor development, because motor experiences are vital to the full development of motor skill. Children who are socialized into motor experiences are more likely to learn motor skills. Increased proficiency in the performance of skills is enjoyable and rewarding in itself and promotes, in turn, continued participation. On the other hand, children who are not exposed to motor experiences are less likely to master motor skills. With limited practice, they are more likely to fail and lose their interest in physical activities (Greendorfer, 1983).

For example, consider a family in which the parents are active. They exercise regularly and join recreational sport leagues. Their children see them in these settings. When they go to the tennis courts, the children come along and get a turn to play tennis. The parents may purchase a tennis racquet for each child and teach them some of the basic tennis skills. It would be of little surprise to find these individuals are active sport participants in adolescence and adulthood.

Concept 9.1   Children and adults are socialized into physically active lifestyles.

Early sport and physical activity socialization is a key factor in both motor development and the likelihood of later participation in physical activities. People and situations continue to influence individuals in their choice of activities over the life span. Peers, for example, influence which recreational activities, active or sedentary, are undertaken and over a period of time whether the lifestyle is active or inactive. Certainly the socialization process and the agents who are influential in the process deserve attention as major environmental influences on motor development.

Three major elements of the socialization process lead to the learning of a societal role: (a) socializing agents (i.e., "significant others"), (b) social situations, and (c) personal attributes (Kenyon & McPherson, 1973). Among the important socializing agents are family members, peers, and teachers/coaches. Of these the family is perhaps the major socializing force, partly because it exerts its influence early in life. Family members expose infants to certain experiences and attitudes, and they reinforce the behaviors deemed appropriate by gestures, praise, and rewards, and they punish inappropriate behaviors. In this way, too, infants learn their gender role. The process is systematic but at times so subtle that family members may hardly realize what and how they communicate to an infant.

Socializing Agents

Family Members

The family is a major influence in the sport (using the term broadly) socialization process (Snyder & Spreitzer, 1973; Kelly, 1974), just as it is in the socialization of children into other pursuits such as music (Snyder & Spreitzer, 1978). The participation of older children, adolescents, and adults in sport reflects in part their parents' interest and encouragement during the early years. Parents can encourage children and reinforce them for engaging in active types of play that involve motor skill, or they can support sedentary play. As the child grows physically active, parents can encourage or discourage games and, eventually, specific sports. There is little doubt that socialization into sport begins in childhood; about 75% of the eventual participants become involved in sport by the age of 8 (Greendorfer, 1976; Snyder & Spreitzer, 1976), and the best predictor of adult sport involvement is childhood and adolescent participation (Greendorfer, 1979; Loy et al., 1978; Snyder & Spreitzer, 1976).

Stereotypical Behavior. Parents and other significant socializing agents can encourage certain children toward different types of behavior. It has been common for societies to socialize boys and girls into different societal roles. This practice is often termed *sex-typing* or *sex role stereotyping*. Traditionally, Western societies have carried sex-typing through to sport involvement. Sports have been considered appropriate, even important, activities for boys but the same beliefs were not necessarily supported for girls. Therefore, vigorous, outgoing play was permitted and encouraged for toddler boys, while girls were discouraged from or even punished for venturing far from parents, running, climbing, and so on (Lewis, 1972). Socializing agents reinforced constrained, sedentary types of play in girls; and thus many girls self-selected away from vigorous play (Greendorfer, 1983), leaving a comparatively small number of girls as active participants in vigorous, skilled play.

With such limited involvement and practice, many girls never developed their motor skills to full potential. Even among the girl participants there could be a feeling that all-out effort and skilled performance are inappropriate to the gender role supported by society. This in turn could affect a girl's or woman's motivation for participating, for training, or for working toward high achievement standards that rival those of men. Thus, this pervasive societal influence on the sport participation of boys and girls is believed to be a factor in measurements of skill and fitness that compare the sexes.

The role family members play in the socialization of children, then, can vary with the sex of the child. Too, the sex of the parent serving as a model for behavior may differentially influence the internalization of the behavior by the child. This influence is true of other socializing agents as well, so that the sex of the socializing agent and the individual person must be kept in mind throughout any discussion of the socializing process.

Individual Roles Affect Sport Involvement. Individual family members probably play differential roles in the sport socialization process. Snyder and Spreitzer (1973) noted that the same-sex parent was most influential in extent of sport involvement, and McPherson (1978) suggested specifically that mothers serve as sport role models for their daughters. Lewko and Ewing (1980) found that boys between the ages of 9 and 11 years who were highly involved in sports were influenced by their fathers and highly involved girls by their mothers. A difference between boys and girls, however, was that girls seemed to need a higher level of encouragement than boys did from their families, and they needed it from many members of the family to become involved (see Table 9.1). This necessity for a higher level of encouragement by more significant others probably reflects the traditional attitude of American society that considers sports to be more appropriate for boys than girls. In contrast to these studies, Greendorfer and Lewko (1978b) identified fathers as a major influence on the sport involvement of both boys and girls, while mothers did not appear to be a factor in sport socialization.

Some investigators feel that siblings are also important agents in the sport socialization process, because they provide the first play group for an infant. Brothers, for example, are often considered important to girls' sport involve-

Table 9.1 Family Members' Influence on Sport Involvement

	Sport Involvement Level							
	Males				Females			
Family	Low		High		Low		High	
Member	M	SD	M	SD	M	SD	M	SD
Father	15.13	4.63	18.46	4.34	14.92	3.53	18.53	4.06
Mother	12.66	3.25	14.48	3.66	13.62	3.59	17.74	3.67
Brother	13.32	6.98	15.61	7.14	14.14	5.71	16.24	7.26
Sister	11.32	5.18	11.21	5.29	11.89	5.22	14.60	6.77

Note. Mean scores (*M*) and standard deviations (*SD*) from a questionnaire are given in the table; higher means reflect stronger influence. From "Sex Differences and Parental Influence in Sport Involvement of Children" by Lewko, J.H., and Ewing, M.E., 1980, *Journal of Sport Psychology*, **2**, 66. Copyright 1980 by Human Kinetics. Adapted by permission.

ment (Weiss & Knoppers, 1982), although sisters can influence girls' participation, too (Lewko & Ewing, 1980). On the other hand, Greendorfer and
Lewko (1978b) found that siblings were not significant agents in the sport
socialization of their study participants.

It is obvious that various research studies reached different conclusions
on the role of family members in sport socialization. Greendorfer and Lewko
(1978a) attempted to clarify these various conclusions by questioning children from a broad range of social backgrounds. They found some differences
in the pattern of significant influences among subsamples of subjects. The
socializing agent who exerted the most influence in sport socialization varied
somewhat among groups of different sex and different social background, race,
and geographic location. The overall pattern of family member influence is
nevertheless clear.

The pattern of significant influences on sport socialization is more consistent among samples of males than females, according to Greendorfer and
Lewko. The family, especially the father, is consistently influential in the sport
involvement of boys. The pattern for girls is more variable across social background. One explanation for the inconsistent pattern of girls' sport involvement is the lack of a specific family member to take responsibility for
socializing a daughter into sport. In comparison, fathers feel responsible for
initiating their sons' interest in sport. Despite the minor inconsistencies in pattern of influence among subsamples of subjects, family members, especially
parents, are clearly important agents in the sport socialization process.

Peers

Peers have the potential to reinforce the sport socialization process begun in the family for both boys and girls (Greendorfer & Lewko, 1978b). The
first peer group encountered is typically a play group. Children become involved in such groups at approximately 3 to 4 years of age and continue in
them during the early school years. During preadolescence, children enter
a more formalized peer group, such as a clique or gang. In childhood and
adolescence, a supportive peer group is usually of the same sex as the participant. In adulthood and particularly after marriage, opposite-sex peers
become more influential in either encouraging or discouraging involvement
in certain activities, especially for women (Loy et al., 1978).

At any age, if a peer group tends to participate in active play or sports,
individual members are drawn to such activities. If, on the other hand, the
group prefers passive activities, individual members tend to follow this lead.
Adult athletes typically report that a peer group or friend influenced the extent
of their participation in sport during the school years, although the strength
of this influence varies among sports. Both boys and girls report that peers

influenced their sport participation (Greendorfer & Lewko, 1978b). In fact, of the women she questioned, Greendorfer (1976) found that the peer group was the only socializing agent that influenced sport involvement throughout all phases of the life cycle studied: childhood, adolescence, and young adulthood. Other socializing agents were important at some ages but not others. Peers are often a stronger influence for participation in team sports than individual sports during childhood and adolescence (Kenyon & McPherson, 1973).

As individuals leave school and enter a new social environment as a member of the work force, they often leave their peer group. If their group had been sport-oriented, a reduction in sport involvement might follow. New peer groups at the work place, on the other hand, could stimulate sport involvement by forming teams for recreational sport leagues or perhaps by participation in company-sponsored exercise and recreation programs (Loy et al., 1978). It is likely that the typical middle-aged adult, even if involved in sport during young adulthood, reduces sport involvement. This trend might be due in part to a lack of programs specifically for middle and older adult age-groups. Renewed emphasis on fitness beginning in the late 1970s has led to exercise and recreation programs for members of these age-groups. Additionally, participation in sport and exercise programs by adults has gained acceptance and even desirability in Western societies. With specific programs now available, peer groups might once again influence recreational involvement at older ages. Once involved, adults maintain their participation to be a part of the peer group.

Despite the strong influence of peer groups on sport participation throughout the life cycle, it is still not clear that membership in a sport-oriented peer group always *precedes* participation, that is, that one is drawn to an activity because of a desire to associate with peers. Possibly individuals first select groups that fit their interests, including an interest in sports (Loy et al., 1978). Although it is not clear which comes first, the interest in sports and the desire to be a part of a peer group make it likely that an individual will continue to participate and to select membership in active groups.

Coaches and Teachers

Coaches and teachers are also socializing agents who influence sport involvement, although probably more so for boys than girls (Greendorfer & Lewko, 1978b). Male athletes consistently report that coaches and teachers were influential in both their participation and their selection of sports, particularly during adolescence and young adulthood (Kenyon & McPherson, 1973). In contrast, female athletes report that teachers and coaches influenced them during adolescence, but not in childhood or young adulthood (Greendorfer, 1976). Thus, for female athletes, teachers and coaches appear to strengthen sport socialization processes begun earlier by the family and friends.

Teachers and coaches should not overlook their potential influence on the sport involvement of students. They can introduce children and adolescents to exciting new activities and stimulate them to learn the skills and attitudes associated with sport. Conversely, teachers and coaches also must recognize the potential they have to turn off their students from sport and physical activity. Bad experiences during the school years can have lifelong consequences for one's overall lifestyle (Snyder & Spreitzer, 1983). Such negative experiences are known as *aversive socialization*, and in the schools it often takes the form of embarrassing children in front of their peers, overemphasizing performance criteria at the expense of enjoyment and programming experiences that result in overwhelming failure rather than success. Children who experience aversive socialization naturally avoid physical activities and fail to learn skills well; consequently, any attempt to participate remains frustrating and discouraging. While teachers and coaches can take pride in students who achieve in sport and dance, they can also strive to make physical activities enjoyable for all students with whom they work.

Social Situations

Play Environments and Games

An adequate environment for play, such as a backyard or playground, can provide the social situation and environment to initiate sport involvement. Play spaces probably influence sport selection as well. Lack of an adequate play space diminishes the opportunity for involvement in activity and practice of skills, thus discouraging participation in sports. Children who grow up in urban areas where playing fields are limited are typically exposed to sports that require little space and equipment, such as basketball. Boys and girls could also be influenced to participate in sex-typed activities in some play environments. A boy might be labeled a "sissy" for jumping rope or a girl a "tomboy" for playing basketball. American society has traditionally considered certain types of games to be appropriate for boys but not girls and vice versa. This labeling is particularly apparent as children enter adolescence.

The influence to participate in gender-role appropriate games has implications for skill practice opportunities. Traditional boys' games are typically complex and involve the use of strategies. They encourage work toward a specific goal and promote negotiation to settle disputes over rules. Traditional girls' games, on the other hand, are typically noncompetitive, and rather than encouraging interdependence among the group, they involve waiting for a turn to perform a simple repetitive task, such as rope-jumping or hop-scotch. Such games rarely provide girls with an opportunity to increase the complexity of the game or develop increasingly more difficult skills. In fact, the games often end because the participants lose interest rather than achieve a goal (Greendorfer, 1983). Fortunately, sex-typing through games has diminished in recent years, but educators should keep in mind that a play environment that channels boys and girls into sex-typed games maintains a situation that fosters skill development for boys but not girls.

Play With Toys

Children's toys are another facet of the socialization process. Toys can encourage children to be active or inactive and can stimulate them to model sport figures. For example, a hockey stick encourages a child to run or skate, dodge obstacles, and develop an accurate shot; board games encourage sedentary play. Obviously, each kind of toy has its advantages, but certainly socialization into sport is facilitated by some toys and not others.

Toys are also a means by which sex-typing can occur in the socialization process. For example, toys marketed for boys tend to be complex and encourage more vigorous activity than those marketed for girls. The typical girls' toy promotes quiet indoor play, such as "playing house" (Greendorfer, 1983). Sex-typing through toys is well entrenched in society. Manufacturers often advertise their products along sex-typed strategies. For example, boys are featured on commercials or packaging for racing car sets, and girls are pictured with toy kitchen sets. Not only are children consumers of these marketing ploys, but so are their parents. In addition, parents enjoy giving their children the same kinds of toys they played with as children, thus tending to perpetuate traditional sex-typing. Moreover, parents can promote sex-typing by negatively reinforcing play with toys they judge to be sex-inappropriate (Fagot, 1978). Such sex-typing is slow to change.

In recent years awareness of the many ways children are sex-typed and the implications of this process have been heightened. Yet little evidence shows substantial change away from sex-typing (Huston, 1984; Kaiser & Phinney, 1983; Langlois & Downs, 1980; Schwartz & Markham, 1985). Teachers must realize they play a role in this aspect of socialization (Fagot, 1984). They can reinforce early sex-typing by continuing to label certain activities as more important or appropriate for one sex than the other, choosing different activities for the two groups, and holding different expectations for the achievements of boys and girls. Or they can make every attempt possible to eliminate such distinctions and allow individuals to explore their full potential. It is likely that such day-to-day decisions and expectations accumulate over time to produce differences in boys' and girls' motor development by channeling practice opportunities (Brundage, 1983; Greendorfer & Brundage, 1984).

Personal Attributes

Socializing agents and situations interact with an individual's personal attributes to influence sport involvement. Certainly perceived ability is one attribute important to choice of activity (Kukla, 1978). One is not likely to continually choose an activity if the expectation is to achieve little success. On the other hand, a person would probably persist in an activity, such as sports, if the perceived ability is high, even in the face of limited real success.

Perceived Sport Ability in Children

Lewko and Ewing (1980) questioned children about their perceived ability in sport and level of involvement. Interestingly, boys as a group perceived their ability as high regardless of their sport involvement level. This may reflect the boys' tendency to respond in accordance with a male stereotype. In contrast, only girls involved in sport perceived their ability as high; girls uninvolved perceived their ability as low. These findings suggest that the sport socialization process can deliver two very different messages to young boys and girls.

Boys are expected to be capable of sport participation. For most boys this is an advantage in that they enter sport participation with a positive expectancy. Of course, boys with low expectancies and subsequent failures in sport are left with a feeling of inadequacy and often withdraw from sport and exercise. The message many girls get through the sport socialization process is that they are incapable of highly-skilled performance. Even though the message is invalid, they approach skills with an expectation of failure. To compound the negative expectancy situation, girls frequently have limited motor experiences and practice opportunities; hence, they have a greater propensity to fail. When this happens, many girls lose their interest in physical activities (Greendorfer, 1983). Even those who develop good skills can have lingering doubts as to their potential or the appropriateness of their sport involvement. While this scenario need not be true, it is important for educators to realize that many girls come to believe they have limited potential for skilled performance, and failure only tends to reinforce this belief. Boys who have low skill can feel they are not living up to their gender role, particularly if pressured by fathers and coaches. This can contribute to a poor self-image that affects many behaviors.

Adult Socialization

As a result of childhood and adolescent socialization, individuals form an identity based upon social roles with certain social expectations. These expectations are the basis of new social learning in adulthood. Changes in identity are a function of new adult roles, such as those associated with a career or parenthood (Brim, 1966). While children are socialized into cultural values transmitted by parents and the school system, adults learn behaviors attached to specific roles (Inkeles, 1969). Individuals also anticipate the roles they will occupy in future years. Hence, children play-act roles they might adopt as adults, young adults anticipate achieving a certain economic standard of living by middle adulthood, middle-age adults anticipate leisure activities in retirement, and so on. These anticipated roles are often formed by conforming to the age-linked behaviors society holds as appropriate for a particular age span. Acting outside the accepted social role often invites negative reactions from others and brings about discord within the individual.

A typical pattern of social behavior in Western societies has been characterized by decreased involvement in active sports throughout the adult years, so that older adults are often considered sedentary, even feeble. The anticipated role of older adulthood often included cessation of vigorous activity. Recently, attitudes have shifted to favor exercise and activity throughout the life span. This change has probably been stimulated by medical research but undoubtedly involves a redefinition of the appropriate age-linked behaviors related to sport and exercise. Hence, in recent years society has come to accept middle-aged and older adults dressed in exercise clothes and running shoes. Activity groups for older adults have emerged, and special sport-related functions for older adults, such as the Senior Olympics, are widely accepted. Whereas older adults might previously have been socialized into a sedentary lifestyle, recent attitude shifts have allowed for socialization into an active lifestyle.

New activity-oriented peer groups are an important aspect of this emerging active lifestyle in the later years. Older adults might join exercise and recreational groups as much for the social benefits as the physical benefits. New friendships and peer groups are established. These activity-oriented friends encourage continued involvement in the activity program. Hence, exercise and activity become a normal characteristic of the lifestyle.

While the active exercising older adult has gained acceptance in recent years, some older adults remain uncomfortable in adopting this role. The extent of sport socialization during youth likely affects one's participation throughout life. Although peer groups and the availability of sport situations undoubtedly play a role in adult sport involvement, they often do so against the backdrop of early sport socialization. Hence, those socialized into a role characterized by a sedentary lifestyle probably persist in this lifestyle, even when exercise and activity become critical to overall health. The older adult who was very active as a younger person finds it easier to become active, even if years of inactivity might have intervened, than someone who had not been active during his or her youth. This emphasizes the importance to lifelong health of socializing both males and females into active lifestyles, if not sport, during their early years.

Summary 9.1—The Socialization Process

Young individuals learn social behavior by observing and internalizing the behavior of significant others, who serve as models. Further, reinforcement from these significant people contributes to the likelihood that certain behaviors will be adopted. Involvement in sport is one of the behaviors influenced by this process. Family members, especially fathers, peer groups, teachers, and coaches can successfully encourage participation in sports. Environmental spaces and objects can also facilitate the development of skill and participation in sport, although sex-typing through games and toys can limit the skill achieved by girls.

The strong influence of social factors on motor development provides much food for thought when males and females are compared on skill achievements. Are differences primarily biological? Or might social factors be so pervasive as to limit the achievements of girls and women more than any relevant biological factors? These questions are difficult to answer because most female athletes are still products of a socialization process that has tended to be different for girls than boys.

In the past the socially acceptable role for middle and older adults lacked participation in exercise and vigorous activity, but recently a new model has emerged for adults. This new role accepts exercise and physical activity as an integral part of the lifestyle. Exercise and recreation programs for middle and older adults foster the formation of new, activity-oriented peer groups, which in turn encourage continued involvement.

We have seen that social values and norms influence sport participation and lifestyle. Certainly these values and social norms differ among various cultures and ethnic groups. So, too, do standards of living, including diet. We will discuss next what effects these and other factors might have on the motor development of various ethnic and cultural groups.

Concept 9.2 **Ethnic and cultural differences in motor development are related to the environmental variables affecting group members.**

Throughout our discussions we have emphasized the influence of environmental factors on motor development. For example, motor development can lag if nutrition is poor pre- or postnatally, if disease is prevalent, and if physical growth is subsequently slowed, but it can be maximized if nutrition and health care are good and the opportunities for skill practice are numerous. Educational programs can stimulate thought and creativity to maximize a child's cognitive development. The activities demonstrated by family members and the childhood behaviors reinforced by persons important to the child can either encourage or discourage an individual's involvement in physical activities. Child-rearing practices can lend themselves to stimulation of active play and skill development or can limit these opportunities. Economic status can influence the amount of play space available and the number and type of toys available, which in turn can affect opportunities to attempt and practice skills. These are just some of the environmental factors that can vary for a developing individual.

Many of these environmental factors are similar for whole groups of people, that is, races, cultures, or ethnic groups. Might this lead to differences among such groups in their pattern or tempo of motor development? Identifying any such differences would have at least two benefits. First, if such differences exist, norms for a particular group can be established and considered by teachers in working with members of the group. Second, if the environmental conditions that vary among groups can be identified, then the effects of environmental factors on the acceleration or deceleration of motor development can be identified. The focus of our discussion is whether differences actually exist in motor performance among racial, ethnic, and cultural groups and which environmental factors could bring about these differences.

Black and White Children

The two ethnic groups in the United States whose motor performance is tested most often are whites of European ancestry and blacks. Sometimes, performance differences between the groups are noted, although at other times and on some tests, no differences are detected. Most of the differences are observed between birth and 2 years of age and consist of *tempo* differences in the emergence of the motor milestones. The *sequence* of motor development is remarkably stable across these two groups (Malina, 1973). The timing differences are usually in favor of black children. For example, Bayley (1965) observed that black infants were ahead of white infants in mean score on the Bayley Scale of Infant Development at every month from age 1 month to age 14 months (see Table 9.2). This advantage existed on most of the 60 test items, so that one type of skill was not responsible for the difference in the scale score. While Bayley's observations are shared by many other investigators,

Table 9.2 Performance on the Bayley Infant Scale of Motor Development for Babies by Race

Age (mos)	White Babies			Black Babies		
	N	M	SD	N	M	SD
1	41	6.34	2.03	41	6.39	2.98
2	45	9.31	2.20	37	9.89	2.22
3	42	12.12	2.57	41	13.39	2.82
4	47	14.57	3.20	31	16.29	2.92
5	41	18.83	3.32	40	21.25	3.46
6	44	25.73	4.40	42	25.76	4.78
7	47	28.47	4.88	41	30.46	4.64
8	61	34.41	5.27	51	35.67	5.02
9	54	37.13	4.06	44	38.95	4.17
10	53	40.11	3.62	40	41.32	3.93
11	43	42.84	3.06	26	44.00	2.97
12	49	44.22	3.16	43	45.88	4.42
13	44	46.45	6.49	36	47.08	3.27
14	48	48.33	3.01	38	48.68	4.03

Note. Mean scores (*M*) and standard deviations (*SD*) on the Bayley Infant Scale of Motor Development are given. From "Comparisons of Mental and Motor Test Scores for Ages 1-15 Months by Sex, Birth Order, Race, Geographic Location, and Education of Parents" by N. Bayley, 1965, *Child Development*, **36**, 405. Copyright 1965 by University of Chicago Press.

a few studies have failed to find significant differences in this age range (see Malina, 1973, for a summary).

Less information on ethnic group differences in motor development is available for the 2- to 6-year age span. Further, the results of the studies on these age-groups tend to be inconclusive. For example, Sessoms (1942) found black 3- and 4-year-olds to be ahead of white children in fine motor task scores, but Rhodes (1937) found no fine motor differences in a sample of preschoolers. More recently, Sandler, Van Campen, Ratner, Stafford, and Weismar (1970) compared the performance of lower class, urban black children at 4 to 6 years to the Denver Developmental Screening Test norms that were established primarily on white children. The black children compared favorably with or scored slightly ahead of the norms on gross motor skill items and some fine motor items. On fine motor items involving "cognitive operations," however, the black children fell below the norms. Thus, no clear ethnic trends emerge from studies of motor development in children during the preschool years.

Comparisons of black and white children at school ages tend to be based on quantitative, or product-oriented, measures, including measures of functional muscle strength. Many of these comparisons also documented higher performance levels by black children and adolescents than their white counterparts. For example, black children scored better than whites on a jump and reach test (boys and girls) and throw for distance (girls) (Temple, 1952), on the 35-yd dash (boys and girls) (Hutinger, 1959; Malina, 1969), and on the vertical jump (boys) (Martino, 1966; Martin, 1966). On the other hand, some studies reported little difference between blacks and whites on motor skills such as softball throw for distance (Malina, 1969), pull-ups, push-ups, or ball-put (Walker, 1938). On occasion, differences in favor of white children were found, such as on the broad jump and the dash (Walker, 1938). Perhaps even more frustrating are repeated measures that show one group ahead at one testing, but the other group ahead at the next (Malina, 1969). The findings are just as variable on measures of functional muscle strength (see Malina, 1973, for a summary). In attempting to summarize these studies, we can only conclude that performance differences among black and white children of school age tend to vary, with few overall trends.

Before turning to the environmental factors that could account for the varied differences between blacks and whites, consider whether or not genetic factors might explain the differences. It is known that the skeletal growth of black infants is ahead of white infants (Malina, 1969), suggesting a faster maturation rate in blacks. Racial differences in body proportions and composition also have implications for performance. The difficulty with attributing all motor development differences to genetic factors is that some studies have found no developmental differences between blacks and whites (Knobloch & Pasamanick, 1958). If innate racial characteristics are operating alone, group differences should be consistently observed. If transient, environmental variables influence the differences, variable results might be obtained by different studies, as is the case. For this reason, environmental factors are emphasized in the explanation of ethnic differences in motor development.

Economics

Many of the environmental conditions that could influence motor development are related to economic factors. For example, poor nutrition often results from the lack of money to buy adequate foods of good nutritional value. Higher incidence of infectious disease can be related to poor nutrition and poor living conditions. A shortage of toys and sport equipment can limit the practice opportunities available to children. Because more black than white families in the United States have been at the lower socioeconomic levels, some performance differences may ultimately be traced to economic factors, particularly on those motor tasks likely to be affected by such factors.

Child-Rearing Practices

Child-rearing practices are believed to influence motor performance. Lower social class families typically permit infants to explore their environment and manipulate objects more freely, facilitating motor development (Williams & Scott, 1953). In contrast, children in upper class families are often placed in play pens or more restricted environments. They are not allowed to "climb on the new furniture," turn the stereo dials, and so on, which limits their opportunities to develop motor skills. If young children spend much of their time in day care centers, the quality of care may reflect what parents can afford. An expensive center might have many toys and more play space than one in a poor urban neighborhood, yet caretakers (in lower supervisor-to-child ratios) might supervise upper class children more closely and restrict children's exploration to meet parents' expectations. Even at older ages, lower social class children may be given more freedom to explore their neighborhoods.

Socialization into Sport

It is likely that socialization into sport differs among races. Greendorfer and Ewing (1981) examined this possibility for black and white children and found that this was indeed the case. White children were more influenced with regard to sport by specific socializing agents. Black children were more influenced by social structure or contextual factors such as values and opportunity. Hence black children receive more diffuse influences. Black athletes successful in professional sports serve as role models to young black children, while models successful in other endeavors are less available and prominent. White children have many role models available in a wider range of careers; their interests may shift to other areas. Success in sport skills, then, takes on relatively more importance for black youths, especially boys, than white children. Sports might be one of the few leisure activities accessible to lower socioeconomic families, in contrast to middle and upper class families who have other activities available to them, such as the theater and concerts. Lower class families, too, can see sports as a chance for fame and fortune and subsequently encourage their children's sport involvement (see Snyder & Spreitzer, 1983, pp. 146-153, for a review). These differences in the sport socialization process could account for differences in practice time, and in turn, differences in motor development among races.

Unanswered Issues

While environmental factors are likely involved in the motor development differences between blacks and whites, many questions remain unexplored. The role of socioeconomic status in motor development is still not clearly understood. Some child-rearing practices in lower social classes favor motor development, but higher socioeconomic levels are often related to advanced development, because better prenatal care, nutrition, and health care are stressed. Certainly child-rearing practices and living conditions have changed over the years since World War II, and consequently the practice of comparing research studies conducted on different cohorts is questionable. Environmental conditions involved in ethnic differences might change from generation to generation, yielding variable results. What is more, an environmental factor in one case can offset differences due to genetic factors or other environmental factors, masking the true nature of group differences. In another case, that same factor might not be strong enough to offset the others.

Other Ethnic Groups

Mexican Americans, other Hispanic Americans, and Americans of Oriental ancestry are sometimes included in studies of ethnic differences in motor development. Unfortunately, data on these groups are limited and even more variable than those comparing black and white children. For example, Thompson and Dove (1942) and Thompson (1944) found that Spanish- and Mexican-American boys in their early teens outperformed white boys on a battery of six quantitative motor tasks (baseball throw, base running, chinning, 60-yard dash, jump-and-reach, and shot put). Miller (1968) reported the opposite results for 13- to 15-year-old boys taking the California Physical Performance Test. Obviously, the same environmental factors that may be responsible for black versus white differences can affect Hispanic and Oriental groups, too. Both groups also tend to be smaller in physical size and stature than whites, possibly accounting for some performance differences, and surely limiting our ability to generalize from the limited number of research studies conducted to date. It is presently impossible to identify any differential trends in the motor development of these ethnic groups.

Summary 9.2—Ethnic Differences in Motor Development

Most of the available information on ethnic differences in motor development compares blacks and whites. Blacks typically reach the motor milestones before whites in the early months of life, but in later years it is difficult to identify trends in group differences. This suggests that a variety of environmental factors might be operating. In a practical sense, an educator must assess the environmental factors influencing a single child on an individual basis. Knowing what factors are likely to influence a member of any ethnic group is valuable as an initial guideline, but further individual assessment allows for a more accurate prescription of motoric activities and experiences.

Suggested Readings

Greendorfer, S. (1983). Shaping the female athlete: The impact of the family. In M.A. Boutilier & L. Sangiovanni, *The sporting woman* (pp. 135-156). Champaign, IL: Human Kinetics.

Kenyon, G.S., & McPherson, B.D. (1973). Becoming involved in physical activity and sport: A process of socialization. In G.L. Rarick (Ed.), *Physical activity: Human growth and development* (pp. 303-332). New York, NY: Academic Press.

Malina, R.M. (1973). Ethnic and cultural factors in the development of motor abilities and strength in American children. In G.L. Rarick (Ed.), *Physical activity: Human growth and development* (pp. 333-363). New York, NY: Academic Press.

Every Person Is Unique

It is natural for persons interested in observing and teaching motor skills to want information about average performances and capabilities of different age groups. Averages serve as a reference point against which individuals may be compared and provide a general idea of what to expect from members of the group. However, the study of developmental processes and the factors influencing those processes repeatedly demonstrates the uniqueness of individuals. Though physical growth and maturation proceed in a consistent pattern dictated by genetic make-up, a variety of environmental factors act throughout the life span to alter motor development patterns and tempos. Factors such as perceptual-motor experiences, cognitive experiences, and socialization experiences have an impact. Differences among individuals are further manifest in the manner in which individuals progress qualitatively from unskilled to skilled performances. Thus, regardless of age, individual motor development is a reflection of genetically inherited attributes coupled with impinging environmental influences that occur throughout life.

The challenge confronting motor developmentalists, teachers, coaches, and parents, then, is to tailor goals and expectations to individual capabilities and characteristics. Optimal motor skill development is likely related to the degree that practice opportunities and insightful instruction are matched to individual capability and potential. And although individualizing motor development goals and instruction in most institutional settings is both complex and time-consuming, findings from motor development research at various stages of the life span point in this direction. Continued research and observation of motor development will undoubtedly yield better understanding of developmental processes, but the task remains to find ways of using these knowledges such that optimal motor development may be realized by every individual.

References

Adams, F.H. (1973). Factors affecting the working capacity of children and adolescents. In G.L. Rarick (Ed.), *Physical activity: Human growth and development* (pp. 80-96). New York, NY: Academic Press.

Adams, G.M., & DeVries, H.A. (1973). Physiological effects of an exercise training regimen upon women aged 52 to 79. *Journal of Gerontology*, **28**, 50-55.

Adams, J.E. (1965). Injury to the throwing arm. *California Medicine*, **102**, 127-132.

Adrian, M.J. (1980). Biomechanics and aging. In J.M. Cooper & B. Haven (Eds.), *Proceedings of the Biomechanics Symposium* (pp. 132-141). Indianapolis, IN: Indiana State Board of Health.

Adrian, M.J. (1981). Flexibility in the aging adult. In E.L. Smith & R.C. Serfass (Eds.), *Exercise and aging: The scientific basis* (pp. 45-57). Hillside, NJ: Enslow Publishers.

Adrian, M.J. (1982, April). *Maintaining movement capabilities in advanced years*. Paper presented at the annual convention of the American Alliance for Health, Physical Education, Recreation and Dance, Houston, TX.

Allon, N. (1973). The stigma of overweight in everyday life. In G.A. Bray (Ed.), *Obesity in perspective* (pp. 83-102) (Fogarty Report No. 017-053-00046-9). Washington, D.C.: U.S. Government Printing Office.

American Alliance for Health, Physical Education, Recreation and Dance. (1976). *Youth Fitness Test Manual, Revised*. Reston, VA: AAHPERD Publications.

Ames, L.B. (1937). The sequential patterning of prone progression in the human infant. *Genetic Psychology Monographs*, **19**, 409-460.

Arenberg, D. (1980). Comments on the processes that account for memory declines with age. In L.W. Poon, J.L. Fozard, L.S. Cermak, D. Arenberg,

& L.W. Thompson (Eds.), *New directions in memory and aging.* Hillsdale, NJ: Lawrence Erlbaum Associates.

Arlin, P.K. (1975). Cognitive development in adulthood: A fifth stage? *Developmental Psychology,* **11**, 602-606.

Arlin, P.K. (1977). Piagetian operations in problem finding. *Developmental Psychology,* **13**, 297-298.

Aronson, E., & Rosenbloom, S. (1971). Space perception in early infancy: Perception within a common auditory visual space. *Science,* **172**, 1161-1163.

Asano, K., Ogawa, S., & Furuta, Y. (1978). Aerobic work capacity in middle- and old-aged runners. In F. Landry & W.A.R. Orban (Eds.), *Exercise physiology: Proceedings of the International Congress of Physical Activity Sciences* (Vol. 4). Quebec: Symposia Specialists.

Asmussen, E. (1973). Growth in muscular strength and power. In G.L. Rarick (Ed.), *Physical activity: Human growth and development* (pp. 60-79). New York, NY: Academic Press.

Asmussen, E., & Heeboll-Nielsen, K. (1955). A dimensional analysis of physical performance and growth in boys. *Journal of Applied Physiology,* **7**, 593-603.

Asmussen, E., & Heeboll-Nielsen, K. (1956). Physical performance and growth in children: Influence of sex, age, and intelligence. *Journal of Applied Physiology,* **8**, 371-380.

Åstrand, P. (1976). The child in sport and physical activity-physiology. In J.G. Albinson & G.M. Andrew (Eds.), *Child in sport and physical activity* (pp. 19-33). Baltimore, MD: University Park Press.

Atkinson, J., & Braddick, O. (1981). Acuity, contrast sensitivity, and accommodation in infancy. In R. Aslin, J. Alberts, & M. Peterson (Eds.), *Development of perception.* New York, NY: Academic Press.

Auerbach, C., & Sperling, P. (1974). A common auditory-visual space: Evidence for its reality. *Perception and Psychophysics,* **16**, 129-135.

Ayres, A.J. (1965). Patterns of perceptual-motor dysfunction in children: A factor analytic study. *Perceptual and Motor Skills,* **20**, 335-368.

Ayres, A.J. (1966). *Southern California sensory-motor integration tests.* Los Angeles, CA: Western Psychological Corporation.

Ayres, A.J. (1969). *Southern California perceptual-motor tests.* Los Angeles, CA: Western Psychological Services.

Ayres, A.J. (1972). *Southern California sensory-motor integration tests manual*. Los Angeles, CA: Western Psychological Services.

Bachman, J.C. (1961). Motor learning and performance as related to age and sex in two measures of balance coordination. *Research Quarterly*, **32**, 123-137.

Bailer, I., Doll, L., & Winsberg, B.G. (1973). *Modified Lincoln-Oseretsky Motor Development Scale*. New York, NY: New York State Department of Mental Hygiene.

Bailey, D.A. (1976). The growing child and the need for physical activity. In J.G. Albinson & G.M. Andrew (Eds.), *Child in sport and physical activity*. Baltimore, MD: University Park Press.

Bailey, D.A., Malina, R.M., & Rasmussen, R.L. (1978). The influence of exercise, physical activity, and athletic performance on the dynamics of human growth. In F. Falkner & J.M. Tanner (Eds.), *Human growth* (Vol. 2) (pp. 475-505). New York, NY: Plenum Press.

Baldwin, B.T. (1920). *The physical growth of children from birth to maturity*. Iowa City, IA: University of Iowa.

Baldwin, K.M. (1984). Muscle development: Neonatal to adult. In R.L. Terjung (Ed.), *Exercise and sport science reviews* (Vol. 12) (pp. 1-19). Lexington, MA: Collamore Press.

Ball, T.S. (1971). *Itard, Sequin, and Kephart: Sensory education—a learning interpretation*. Columbus, OH: Charles E. Merrill.

Bandura, A. (1969). Social learning theory of identificatory process. In D. Goslin (Ed.), *Handbook of socialization theory and research*. Chicago, IL: Rand McNally.

Bandura, A. (1977). *Social learning theory*. Englewood Cliffs, NJ: Prentice-Hall.

Bandura, A., & Walters, R.H. (1963). *Social learning and personality development*. New York, NY: Holt, Rinehart, and Winston.

Bar-or, O., Shephard, R.J., & Allen, C.L. (1971). Cardiac output of 10- to 13-year-old boys and girls during submaximal exercise. *Journal of Applied Physiology*, **30**, 219-223.

Barrett, K.R. (1979). Observation for teaching and coaching. *Journal of Physical Education and Recreation*, **50**, 23-25.

Barsch, R.H. (1965). *Achieving perceptual-motor efficiency*. Seattle, WA: Special Child Publications.

Bayley, N. (1935). The development of motor abilities during the first three years. *Society for Research in Child Development Monograph*, **1**, 1.

Bayley, N. (1965). Comparisons of mental and motor test scores for ages 1-15 months by sex, birth order, race, geographical location and education of parents. *Child Development*, **36**, 379-411.

Bayley, N. (1969). *Manual for the Bayley scales of infant development*. New York, NY: The Psychological Corporation.

Beck, M. (1966). *The path of the center of gravity during running in boys grades one to six*. Unpublished doctoral dissertation, University of Wisconsin, Madison, WI.

Becklake, M.R., Frank, H., Dagenais, G.R., Ostiguy, G.L., & Guzman, G.A. (1965). Influence of age and sex on exercise cardiac output. *Journal of Applied Physiology*, **20**, 938-947.

Belmont, J.M., & Butterfield, E.C. (1971). What the development of short-term memory is. *Human Development*, **14**, 236-248.

Birch, L.L. (1976). Age trends in children's time-sharing performance. *Journal of Experimental Child Psychology*, **22**, 331-345.

Birren, J.E. (1964a). *The psychology of aging*. Englewood Cliffs, NJ: Prentice-Hall.

Birren, J.E. (1964b). The psychology of aging in relation to development. In J.E. Birren (Ed.), *Relations of development and aging* (pp. 99-120). Springfield, IL: Charles C. Thomas.

Boone, P.C., & Azen, S.P. (1979). Normal range of motion of joints in male subjects. *Journal of Bone and Joint Surgery*, **61A**, 756-759.

Botwinick, J. (1970). Learning in children and in older adults. In L.R. Goulet & P.B. Baltes (Eds.), *Life-span developmental psychology* (pp. 257-284). New York, NY: Academic Press.

Bower, T.G.R. (1972). Object perception in infants. *Perception*, **1**, 15-30.

Bower, T.G.R. (1977). *A primer of infant development*. San Francisco, CA: W.H. Freeman.

Bower, T.G.R., Broughton, J.M., & Moore, M.K. (1970). The co-ordination of visual and tactual input in infants. *Perception and Psychophysics*, **8**, 51-53.

Bowlby, J. (1978). Evidence on effects of deprivation. In J.P. Scott (Ed.), *Critical periods*. Stroudsburg, PA: Dowden, Hutchinson, & Ross.

Boyd, E. (1929). The experimental error inherent in measuring the growing human body. *American Journal of Physical Anthropology*, **13**, 389-432.

Braddick, O., & Atkinson, J. (1979). Accommodation and acuity in the human infant. In R.D. Freeman (Ed.), *Developmental neurobiology of vision*. New York, NY: Plenum.

Brandfonbrener, M., Landowne, M., & Shock, N.W. (1955). Changes in cardiac output with age. *Circulation*, **12**, 557-566.

Brandt, I. (1978). Growth dynamics of low-birth-weight infants with emphasis on the perinatal period. In F. Falkner & J.M. Tanner (Eds.), *Human growth: Vol. 2. Postnatal growth*. New York, NY: Plenum.

Branta, C., Haubenstricker, J., & Seefeldt, V. (1984). Age changes in motor skill during childhood and adolescence. In R.L. Terjung (Ed.), *Exercise and sport science reviews: Vol. 12* (pp. 467-520). Lexington, MA: Collamore Press.

Braun, H.W., & Geiselhart, R. (1959). Age differences in the acquisition and extinction of the conditioned eye-lid response. *Journal of Experimental Psychology*, **57**, 386-388.

Brewer, V., Meyer, B.M., Kele, M.S., Upton, S.J., & Hagan, R.D. (1983). Role of exercise in prevention of involutional bone loss. *Medicine and Science in Sports and Exercise*, **15**, 445-449.

Brim, O.G. (1966). Socialization through the life cycle. In O.G. Brim & S. Wheeler (Eds.), *Socialization after childhood*. New York, NY: John Wiley & Sons.

Bruce, R. (1966). *The effects of variations in ball trajectory upon the catching performance of elementary school children*. Unpublished doctoral dissertation, University of Wisconsin, Madison, WI.

Bruininks, R.H. (1978). *Bruininks-Oseretsky test of motor proficiency*. Circle Pines, MN: American Guidance Service.

Brundage, C.L. (1983). *Parent/Child play behaviors as they relate to children's later socialization into sport*. Unpublished master's thesis, University of Illinois, Urbana, IL.

Burke, W.E., Tuttle, W.W., Thompson, C.W., Janney, C.D., & Weber, R.J. (1953). The relation of grip strength and grip-strength endurance to age. *Journal of Applied Physiology*, **5**, 628-630.

Burnett, C.N., & Johnson, E.W. (1971). Development of gait in childhood, Part II. *Developmental Medicine and Child Neurology*, **13**, 207-215.

Buros, O.K. (Ed.). (1972). *The seventh mental measurement yearbook*. Highland Park, NJ: Gryphon.

Bushnell, E.W. (1982). The ontogeny of intermodal relations: Visions and touch in infancy. In R. Walk & H. Pick (Ed.), *Intersensory perception and sensory integration* (pp. 5-36). New York, NY: Plenum.

Campbell, W.R., & Pohndorf, R.H. (1961). Physical fitness of British and United States children. In L.A. Larson (Ed.), *Health and fitness in the modern world* (pp. 8-16). Chicago, IL: Athletic Institute.

Carron, A.V., & Bailey, D.A. (1974). Strength development in boys from 10 through 16 years. *Monograph of the Society for Research in Child Development*, **39**.

Carson, L.M., & Wiegand, R.L. (1979). Motor schema formation and retention in young children: A test of Schmidt's schema theory. *Journal of Motor Behavior*, **11**, 247-252.

Case, R. (1972a). Learning and development: A neo-Piagetian interpretation. *Human Development*, **15**, 339-358.

Case, R. (1972b). Validation of a neo-Piagetian mental capacity construct. *Journal of Experimental Child Psychology*, **14**, 287-302.

Case, R. (1974a). Mental strategies, mental capacity, and instruction. *Journal of Experimental Child Psychology*, **18**, 382-397.

Case, R. (1974b). Structures and strictures: Some functional limitations on the course of cognitive growth. *Cognitive Psychology*, **6**, 544-573.

Case, R., & Globerson, T. (1974). Field independence and central computing space. *Child Development*, **45**, 772-778.

Chapman, E.A., DeVries, H.A., & Swezey, R. (1972). Joint stiffness: The effects of exercise on young and old men. *Journal of Gerontology*, **27**, 218-221.

Chi, M. (1976). Short-term memory limitations in children: Capacity or processing deficits? *Memory and Cognition*, **4**, 559-572.

Chi, M. (1977a). Age differences in memory span. *Journal of Experimental Child Psychology*, **23**, 266-281.

Chi, M. (1977b). Age differences in the speed of processing: A critique. *Developmental Psychology*, **13**, 543-544.

Clark, J.E. (1982). Developmental differences in response processing. *Journal of Motor Behavior*, **14**, 247-254.

Clark, J.E., Phillips, S.J., Peterson, R., & Welker, H. (1982, May). *Developmental changes in coordination patterns of the standing long jump*. Paper presented at the meeting of the North American Society for Psychology of Sport and Physical Activity, College Park, MD.

Clarke, H.E. (1966). *Muscular strength and endurance in man*. Englewood Cliffs, NJ: Prentice-Hall.

Clarke, H.H. (Ed.). (1975). Joint and body range of movement. *Physical Fitness Research Digest*, **5**, 16-18.

Clouse, F. (1959). *A kinematic analysis of the development of the running pattern of preschool boys*. Unpublished doctoral dissertation, University of Wisconsin, Madison, WI.

Colling-Saltin, A.S. (1980). Skeletal muscle development in the human fetus and during childhood. In K. Berg & B.O. Eriksson (Eds.), *Children and exercise IX*. Baltimore, MD: University Park Press.

Collins, J.K. (1976). Distance perception as a function of age. *Australian Journal of Psychology*, **28**, 109-113.

Corbin, C.B. (1980). *A textbook of motor development* (2nd ed.). Dubuque, IA: Brown Company.

Corso, J.F. (1977). Auditory perception and communication. In J.E. Birren & K.W. Schaie (Eds.), *Handbook of the psychology of aging* (pp. 535-553). New York, NY: Van Nostrand Reinhold.

Craik, F.I.M. (1977). Age differences in human memory. In J.E. Birren & K.W. Schaie (Eds.), *Handbook of the psychology of aging*. New York, NY: Van Nostrand Reinhold.

Craik, F.I.M., & Simon, E. (1980). Age differences in memory: The roles of attention and depth of processing. In L.W. Poon, J.L. Fozard, L.S. Cermak, D. Arenberg, & L.W. Thompson (Eds.), *New directions in memory and aging*. Hillsdale, NJ: Lawrence Erlbaum Associates.

Cratty, B.J. (1979). *Perceptual and motor development in infants and children* (2nd ed.). Englewood Cliffs, NJ: Prentice-Hall.

Crossman, E.R.F.W., & Szafran, J. (1956). Changes with age in the speed of information intake and discrimination. *Experientia (Suppl.)*, **4**, 128-135.

DaCosta, M.I. (1946). The Oseretsky tests. (E.J. Fosa, Trans.). *Training School Bulletin*, **43**, 1-13, 27-38, 50-59, 62-74.

Daehler, M.W., Horowitz, A.B., Wynns, F.C., & Flavell, J.H. (1969). Verbal and non-verbal rehearsal in children's recall. *Child Development*, **40**, 443-452.

Davies, C.T.M. (1972). The oxygen transporting system in relation to age. *Clinical Science*, **42**, 1-13.

Deach, D. (1950). *Genetic development of motor skills in children two through six years of age*. Unpublished doctoral dissertation, University of Michigan, Ann Arbor, MI.

de Garay, A.L., Levine, L., & Carter, J.E.L. (1974). *Genetic and anthropological studies of Olympic athletes*. New York, NY: Academic Press.

Dehn, M.M., & Bruce, R.A. (1972). Longitudinal variations in maximum oxygen intake with age and activity. *Journal of Applied Physiology*, **33**, 805-807.

Dekaban, A. (1970). *Neurology of early childhood*. Baltimore, MD: Williams and Wilkins.

Delacato, C.H. (1959). *Treatment and prevention of reading problems*. Springfield, IL: Charles C. Thomas.

Delacato, C.H. (1966). *Neurological organization and reading*. Springfield, IL: Charles C. Thomas.

Dennis, W. (1940). The effect of cradling practices upon the onset of walking in Hopi children. *Journal of Genetic Psychology*, **56**, 77-86.

Dennis, W. (1963). Environmental influences upon motor development. In W. Dennis (Ed.), *Readings in child psychology* (2nd ed.). Englewood Cliffs, NJ: Prentice-Hall.

DeOreo, K.L. (1971). *Dynamic and static balance in preschool children*. Unpublished doctoral dissertation, University of Illinois, Urbana, IL.

DeOreo, K.L. (1974). The performance and development of fundamental motor skills in preschool children. In D.M. Landers (Ed.), *Psychology of motor behavior and sport*. Champaign, IL: Human Kinetics.

DeOreo, K., & Keogh, J. (1980). Performance of fundamental motor tasks. In C.B. Corbin (Ed.), *A textbook of motor development* (2nd ed.) (pp. 76-91). Dubuque, IA: William C. Brown.

DeOreo, K., & Wade, M.G. (1971). Dynamic and static balancing ability of preschool children. *Journal of Motor Behavior, 3*, 326-335.

DeOreo, K.L., & Williams, H.G. (1980). Characteristics of kinesthetic perception. In C.B. Corbin (Ed.), *A textbook of motor development* (2nd ed.) (pp. 174-196). Dubuque, IA: William C. Brown.

DeVries, H.A. (1970). Physiological effects of an exercise training regimen upon men aged 52 to 88. *Journal of Gerontology, 25*, 325-336.

DeVries, H.A. (1980). *Physiology of exercise for physical education and athletics* (3rd ed.). Dubuque, IA: William C. Brown.

Dickinson, J. (1974). *Proprioceptive control of human movement.* Princeton, NJ: Princeton Book Company.

DiNucci, J.M. (1976). Gross motor performance: A comprehensive analysis of age and sex differences between boys and girls ages six to nine years. In J. Broekhoff (Ed.), *Physical education, sports, and the sciences.* Eugene, OR: Microform Publications.

DiSimoni, F.G. (1975). Perceptual and perceptual-motor characteristics of phonemic development. *Child Development, 46*, 243-246.

Dittmer, J. (1962). *A kinematic analysis of the development of the running pattern of grade school girls and certain factors which distinguish good from poor performance at the observed ages.* Unpublished master's thesis, University of Wisconsin, Madison, WI.

Doty, D. (1974). Infant speech perception. *Human Development, 17*, 74-80.

Drinkwater, B.L., Horvath, S.M., & Wells, C.L. (1975). Aerobic power of females, age 10-68. *Journal of Gerontology, 30*, 385-394.

Drowatzky, J.N., & Zuccato, F.C. (1967). Interrelationship between static and dynamic balance. *Research Quarterly, 38*, 509-510.

Dwyer, J., & Mayer, J. (1973). The dismal condition: Problems faced by obese adolescent girls in American society. In G.A. Bray (Ed.), *Obesity in perspective* (pp. 103-110) (Fogarty Report No. 017-053-00046-9). Washington, D.C.: U.S. Government Printing Office.

Edwards, R.G. (1981). *The beginnings of human life.* Burlington, NC: Carolina Biological Supply.

Elkind, D. (1975). Perceptual development in children. *American Scientist, 63*, 533-541.

Elkind, D., Koegler, R., & Go, E. (1964). Studies in perceptual development: Whole-part perception. *Child Development, 35*, 81-90.

Elliott, R. (1972). Simple reaction time in children: Effects of incentive, incentive shift, and other training variables. *Journal of Experimental Child Psychology, 13*, 540-557.

Endler, N.S., Boulter, L.R., & Osser, H. (1976). *Contemporary issues in developmental psychology* (2nd ed.). New York, NY: Holt, Rinehart, and Winston.

Eriksson, B.O. (1978). Physical activity from childhood to maturity: Medical and pediatric considerations. In F. Landry & W.A.R. Orban (Eds.), *Physical activity and human well-being*. Miami, FL: Symposia Specialists.

Espenschade, A.S. (1940). Motor performance in adolescence including the study of relationships with measures of physical growth and maturity. *Monograph of the Society for Research in Child Development, 5*, 1-126.

Espenschade, A.S. (1947). Development of motor coordination in boys and girls. *Research Quarterly, 18*, 30-44.

Espenschade, A.S. (1960). Motor development. In W.R. Johnson (Ed.), *Science and medicine of exercise and sports*. New York, NY: Harper & Row.

Espenschade, A., Dable, R.R., & Schoendube, R. (1953). Dynamic balance in adolescent boys. *Research Quarterly, 24*, 270-274.

Espenschade, A., & Eckert, H. (1974). Motor development. In W.R. Johnson & E.R. Buskirk (Eds.), *Science and medicine of exercise and sport* (2nd ed.). New York, NY: Harper & Row.

Espenschade, A.S., & Eckert, H.D. (1980). *Motor development* (2nd ed.). Columbus, OH: Charles E. Merrill.

Fagot, B.I. (1978). The influence of sex of child on parental reactions to toddler children. *Child Development, 49*, 459-465.

Fagot, B.I. (1984). Teacher and peer reactions to boys' and girls' play styles. *Sex Roles, 11*, 691-702.

Fakouri, M.E. (1976). Cognitive development in adulthood: A fifth stage? A critique. *Developmental Psychology, 12*, 472.

Falkner, F., & Tanner, J.M. (Eds.). (1978). *Human growth* (Vols. 1-3). New York, NY: Plenum Press.

Fieandt, K. von, Huhtala, A., Kullberg, P., & Saari, K. (1956). *Personal tempo and phenomenal time at different age levels* (Report No. 2). Psychological Institute, University of Helsinki.

Fox, E.L., & Mathews, D.K. (1981). *The physiological basis of physical education and athletics* (3rd ed.). Philadelphia, PA: Saunders College.

Frankenburg, W.K., & Dodds, J.B. (1967). The Denver developmental screening test. *Journal of Pediatrics, 71*, 181-191.

Frisch, R.E. (1972). Weight at menarche: Similarity for well-nourished and undernourished girls at differing ages, and evidence for historical constancy. *Pediatrics, 50*, 445-450.

Frostig, M. (1969). *Move, grow and learn*. Chicago, IL: Follett.

Frostig, M., Lefever, W., & Whittlesey, J. (1966). *Administration and scoring manual: Marianne Frostig developmental test of visual perception*. Palo Alto, CA: Consulting Psychologists Press.

Gaines, G.J., & Raskin, L.M. (1970). Comparison of cross-modal and intra-modal form recognition in children with learning disabilities. *Journal of Learning Disabilities, 3*, 243-246.

Gallagher, J.D., & Thomas, J.R. (1980a, April). *Adult-child differences in movement reproduction: Effects of kinesthetic sensory store and organization of memory*. Paper presented at the annual convention of the American Alliance for Health, Physical Education, Recreation, and Dance, Detroit, MI.

Gallagher, J.D., & Thomas, J.R. (1980b). Effects of varying post-KR intervals upon children's motor performance. *Journal of Motor Behavior, 12*, 41-46.

Gallahue, D.L. (1982). *Understanding motor development in children*. New York, NY: John Wiley & Sons.

Gallahue, D.L. (1983, April). *Perceptual aspects of motor performance*. Paper presented at the annual convention of the American Alliance for Health, Physical Education, Recreation, and Dance, Houston, TX.

Gatev, G. (1972). Role of inhibition in the development of motor coordination in early childhood. *Developmental Medicine and Child Psychology, 14*, 336-341.

Gesell, A. (1954). The ontogenesis of infant behavior. In L. Carmichael (Ed.), *Manual of child psychology* (2nd ed.). New York, NY: John Wiley & Sons.

Gesell, A., & Amatruda, C.S. (1949). *Gesell developmental schedules*. New York, NY: Psychological Company.

Gesell, A., & Ames, L.B. (1940). The ontogenetic organization of prone behavior in human infancy. *Journal of Genetic Psychology, 56*, 247-263.

Getman, G.N. (1952). *How to develop your child's intelligence, a research publication*. Lucerne, MN: Author.

Getman, G.N. (1963). *The physiology of readiness experiment*. Minneapolis, MN: P.A.S.S.

Gibson, J. (1966). *The senses considered as perceptual systems*. New York, NY: Houghton Mifflin.

Gilliam, T.B., Katch, V.L., Thorland, W., & Weltman, A. (1977). Prevalence of coronary heart disease risk factors in active children, 7 to 12 years of age. *Medicine and Science in Sports, 9*, 21-25.

Glassow, R.B., & Kruse, P. (1960). Motor performance of girls age 6 to 14 years. *Research Quarterly, 31*, 426-433.

Goodman, L., & Hamill, D. (1973). The effectiveness of the Kephart Getman activities in developing perceptual-motor and cognitive skills. *Focus on Exceptional Children, 4*, 1-9.

Goodnow, J.J. (1971a). Eye and hand: Differential memory and its effect on matching. *Neuropsychologica, 9*, 89-95.

Goodnow, J.J. (1971b). Matching auditory and visual series: Modality problem or translation problem? *Child Development, 42*, 1187-1201.

Gotts, E.E. (1972). Letter to the editor: Newborn walking. *Science, 177*, 1057-1058.

Greendorfer, S.L. (1976, September). *A social learning approach to female sport involvement*. Paper presented at the annual convention of the American Psychological Association, Washington, D.C.

Greendorfer, S.L. (1979). Childhood sport socialization influences of male and female track athletes. *Arena Review, 3*, 39-53.

Greendorfer, S.L. (1983). Shaping the female athlete: The impact of the family. In M.A. Boutilier & L. Sangiovanni (Eds.), *The sporting woman*. Champaign, IL: Human Kinetics.

Greendorfer, S.L., & Brundage, C.L. (1984, July). *Sex differences in children's motor skills: Toward a cross-disciplinary perspective*. Paper presented at the 1984 Olympic Scientific Congress, Eugene, OR.

Greendorfer, S.L., & Ewing, M.E. (1981). Race and gender differences in children's socialization into sport. *Research Quarterly for Exercise and Sport,* **52**, 301-310.

Greendorfer, S.L., & Lewko, J.H. (1978a). *Children's socialization into sport: A conceptual and empirical analysis.* Paper presented at the meeting of the 9th World Congress of Sociology, Uppsala, Sweden.

Greendorfer, S.L., & Lewko, J.H. (1978b). Role of family members in sport socialization of children. *Research Quarterly,* **49**, 146-152.

Greulich, W.W., & Pyle, S.I. (1959). *Radiographic atlas of skeletal development of the hand and wrist* (2nd ed.). Stanford, CA: Stanford University Press.

Grillner, S. (1975). Locomotion in vertebrates: Central mechanisms and reflex interaction. *Physiological Review,* **55**, 247-304.

Grimby, G., Nilsson, N.J., & Saltin, B. (1966). Cardiac output during submaximal and maximal exercise in active middle-aged athletes. *Journal of Applied Physiology,* **21**, 1150-1156.

Grodjinovsky, A., Inbar, O., Dotan, R., & Bar-or, O. (1980). Training effect on the anaerobic performance of children as measured by the Wingate anaerobic test. In K. Berg & B.O. Eriksson (Eds.), *Children and exercise IX* (pp. 139-145). Baltimore, MD: University Park Press.

Gutteridge, M. (1939). A study of motor achievements of young children. *Archives of Psychology,* **244**, 1-178.

Haith, M.M. (1966). The response of the human newborn to visual movement. *Journal of Experimental Child Psychology,* **3**, 235-243.

Halverson, H.M. (1931). An experimental study of prehension in infants by means of systematic cinema records. *Genetic Psychology Monographs,* **10**, 107-286.

Halverson, L. (1983). *Observing children's motor development in action.* Symposium papers from the annual conference of the American Alliance for Health, Physical Education, Recreation, and Dance. Eugene, OR: Microform Publications.

Halverson, L.E., & Roberton, M.A. (1979). The effects of instruction on overhand throwing development in children. In K. Newell & G. Roberts (Eds.), *Psychology of motor behavior and sport—1978* (pp. 258-269). Champaign, IL: Human Kinetics.

Halverson, L.E., Roberton, M.A., & Langendorfer, S. (1982). Development of the overarm throw: Movement and ball velocity changes by seventh grade. *Research Quarterly for Exercise and Sport*, **53**, 198-205.

Halverson, L.E., & Williams, K. (1985). Developmental sequences for hopping over distance: A prelongitudinal screening. *Research Quarterly for Exercise and Sport*, **56**, 37-44.

Harris, G.J., & Burke, D. (1972). The effects of grouping on short-term serial recall of digits by children: Developmental trends. *Child Development*, **43**, 710-716.

Harrison, T.R., Dixon, K., Russell, R.O., Bidwai, P.S., & Coleman, H.N. (1964). The relation of age to the duration of contraction, ejection, and relaxation of the normal human heart. *American Heart Journal*, **67**, 189-199.

Hasselkus, B.R., & Shambes, G.M. (1975). Aging and postural sway in women. *Journal of Gerontology*, **30**, 661-667.

Haubenstricker, J.L., Branta, C.F., & Seefeldt, V.D. (1983). *Standards of performance for throwing and catching.* Proceedings of the Annual Conference of the North American Society for Psychology in Sport and Physical Activity, Assimilar, CA.

Haubenstricker, J.L., Seefeldt, V.D., & Branta, C.F. (1983). *Preliminary validation of a developmental sequence for the standing long jump.* Paper presented at the meeting of the American Alliance for Health, Physical Education, Recreation and Dance.

Hay, J.G., & Reid, J.G. (1982). *The anatomical and mechanical bases of human motion.* Englewood Cliffs, NJ: Prentice-Hall.

Hay, L. (1978). Accuracy of children on an open-loop pointing task. *Perceptual and Motor Skills*, **47**, 1079-1082.

Hay, L. (1979). Spatial-temporal analysis of movements in children: Motor programs. *Journal of Motor Behavior*, **11**, 189-200.

Haywood, K.M. (1977). Eye movements during coincidence-anticipation performance. *Journal of Motor Behavior*, **9**, 313-318.

Haywood, K.M., Greenwald, G., & Lewis, C. (1981). Contextual factors and age group differences in coincidence-anticipation performance. *Research Quarterly for Exercise and Sport*, **52**, 458-464.

Haywood, K.M., & Patryla, V. (1978, May). *Relationship between growth and balance performance among normal and learning disabled children.* Paper presented at the meeting of the North American Society for Psychology of Sport and Physical Activity, Tallahassee, FL.

Haywood, K.M., Teeple, J., Givens, M., & Patterson, J. (1977). Young children's rod-and-frame test performance. *Perceptual and Motor Skills, 45,* 163-169.

Haywood, K.M., & Trick, L.R. (1983). *Age-related visual changes and their implications for the motor skill performance of older adults.* Paper presented at the annual convention of the American Alliance for Health, Physical Education, Recreation and Dance. (ERIC Document Reproduction Service No. ED 230 538)

Hecaen, H., & de Ajuriaguerra, J. (1964). *Left-handedness: Manual superiority and cerebral dominance.* New York, NY: Grune & Stratton.

Held, R., & Hein, A. (1963). Movement-produced stimulation in the development of visually guided behavior. *Journal of Comparative and Physiological Psychology, 56,* 872-876.

Hellebrandt, F.A., & Braun, G.L. (1939). The influence of sex and age on the postural sway of man. *American Journal of Physical Anthropology, 24,* Series 1, 347-360.

Herkowitz, J. (1978a). Assessing the motor development of children: Presentation and critique of tests. In M.V. Ridenour (Ed.), *Motor development* (pp. 165-187). Princeton, NJ: Princeton Book.

Herkowitz, J. (1978b). Developmental task analysis: The design of movement experiences and evaluation of motor development status. In M.V. Ridenour (Ed.), *Motor development.* Princeton, NJ: Princeton Book.

Herkowitz, J. (1978c). Instruments which assess the efficiency/maturity of children's fundamental motor pattern performance. In D.M. Landers & R.W. Christina (Eds.), *Psychology of motor behavior and sport-1977* (pp. 529-535). Champaign, IL: Human Kinetics.

Heyward, V.H. (1984). *Designs for fitness.* Minneapolis, MN: Burgess Publishing.

Hirsch, J., & Knittle, J.L. (1970). Cellularity of obese and nonobese human adipose tissue. *Federation Proceedings, 29,* 1516-1521.

Horine, L.E. (1968). An investigation of the relationship of laterality to performance on selected motor ability tests. *Research Quarterly, 39,* 90-95.

Howell, M.L., Loiselle, D.S., & Lucas, W.G. (1966). *Strength of Edmonton schoolchildren.* Unpublished manuscript, University of Alberta Fitness Research Unit, Edmonton, Alberta, Canada.

Howell, M.L., & MacNab, R. (1966). *The physical work capacity of Canadian children.* Ottawa: Canadian Association for Physical Health Education and Recreation.

Hupprich, F.L., & Sigerseth, P.O. (1950). The specificity of flexibility in girls. *Research Quarterly*, **21**, 25-33.

Huston, A. (1984). Sex typing. In P.H. Mussen (Ed.), *Carmichael's handbook of child psychology* (Vol. 4, pp. 387-469). New York, NY: John Wiley & Sons.

Hutinger, P.A. (1959). Differences in speed between American Negro and white children in performance of the 35-yard dash. *Research Quarterly*, **30**, 366-367.

Ikai, M. (1967). Trainability of muscular endurance as related to age. *Proceedings of ICHPER 10th International Congress* (pp. 29-35). Vancouver, British Columbia, Canada.

Inkeles, A. (1969). Social structure and socialization. In D.A. Goslin (Ed.), *Handbook of socialization theory and research*. Skokie, IL: Rand McNally.

Jenkins, L.M. (1930). *A comparative study of motor achievements of children five, six, and seven years of age*. New York, NY: Teacher's College, Columbia University.

Jones, H.E. (1947). Sex differences in physical abilities. *Human Biology*, **19**, 12-25.

Julius, S., Amery, A., Whitlock, L.S., & Conway, J. (1967). Influence of age on the hemodynamic response to exercise. *Circulation*, **36**, 222-230.

Kaiser, S.B., & Phinney, J.S. (1983). Sex typing of play activities by girls' clothing style: Pants versus skirts. *Child Study Journal*, **13**, 115-132.

Karpovich, P.V. (1937). Textbook fallacies regarding the development of the child's heart. *Research Quarterly*, **8**, 33-37.

Kasch, F.W., & Wallace, J.P. (1976). Physiological variables during 10 years of endurance exercise. *Medicine and Science in Sports*, **8**, 5-8.

Kausler, D.H. (1982). *Experimental psychology and human aging*. New York, NY: John Wiley & Sons.

Kavanagh, T., & Shephard, R.J. (1977). The effects of continued training on the aging process. *Annals of the New York Academy of Sciences*, **301**, 656-670.

Kelly, J.R. (1974). Socialization toward leisure: A developmental approach. *Journal of Leisure Research*, **6**, 181-193.

Kelso, J.A.S., Holt, K.G., Kugler, P.N., & Turvey, M.T. (1980). On the concept of coordinative structures in dissipative structures: II. Empirical lines of convergence. In G.E. Stelmach & J. Requin (Eds.), *Tutorials in motor behavior*. New York, NY: North-Holland.

Kenshalo, D.R. (1977). Age changes in touch, vibration, temperature, kines-thesis, and pain sensitivity. In J.E. Birren & K.W. Schaie (Eds.), *Handbook of the psychology of aging* (pp. 562-579). New York, NY: Van Nostrand Reinhold.

Kenyon, G.S., & McPherson, B.D. (1973). Becoming involved in physical activity and sport: A process of socialization. In G.L. Rarick (Ed.), *Physical activity: Human growth and development* (pp. 301-332). New York, NY: Academic Press.

Kephart, N.C. (1964). Perceptual-motor aspects of learning disabilities. *Exceptional Children, 31*, 201-206.

Kephart, N.C. (1971). *The slow learner in the classroom* (2nd ed.). Columbus, OH: Charles E. Merrill.

Kerr, R., & Booth, B. (1977). Skill acquisition in elementary school children and schema theory. In R.W. Christina & D.M. Landers (Eds.), *Psychology of motor behavior and sport-1976* (pp. 243-247). Champaign, IL: Human Kinetics.

Kidd, A.H., & Kidd, R.M. (1966). The development of auditory perception in children. In A.H. Kidd & J.L. Rivoire (Eds.), *Perceptual development in children*. New York, NY: International Universities Press.

Klinger, A., Masataka, T., Adrian, M., & Smith, E. (1980, April). *Temporal and spatial characteristics of movement patterns of women over 60*. (Cited in Adrian, 1982.) AAHPERD Research Symposium, Detroit, MI.

Knittle, J.L. (1978). Adipose tissue development in man. In F. Falkner & J.M. Tanner (Eds.), *Human growth: Vol. 2. Postnatal growth*. New York, NY: Plenum Press.

Knittle, J.L., & Hirsch, J. (1968). Effect of early nutrition on the development of rat epididymal fat pads: Cellularity and metabolism. *Journal of Clinical Investigation, 47*, 2091-2098.

Knobloch, H., & Pasamanick, B. (1958). The relationship of race and socio-economic status to the development of motor behavior patterns in infancy. *Psychiatric Research Reports of the American Psychiatric Association, 10*, 123-133.

Komi, P.V. (1984). Physiological and biomechanical correlates of muscle func-tion: Effects of muscle structure and stretch-shortening cycle on force and speed. In R.J. Terjung (Ed.), *Exercise and sport sciences reviews, Vol. 12* (pp. 81-121). Lexington, MA: The Collamore Press.

Krahenbuhl, G.S., & Martin, S.L. (1977). Adolescent body size and flexibility. *Research Quarterly, 48*, 797-799.

Krahenbuhl, G.S., Pangrazi, R.P., Petersen, G.W., Burkett, L.N., & Schneider, M.J. (1978). Field testing of cardiorespiratory fitness in primary school children. *Medicine and Science in Sports*, **10**, 208-213.

Kreighbaum, E., & Barthels, K.M. (1985). *Biomechanics* (2nd ed.). Minneapolis, MN: Burgess.

Kuczaj, S.A., II, & Maratsos, M.P. (1975). On the acquisition of front, back, and side. *Child Development*, **46**, 202-210.

Kuffler, S.W., Nicholls, J.G., & Martin, A.R. (1984). *From neuron to brain* (2nd ed.). Sunderland, MA: Sinauer Associates.

Kugler, P.N., Kelso, J.A.S., & Turvey, M.T. (1980). On the concept of coordinative structures in dissipative structures. I. Theoretical lines of convergence. In G.E. Stelmach & J. Requin (Eds.), *Tutorials in motor behavior*. New York, NY: North-Holland.

Kugler, P.N., Kelso, J.A.S., & Turvey, M.T. (1982). On the control and coordination of naturally developing systems. In J.A.S. Kelso & J.E. Clark (Eds.), *The development of movement control and coordination*. New York, NY: John Wiley & Sons.

Kukla, A. (1978). An attributional theory of choice. In L. Berkowitz (Ed.), *Advances in experimental social psychology* (Vol. 2). New York, NY: Academic Press.

Laidlaw, R.W., & Hamilton, M.A. (1937). A study of thresholds in appreciation of passive movement among normal control subjects. *Bulletin of the Neurological Institute*, **6**, 268-273.

Landahl, H.D., & Birren, J.E. (1959). Effects of age on the discrimination of lifted weights. *Journal of Gerontology*, **14**, 48-55.

Langendorfer, S. (1980). *Longitudinal evidence for developmental changes in the preparatory phase of the overarm throw for force*. Paper presented at the annual convention of the American Alliance for Health, Physical Education, Recreation, and Dance, Detroit, MI.

Langendorfer, S. (1982). *Developmental relationships between throwing and striking: A pre-longitudinal test of motor stage theory*. Unpublished doctoral dissertation, University of Wisconsin, Madison, WI.

Langlois, J.H., & Downs, A.C. (1980). Mothers, fathers, and peers as socialization agents of sex-typed play behaviors in young children. *Child Development*, **51**, 1237-1247.

Lasky, R.E. (1977). The effect of visual feedback of the hand on the reaching and retrieval behavior of young infants. *Child Development*, **48**, 112-117.

Lawrence, D.G., & Hopkins, D.A. (1972). Developmental aspects of pyramidal motor control in the rhesus monkey. *Brain Research*, **40**, 117-118.

Lawrence, D.G., & Kuypers, H.G.J.M. (1968). The functional organization of the motor system in the monkey. I. The effects of bilateral pyramidal lesions. *Brain*, **91**, 1-14.

Lehman, H.C. (1953). *Age and achievement*. Princeton, NJ: Princeton University Press.

Leme, S., & Shambes, G. (1978). Immature throwing patterns in normal adult women. *Journal of Human Movement Studies*, **4**, 85-93.

Lewis, M. (1972). Culture and gender roles: There is no unisex in the nursery. *Psychology Today*, **5**, 54-57.

Lewko, J.H., & Ewing, M.E. (1980). Sex differences and parental influences in sport involvement of children. *Journal of Sport Psychology*, **2**, 62-68.

Liberty, C., & Ornstein, P.A. (1973). Age differences in organization and recall: The effects of training in categorization. *Journal of Experimental Child Psychology*, **15**, 169-186.

Little, M.A., & Hochner, D.H. (1973). *Human Thermoregulation, Growth, and Mortality* (Module in Anthropology No. 36). Reading, MA: Addison-Wesley.

Long, A.B., & Looft, W.R. (1972). Development of directionality in children: Ages six through twelve. *Developmental Psychology*, **6**, 375-380.

Loovis, E.M. (1976). Model for individualizing physical education experiences for the preschool moderately retarded child (Doctoral dissertation, The Ohio State University, 1975). *Dissertation Abstracts International*, **36**, 5126A. (University Microfilms No. 76-3485)

Lowrey, G.H. (1973). *Growth and development of children*. Chicago, IL: Year Book Medical Publishers.

Loy, J.W., McPherson, B.D., & Kenyon, G. (1978). *Sport and social systems*. Reading, MA: Addison-Wesley.

Malina, R.M. (1969). Growth, maturation, and performance of Philadelphia Negro and white elementary school children (Doctoral dissertation, University of Pennsylvania, 1968). *Dissertation Abstracts International*, 30-03-B. (University Microfilms No. 69-15091)

Malina, R.M. (1973). Ethnic and cultural factors in the development of motor abilities and strength in American children. In G.L. Rarick (Ed.), *Physical activity: Human growth and development* (pp. 333-363). New York, NY: Academic Press.

Malina, R.M. (1975). *Growth and development: The first twenty years in man.* Minneapolis, MN: Burgess Publishing.

Malina, R.M. (1978). Growth of muscle tissue and muscle mass. In F. Falkner & J.M. Tanner (Eds.), *Human growth: Vol. 2. Postnatal growth* (pp. 273-294). New York, NY: Plenum Press.

Malina, R.M. (1980). Adolescent growth, maturity, and development. In C.B. Corbin (Ed.), *A textbook of motor development* (2nd ed.). Dubuque, IA: Brown Company.

Malina, R.M., Bouchard, C., Shoup, R.F., & Lariviere, G. (1982). Age, family size and birth order in Montreal Olympic athletes. In J.E.L. Carter (Ed.), *Physical structure of Olympic athletes, Part I.* Basel, Switzerland: S. Karger.

Martin, R.W. (1966). *Selected anthropometric, strength, and power characteristics of white and Negro boys.* Unpublished master's thesis, University of Toledo, Toledo, OH.

Martino, A. (1966). *Anthropometric measurements in the lower leg of white and Negro high school boys in relation to vertical jumping ability.* Unpublished master's thesis, University of Oklahoma, Norman, OK.

Mathews, D.K. (1963). *Measurement in physical education.* Philadelphia, PA: W.B. Saunders.

Mayer, J. (1968). *Overweight: Causes, cost, and control.* Englewood Cliffs, NJ: Prentice Hall.

McCarver, R.B. (1972). A developmental study of the effect of organization cues on short-term memory. *Child Development, 43,* 1317-1325.

McCaskill, C.L., & Wellman, B.L. (1938). A study of common motor achievements at the preschool ages. *Child Development, 9,* 141-150.

McClenaghan, B.A., & Gallahue, D.L. (1978). *Fundamental movement: A developmental and remedial approach.* Philadelphia, PA: W.B. Saunders.

McDonnell, P.M. (1975). The development of visually guided reaching. *Perception and Psychophysics, 18,* 181-185.

McDonnell, P.M. (1979). Patterns of eye-hand coordination in the first year of life. *Canadian Journal of Psychology, 33,* 253-267.

McGraw, M.B. (1935). *Growth: A study of Johnny and Jimmy.* New York, NY: Appleton-Century. (Reprinted by Arno Press, 1975)

McGraw, M.B. (1939). Later development of children specially trained during infancy. *Child Development, 10,* 1-19.

McGraw, M.B. (1940). Neuromuscular development of the human infant as exemplified in the achievement of erect locomotion. *Journal of Pediatrics*, **17**, 747-771.

McGraw, M.B. (1943). *The neuromuscular maturation of the human infant.* New York, NY: Columbia University Press. (Reprinted by Hafner, 1963)

McGraw, M.B. (1946). Maturation of behavior. In L. Carmichael (Ed.), *Manual of child psychology.* New York, NY: John Wiley & Sons.

McPherson, B.D. (1978). The child in competitive sport: Influence of the social milieu. In R.A. Magill, M.J. Ash, & F.L. Smoll (Eds.), *Children in sport: A contemporary anthology* (pp. 219-249). Champaign, IL: Human Kinetics.

Milani Comparetti, A. (1981). The neurophysiologic and clinical implications of studies on fetal motor behavior. *Seminars in Perinatology*, **5**, 183-189.

Miller, F.S. (1968). *A comparative analysis of physical performance between male Caucasian and non-Caucasian (Mexican) students at the seventh and eighth grade level.* Unpublished master's thesis, California State College at Long Beach.

Miller, P.H. (1983). *Theories of developmental psychology.* San Francisco, CA: W.H. Freeman.

Milne, C., Seefeldt, V., & Reuschlein, P. (1976). Relationship between grade, sex, race, and motor performance in young children. *Research Quarterly*, **47**, 726-730.

Molnar, G. (1978). Analysis of motor disorder in retarded infants and young children. *American Journal of Mental Deficiency*, **83**, 213-222.

Moritani, T., & DeVries, H.A. (1980). Potential for gross muscle hypertrophy in older men. *Journal of Gerontology*, **35**, 672-682.

Morris, G.S.D. (1976). Effects ball and background color have upon the catching performance of elementary school children. *Research Quarterly*, **47**, 409-416.

Munns, K. (1981). Effects of exercise on the range of joint motion in elderly subjects. In E.L. Smith & R.C. Serfass (Eds.), *Exercise and aging: The scientific basis* (pp. 149-166). Hillside, NJ: Enslow Publishers.

Murray, M.P., Drought, A.B., & Kory, R.C. (1964). Walking patterns of normal men. *Journal of Bone and Joint Surgery*, **46-A**, 335-360.

Murray, M.P., Kory, R.C., Clarkson, B.H., & Sepic, S.B. (1966). Comparison of free and fast speed walking patterns of normal men. *American Journal of Physical Medicine*, **45**, 8-24.

Murray, M.P., Kory, R.C., & Sepic, S.B. (1970). Walking patterns of normal women. *Archives of Physical Medicine and Rehabilitation*, **51**, 637-650.

Napier, J. (1956). The prehensile movements of the human hand. *Journal of Bone and Joint Surgery*, **38B**, 902-913.

Naus, M., & Shillman, R. (1976). Why a Y is not a V: A new look at the distinctive features of letters. *Journal of Experimental Psychology: Human Perception and Performance*, **2**, 394-400.

Nelson, C.J. (1981). *Locomotor patterns of women over 57*. Unpublished master's thesis, Washington State University, Pullman, WA.

Nilsson, B.E., & Westlin, N.E. (1971). Bone density in athletes. *Clinical Orthopedics*, **77**, 179-182.

Norris, A.H., Shock, N.W., Landowne, M., & Falzone, J.A. (1956). Pulmonary function studies: Age differences in lung volume and bellows function. *Journal of Gerontology*, **11**, 379-387.

Northman, J.E., & Black, K.N. (1976). An examination of errors in children's visual and haptic-tactual memory for random forms. *Journal of Genetic Psychology*, **129**, 161-165.

Ornstein, P.A., & Naus, M.J. (1978). Rehearsal processes in children's memory. In P.A. Ornstein (Ed.), *Memory development in children*. Hillsdale, NJ: Lawrence Erlbaum Associates.

Oscai, L.B., Babirak, S.P., Dubach, F.B., McGarr, J.A., & Spirakis, C.N. (1974). Exercise or food restriction: Effect on adipose tissue cellularity. *American Journal of Physiology*, **227**, 901-904.

Oyster, N., Morton, M., & Linnell, S. (1984). Physical activity and osteoporosis in post-menopausal women. *Medicine and Science in Sports and Exercise*, **16**, 44-50.

Papalia, D.E. (1972). The status of several conservation abilities across the life span. *Human Development*, **15**, 229-243.

Parizkova, J. (1963). Impact of age, diet, and exercise on man's body composition. *Annals of the New York Academy of Sciences*, **110**, 661-674.

Parizkova, J. (1968). Longitudinal study of the development of body composition and body build in boys of various physical activity. *Human Biology*, **40**, 212-225.

Parizkova, J. (1972). Somatic development and body composition changes in adolescent boys differing in physical activity and fitness: A longitudinal study. *Anthropologie*, **10**, 3-36.

Parizkova, J. (1973). Body composition and exercise during growth and development. In G.L. Rarick (Ed.), *Physical activity: Human growth and development* (pp. 97-124). New York, NY: Academic Press.

Parizkova, J. (1977). *Body fat and physical fitness*. The Hague, The Netherlands: Martinus Nijhoff B.V.

Parizkova, J., & Eiselt, E. (1968). Longitudinal study of changes in anthropometric indicators and body composition in old men of various physical activity. *Human Biology, 40*, 331-344.

Pascual-Leone, J. (1970). A mathematical model for the transition rule in Piaget's developmental stages. *Acta Psychologica, 32*, 301-345.

Pascual-Leone, J. (1976). Metasubjective problems of constructive cognition: Forms of knowing and their psychological mechanism. *Canadian Psychological Review, 17*, 110-125.

Pascual-Leone, J., & Smith, J. (1969). The encoding and decoding of symbols by children: A new experimental paradigm and a neo-Piagetian model. *Journal of Experimental Child Psychology, 8*, 328-355.

Patterson, C.J., & Mischel, W. (1975). Plans to resist distraction. *Developmental Psychology, 11*, 369-378.

Peiper, A. (1963). *Cerebral function in infancy and childhood*. New York, NY: Consultants Bureau.

Perelle, I.B. (1975). Difference in attention to stimulus presentation mode with regard to age. *Developmental Psychology, 11*, 403-404.

Pew, R.W., & Rupp, G. (1971). Two quantitative measures of skill development. *Journal of Experimental Psychology, 90*, 1-7.

Phillips, M., Bookwalter, C., Denman, C., McAuley, J., Sherwin, H., Summers, D., & Yeakel, H. (1955). Analysis of results from the Kraus-Weber test of minimum muscular fitness in children. *Research Quarterly, 26*, 314-323.

Piaget, J. (1952). *The origins of intelligence in children*. New York, NY: International Universities Press.

Pick, A.D. (Ed.). (1979). *Perception and its development: A tribute to Eleanor J. Gibson*. Hillsdale, NJ: Lawrence Erlbaum Associates.

Pikler, E. (1968). Some contributions to the study of gross motor development in children. *Journal of Genetic Psychology, 113*, 27-39.

Pollock, M.L. (1974). Physiological characteristics of older champion track athletes. *Research Quarterly, 45*, 363-373.

Pomerance, A. (1965). Pathology of the heart with and without failure in the aged. *British Heart Journal*, **27**, 697-710.

Pontius, A.A. (1973). Neuro-ethics of "walking" in the newborn. *Perceptual and Motor Skills*, **37**, 235-245.

Prader, A., Tanner, J.M., & von Harnack, G.A. (1963). Catch-up growth following illness or starvation: An example of developmental canalization in man. *Journal of Pediatrics*, **62**, 646-659.

Prudden, B. (1964). *How to keep your child fit from birth to six*. New York, NY: Harper & Row.

Rabbitt, P. (1965). An age decrement in the ability to ignore irrelevant information. *Journal of Gerontology*, **20**, 233-238.

Rarick, G.L. (Ed.). (1973). *Physical activity: Human growth and development*. New York, NY: Academic Press.

Rarick, G.L., & Smoll, F.L. (1967). Stability of growth in strength and motor performance from childhood to adolescence. *Human Biology*, **39**, 295-306.

Reid, L. (1967). *The pathology of emphysema*. London: Lloyd-Luke.

Rhodes, A. (1937). A comparative study of motor abilities of Negroes and whites. *Child Development*, **8**, 369-371.

Rhodes, P. (1981). *Childbirth*. Burlington, NC: Carolina Biological Supply.

Ridenour, M.V. (1978). Programs to optimize infant motor development. In M.V. Ridenour (Ed.), *Motor development: Issues and applications* (pp. 39-61). Princeton, NJ: Princeton Book Company.

Riegel, K.F. (1976). The dialectics of human development. *American Psychologist*, **31**, 689-700.

Roach, E.G., & Kephart, N.C. (1966). *The Purdue perceptual-motor survey*. Columbus, OH: Charles E. Merrill.

Roberton, M.A. (1977). Stability of stage categorizations across trials: Implications for the "stage theory" of overarm throw development. *Journal of Human Movement Studies*, **3**, 49-59.

Roberton, M.A. (1978a). Longitudinal evidence for developmental stages in the forceful overarm throw. *Journal of Human Movement Studies*, **4**, 167-175.

Roberton, M.A. (1978b). Stability of stage categorizations in motor development. In D.M. Landers & R.W. Christina (Eds.), *Psychology of motor behavior and sport-1977* (pp. 494-506). Champaign, IL: Human Kinetics.

Roberton, M.A. (1978c). Stages in motor development. In M.V. Ridenour (Ed.), *Motor development: Issues and applications* (pp. 63-81). Princeton, NJ: Princeton Book Company.

Roberton, M.A. (1984). Changing motor patterns during childhood. In J.R. Thomas (Ed.), *Motor development during childhood and adolescence*. Minneapolis, MN: Burgess Publishing.

Roberton, M.A., & DiRocco, P. (1981). Validating a motor skill sequence for mentally retarded children. *American Corrective Therapy Journal, 35,* 148-154.

Roberton, M.A., & Halverson, L.E. (1984). *Developing children—Their changing movement*. Philadelphia, PA: Lea & Febiger.

Roberton, M.A., Halverson, L., Langendorfer, S., & Williams, K. (1979). Longitudinal changes in children's overarm throw ball velocities. *Research Quarterly, 50,* 256-264.

Roberton, M.A., & Langendorfer, S. (1980). Testing motor development sequences across 9-14 years. In D. Nadeau, W. Halliwell, K. Newell, & G. Roberts (Eds.), *Psychology of Motor Behavior and Sport-1979*. Champaign, IL: Human Kinetics.

Rogers, D. (1982). *Life-span human development*. Monterey, CA: Brooks/Cole Publishing.

Rosinski, R.R. (1977). *The development of visual perception*. Santa Monica, CA: Goodyear Publishing.

Ross, A.O. (1976). *Psychological aspects of learning disabilities and reading disorders*. New York, NY: McGraw-Hill.

Rothstein, A.L. (1977). Information processing in children's skill acquisition. In R.W. Christina & D.M. Landers (Eds.), *Psychology of motor behavior and sport-1976* (pp. 218-227). Champaign, IL: Human Kinetics.

Rubin, K.H. (1976). Extinction of conservation: A life span investigation. *Developmental Psychology, 12,* 51-56.

Rudel, R., & Teuber, H. (1971). Pattern recognition within and across sensory modalities in normal and brain injured children. *Neuropsychologia, 9,* 389-400.

Sabatino, D.A., & Becker, J.T. (1971). Relationship between lateral preference and selected behavioral variables for children failing academically. *Child Development, 42,* 2055-2060.

Salkind, N.J. (1981). *Theories of human development*. New York, NY: D. Van Nostrand Company.

Salthouse, T.A. (1980). Age and memory: Strategies for localizing the loss. In L.W. Poon, J.L. Fozard, L.S. Cermak, D. Arenberg, & L.W. Thompson (Eds.), *New directions in memory and aging*. Hillsdale, NJ: Lawrence Erlbaum Associates.

Saltin, B., & Grimby, G. (1968). Physiological analysis of middle-aged and old former athletes: Comparison with still active athletes of the same ages. *Circulation*, **38**, 1104-1115.

Sandler, L., Van Campen, J., Ratner, G., Stafford, C., & Weismar, R. (1970). Responses of urban preschool children to a developmental screening test. *Journal of Pediatrics*, **77**, 775-781.

Schaie, K.W. (1965). A general model for the study of developmental problems. *Psychological Bulletin*, **64**, 92-107.

Schmidt, R.A. (1977). Schema theory: Implications for movement education. *Motor Skills: Theory Into Practice*, **2**, 36-48.

Schwanda, N.A. (1978). *A biomechanical study of the walking gait of active and inactive middle-age and elderly men*. Unpublished doctoral dissertation, Springfield College, Springfield, MA.

Schwartz, L.A., & Markham, W.T. (1985). Sex stereotyping in children's toy advertisements. *Sex Roles*, **12**, 157-170.

Scott, J.P. (Ed.). (1978). *Critical periods*. Stroudsburg, PA: Dowden, Hutchinson, & Ross.

Seefeldt, V. (1973). *Developmental sequences in fundamental motor skills*. Unpublished paper, Michigan State University, East Lansing, MI.

Seefeldt, V., & Haubenstricker, J. (1982). Patterns, phases, or stages: An analytical model for the study of developmental movement. In J.A.S. Kelso & J.E. Clark (Eds.), *The development of movement control and coordination*. New York, NY: John Wiley & Sons.

Seefeldt, V., Reuschlein, S., & Vogel, P. (1972, April). *Sequencing motor skills within the physical education curriculum*. Paper presented at the annual convention of the American Association for Health, Physical Education, and Recreation, Houston, TX.

Seils, L.G. (1951). The relationship between measures of physical growth and gross motor performance of primary-grade school children. *Research Quarterly*, **22**, 244-260.

Serfass, R.C. (1981). Exercise for the elderly: What are the benefits and how do we get started? In E.L. Smith & R.C. Serfass (Eds.), *Exercise and aging: The scientific basis*. Hillside, NJ: Enslow Publishers.

Sessoms, J.E. (1942). *Common motor abilities of Negro preschool children.* Unpublished master's thesis, Iowa State University, Ames, IA.

Shambes, G.M. (1976). Static postural control in children. *American Journal of Physical Medicine, 55,* 221-252.

Sharkey, B.J. (1984). *Physiology of fitness* (2nd ed.). Champaign, IL: Human Kinetics.

Sheffield, L.T., & Roitman, D. (1973). Systolic blood pressure, heart rate, and treadmill work at anginal threshold. *Chest, 63,* 327-335.

Shephard, R.J. (1978a). Human physiological work capacity. In IBP Human Adaptability Project, *Synthesis: Vol. 4.* New York, NY: Cambridge University Press.

Shephard, R.J. (1978b). *Physical activity and aging.* Chicago, IL: Year Book Medical Publishers.

Shephard, R.J. (1979). Recurrence of myocardial infarction. *British Heart Journal, 42,* 133-138.

Shephard, R.J. (1981). Cardiovascular limitations in the aged. In E.L. Smith & R.C. Serfass (Eds.), *Exercise and aging: The scientific basis* (pp. 19-29). Hillside, NJ: Enslow Publishers.

Shephard, R.J. (1982). *Physical activity and growth.* Chicago, IL: Year Book Medical Publishers.

Shephard, R.J., Jones, G., & Ishii, K. (1969). Factors affecting body density and thickness of subcutaneous fat: Data on 518 Canadian city dwellers. *American Journal of Clinical Nutrition, 22,* 1175-1189.

Shephard, R.J., Lavallee, H., & Jacquier, J.C. (1977). Un programme complementaire d'education physique. Etude preliminaire de l'experience pratiquee dans le district de Trois Rivieres. In J.R. LaCour (Ed.), *Facteurs limitant l'endurance humaine. Les techniques d'amelioration de la performance* (pp. 43-54). France: Universite de St. Etienne.

Shirley, M.M. (1931). *The first two years: A study of twenty-five babies. Postural and locomotor development* (Vol. 1). Minneapolis, MN: University of Minnesota Press.

Shirley, M.M. (1933). *The first two years: A study of twenty-five babies. Intellectual development* (Vol. 2). Minneapolis, MN: University of Minnesota Press.

Shirley, M.M. (1963). The motor sequence. In D. Wayne (Ed.), *Readings in child psychology.* Englewood Cliffs, NJ: Prentice-Hall.

Shock, N.W., & Norris, A.H. (1970). Neuromuscular coordination as a factor in age changes in muscular exercise. In D. Brunner & E. Jokl (Eds.), *Physical activity and aging*. Baltimore, MD: University Park Press.

Sidney, K.H., Shephard, R.J., & Harrison, J.E. (1977). Endurance training and body composition of the elderly. *American Journal of Clinical Nutrition*, **30**, 326-333.

Simard, T. (1969). Fine sensorimotor control in healthy children. *Pediatrics*, **43**, 1035-1041.

Sinclair, C. (1971). Dominance pattern of young children, a follow-up study. *Perceptual and Motor Skills*, **32**, 142.

Sinclair, C.B. (1973). *Movement of the young child: Ages two to six.* Columbus, OH: Merrill.

Singleton, W.T. (1955). Age and performance timing on simple skills. In *Old age and the modern world* (Report of the Third Congress of the International Association of Gerontology). London: E. & S. Livingstone.

Sloan, W. (1955). The Lincoln-Oseretsky motor development scale. *Genetic Psychology Monographs*, **51**, 183-252.

Smith, A.D. (1980). Age differences in encoding, storage, and retrieval. In L.W. Poon, J.L. Fozard, L.S. Cermak, D. Arenberg, & L.W. Thompson (Eds.), *New directions in memory and aging*. Hillsdale, NJ: Lawrence Erlbaum Associates.

Smith, E.L., Sempos, C.T., & Purvis, R.W. (1981). Bone mass and strength decline with age. In E.L. Smith & R.C. Serfass (Eds.), *Exercise and aging: The scientific basis* (pp. 59-87). Hillside, NJ: Enslow Publishers.

Smith, E.L., & Serfass, R.C. (Eds.). (1981). *Exercise and aging: The scientific basis*. Hillside, NJ: Enslow Publishers.

Smith, L.B., Kemler, D.G., & Aronfried, J. (1975). Developmental trends in voluntary selective attention: Differential aspects of source distinctiveness. *Journal of Experimental Child Psychology*, **20**, 353-362.

Snyder, E.E., & Spreitzer, E.A. (1973). Family influence and involvement in sports. *Research Quarterly*, **44**, 249-255.

Snyder, E., & Spreitzer, E. (1976). Correlates of sport participation among adolescent girls. *Research Quarterly*, **47**, 804-809.

Snyder, E.E., & Spreitzer, E. (1978). Socialization comparisons of adolescent female athletes and musicians. *Research Quarterly*, **49**, 342-350.

Snyder, E.E., & Spreitzer, E.A. (1983). *Social aspects of sport* (2nd ed.). Englewood Cliffs, NJ: Prentice-Hall.

Spelke, E.S. (1979). Exploring audible and visible events in infancy. In A.D. Pick (Ed.), *Perception and its development: A tribute to Eleanor J. Gibson.* Hillsdale, NJ: Lawrence Erlbaum Associates.

Stafanik, P.A., Heald, F.P., & Mayer, J. (1959). Caloric intake in relation to energy output of obese and non-obese adolescent boys. *American Journal of Clinical Nutrition, 7,* 55-62.

Stanish, W.D. (1984). Overuse injuries in athletes: A perspective. *Medicine and Science in Sport and Exercise,* **16,** 1-7.

Sterritt, G., Martin, V., & Rudnick, M. (1971). Auditory-visual and temporal-spatial integration as determinants of test difficulty. *Psychonomic Science,* **23,** 289-291.

Stewart, K.J., & Gutin, B. (1976). Effects of physical training on cardiorespiratory fitness in children. *Research Quarterly,* **47,** 110-120.

Stolz, H.R., & Stolz, L.M. (1951). *Somatic development of adolescent boys.* New York, NY: The Macmillan Company.

Stratton, R.K. (1978a). Information processing deficits in children's motor performance: Implications for instruction. *Motor Skills: Theory into Practice,* **3,** 49-55.

Stratton, R.K. (1978b, May). *Selective attention deficits in children's motor performance: Can we help?* Paper presented at the annual conference of the North American Society for Psychology of Sport and Physical Activity, Tallahassee, FL.

Stunkard, A., & Mendelson, M. (1967). Obesity and the body image. I. Characteristics of disturbances in the body image of some obese persons. *American Journal of Psychiatry,* **123,** 1296-1300.

Swanson, R., & Benton, A.L. (1955). Some aspects of the genetic development of right-left discrimination. *Child Development,* **26,** 123-133.

Szafran, J. (1951). Changes with age and with exclusion of vision in performance at an aiming task. *Quarterly Journal of Experimental Psychology,* **3,** 111-118.

Tanner, J. (1961). *Education and physical growth.* London: University of London Press.

Tanner, J.M. (1962). *Growth at adolescence* (2nd ed.). Oxford: Blackwell Scientific Publications.

Teeple, J.B. (1978). Physical growth and maturation. In M.V. Ridenour (Ed.), *Motor development: Issues and applications* (pp. 3-27). Princeton, NJ: Princeton Book.

Temple, A.L. (1952). *Motor abilities of white and Negro children seven, eight, and nine years of age.* Unpublished master's thesis, University of California-Berkeley.

Temple, I.G., Williams, H.G., & Bateman, N.J. (1979). A test battery to assess intrasensory and intersensory development of young children. *Perceptual and Motor Skills, 48,* 643-659.

Thelen, E. (1983). Learning to walk is still an "old" problem: A reply to Zelazo. *Journal of Motor Behavior, 15,* 139-161.

Thomas, J.R. (1980). Acquisition of motor skills: Information processing differences between children and adults. *Research Quarterly for Exercise and Sport, 51,* 158-173.

Thomas, J.R. (Ed.). (1984). *Motor development during childhood and adolescence* (p. 69). Minneapolis, MN: Burgess.

Thomas, J.R., & Bender, P.R. (1977). A developmental explanation for children's motor behavior: A neo-Piagetian interpretation. *Journal of Motor Behavior, 9,* 81-93.

Thomas, J.R., Mitchell, B., & Solomon, M.A. (1979). Precision knowledge of results and motor performance: Relationship to age. *Research Quarterly, 50,* 687-698.

Thomas, J.R., Thomas, K.T., & Gallagher, J.D. (1981). Children's processing of information in physical activity and sport. *Motor Skills: Theory into Practice* [Monograph No. 3], 1-8.

Thompson, M.E. (1944). An experimental study of racial differences in general motor ability. *Journal of Educational Psychology, 35,* 49-54.

Thompson, M.E., & Dove, C.C. (1942). A comparison of physical achievement of Anglo and Spanish American boys in junior high school. *Research Quarterly, 13,* 341-346.

Timiras, P.S. (1972). *Developmental physiology and aging.* New York, NY: The Macmillan Company.

Todor, J.I. (1978). A neo-Piagetian theory of constructive operators: Applications to perceptual-motor development and learning. In D.M. Landers & R.W. Christina (Eds.), *Psychology of motor behavior and Sport-1977.* Champaign, IL: Human Kinetics.

Turner, J.M., Mead, J., & Wohl, M.E. (1968). Elasticity of human lungs in relation to age. *Journal of Applied Physiology*, **35**, 664-671.

Vaccaro, P., & Clarke, D.H. (1978). Cardiorespiratory alterations in 9- to 11-year-old children following a season of competitive swimming. *Medicine and Science in Sports*, **10**, 204-207.

Van Duyne, H.J. (1973). Foundations of tactical perception in three to seven year olds. *Journal of the Association for the Study of Perception*, **8**, 1-9.

VanSant, A. *Development of the standing long jump*. Manuscript in progress.

Van Wieringen, J.C. (1978). Secular growth changes. In F. Falkner & J.M. Tanner (Eds.), *Human growth. Vol. 2: Postnatal growth* (pp. 445-473). New York, NY: Plenum Press.

Victors, E. (1961). *A cinematrographical analysis of catching behavior of a selected group of seven and nine year old boys*. Unpublished doctoral dissertation, University of Wisconsin, Madison, WI.

Von Hofsten, C. (1982). Eye-hand coordination in the newborn. *Developmental Psychology*, **18**, 450-461.

Walk, R.D. (1969). Two types of depth discrimination by the human infant. *Psychonomic Science*, **14**, 253-254.

Walker, L. (1938). *Comparison of selected athletic abilities of white and Negro boys*. Unpublished master's thesis, George Peabody College for Teachers, Nashville, TN.

Walker, R. (1965). *The effect of a controlled program of physical activity on the physical efficiency, respiratory function, airway obstruction and dependency on drugs of the asthmatic child. Report I. Physical work capacity and respiratory function*. Toronto, Ontario: Tuberculosis and Respiratory Disease Association.

Weiner, J., & Lourie, J.A. (1969). *Human biology—A guide to field methods*. Oxford: Blackwell Scientific Publications.

Weiner, J., & Lourie, J.A. (1981). *Practical human biology*. New York, NY: Academic Press.

Weiss, M.R. (1983). Modeling and motor performance: A developmental perspective. *Research Quarterly for Exercise and Sport*, **54**, 190-197.

Weiss, M.R., & Knoppers, A. (1982). The influence of socializing agents on female collegiate volleyball players. *Journal of Sport Psychology*, **4**, 267-279.

Welford, A.T. (1977a). Causes of slowing of performance with age. *Interdisciplinary Topics in Gerontology*, **11**, 23-51.

Welford, A.T. (1977b). Motor performance. In J.E. Birren & K.W. Schaie (Eds.), *Handbook of the psychology of aging*. New York, NY: Van Nostrand Reinhold.

Welford, A.T. (1977c). Serial reaction times, continuity of task, single-channel effects, and age. In S. Dornic (Ed.), *Attention and performance VI*. Hillside, NJ: Lawrence Erlbaum Associates.

Welford, A.T. (1980a). Memory and age: A perspective view. In L.W. Poon, J.L. Fozard, L.S. Cermak, D. Arenberg, & L.W. Thompson (Eds.), *New directions in memory and aging*. Hillside, NJ: Lawrence Erlbaum Associates.

Welford, A.T. (1980b). Motor skill and aging. In C.H. Nadeau, W.R. Halliwell, K.M. Newell, & G.C. Roberts (Eds.), *Psychology of motor behavior and sport-1979* (pp. 253-268). Champaign, IL: Human Kinetics.

Welford, A.T., Norris, A.H., & Shock, N.W. (1969). Speed and accuracy of movement and their changes with age. *Acta Psychologica*, **30**, 3-15.

White, B.L., Castle, P., & Held, R. (1964). Observations on the development of visually-directed reaching. *Child Development*, **35**, 349-364.

Wickens, C.D. (1974). Temporal limits of human information processing: A developmental study. *Psychological Bulletin*, **81**, 739-755.

Wickstrom, R.L. (1983). *Fundamental motor patterns* (3rd ed.). Philadelphia, PA: Lea & Febiger.

Wild, M. (1937). *The behavior pattern of throwing and some observations concerning its course of development in children*. Unpublished doctoral dissertation, University of Wisconsin, Madison, WI.

Wild, M. (1938). The behavior pattern of throwing and some observations concerning its course of development in children. *Research Quarterly*, **9**, 20-24.

Williams, H. (1968). *Effects of systematic variation of speed and direction of object flight and of age and skill classification on visuo-perceptual judgments of moving objects in three-dimensional space*. Unpublished doctoral dissertation, University of Wisconsin-Madison.

Williams, H. (1973). Perceptual-motor development in children. In C. Corbin (Ed.), *A textbook of motor development*. Dubuque, IA: William C. Brown.

Williams, H.G. (1981). Neurophysiological correlates of motor development: A review for practitioners. *Motor skills: Theory into practice* [Monograph No. 3], 31-40.

Williams, H. (1983). *Perceptual and motor development*. Englewood Cliffs, NJ: Prentice-Hall.

Williams, J.R., & Scott, R.B. (1953). Growth and development of Negro infants: IV. Motor development and its relationship to child rearing practices in two groups of Negro infants. *Child Development, 24*, 103-121.

Winterhalter, C. (1974). *Age and sex trends in the development of selected balancing skills*. Unpublished master's thesis, University of Toledo, Toledo, OH.

Witkin, H.A., Oltman, P.K., Rasben, E., & Karp, S.A. (1971). *A manual for the embedded figures tests*. Palo Alto, CA: Consulting Psychologists Press.

Wohlwill, J.F. (1973). *The study of behavioral development*. New York, NY: Academic Press.

Woollacott, M.H. (1983). *Children's changing capacity to process information*. Symposium paper presented at the annual convention of the American Alliance for Health, Physical Education, Recreation and Dance. Eugene, OR: Microform Publications.

Yarmolenko, A. (1933). The motor sphere of school age children. *Journal of Genetic Psychology, 42*, 298-318.

Zaichkowsky, L.D., Zaichkowsky, L.B., & Martinek, T.J. (1980). *Growth and development: The child and physical activity*. St. Louis, MO: The C.V. Mosby Company.

Zelazo, P.R. (1983). The development of walking: New findings and old assumptions. *Journal of Motor Behavior, 15*, 99-137.

Zelazo, P.R., Konner, M., Kolb, S., & Zelazo, N.A. (1974). Newborn walking: A reply to Pontius. *Perceptual and Motor Skills, 39*, 423-428.

Zelazo, P.R., Zelazo, N.A., & Kolb, S. (1972a). Newborn walking. *Science, 177*, 1058-1059.

Zelazo, P.R., Zelazo, N.A., & Kolb, S. (1972b). "Walking" in the newborn. *Science, 176*, 314-315.

Zimmerman, H.M. (1956). Characteristic likenesses and differences between skilled and non-skilled performance of the standing broad jump. *Research Quarterly, 27*, 352.

Author Index

Subject Index

Acceleration curve, 33, 34
Accommodation, 170
Action and reaction, 97
Adipose tissue, 24, 56
Agility run, 142-144
Aging
  and body composition, 56, 236-237
  defined, 7
Anaerobic capacity, 204-205
Anaerobic power, 204-205
Androgens, 57-58, 221
Anorexia nervosa, 67
Anthropometry, 20
Arm lag in throwing, 122-125, 127-128
Arteriosclerosis, 216, 230
Assessment of basic skills, 146-150
Asthma, 217
Atherosclerosis, 216, 230
Atrophy, 224-225
Attention, 242-243
Audition, 184-186
Auditory-kinesthetic integration, 187
Balance, 182-183, 199-200
Ballistic skills, 121-135, 145-146
Bandura's social learning theory, 12, 263-264
Bayley Scale of Infant Development, 83-85, 87, 148, 274-275
Behavioral theories, 11-12
Biacromial distance, 28-29
Bicristal distance, 29
Biiliac distance, 29
Biodynamic theory, 81-82, 90
Biological perspective, 10
Birth, 65-66
Blastocyst, 36-37
Block rotation of the trunk, 122-124, 127, 134
Blood pressure, 210, 215
Body awareness, 180-181, 198
Body composition, 22-26, 230-238

Body part identification, 180-181
Body proportions, 47-48
Breadth measures, 29-30
Bronchitis, 217
Bruininks-Osteretsky Test of Motor Proficiency, 148
Cardiac output, 205-210
Catch-up growth, 44-45, 67
Catching, 135-138
Chicken pox, 217
Child-rearing practices, 277
Children's Embedded Figures Test, 258
Chromosomes, 36
Chunking, 250
Circumference measures, 27-28
Climate, 68
Co-twin method, 11, 92-93
Cognitive theory, 12-13
Cohorts, 15-16
Component model, 100-101
Conception, 35-36
Congenital defects, 39
Consolidation process, 17
Contrast sensitivity, 170-172
Control processes in memory, 249-250
Crawling, 83-86
Creeping, 83-86
Critical period, 14, 41, 90-93
Cross-sectional research, 15
Cultural differences, 274-279
Cutaneous receptors, 179
Cyanotic congenital heart disease, 216
Cystic fibrosis, 217
Dental eruption, 32
Denver Developmental Screening Test, 148, 275
DeOreo's Fundamental Motor Skills Inventory, 148
Deprivation, 91-92